MCQs POINTS

FOR FMGE, DNB, NEET-PG, UPSC-CMS and INI-CET EXAMS

Eighth Edition

Dr. Kamal KV

MBBS, MS (Orthopedics)

Foreign (Academic) Trips (Countries and Cities)

Georgia (Tbilisi, Batumi)
Russia (Nalchik, Cheboksary, Stavropol, Kazan)
Kyrgyzstan (Jalalabad, Osh, Bishkek)
Nepal (Bharatpur, Bhairahawa, Dharan)
Ukraine (Vinnytsia, Kiev)
China (Ningbo, Nanchang, Nanning, Dali, Fuzhou, Guangzhou)
Belarus (Minsk)
Kazakhstan (Almaty, Shymkent)
Uzbekistan (Fergana)

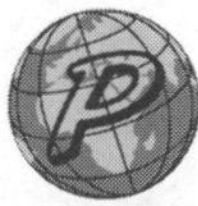

Peepee Publishers and Distributors Private Limited ®

MCQs Points

Published by
Pawaninder P. Vij and Anupam Vij

Peepee Publishers and Distributors Private Limited
Head Office: 160, Shakti Vihar, Pitam Pura
Delhi-110 034 (India)

Correspondence Address:

7/31, First Floor, Ansari Road, Daryaganj
New Delhi-110002 (India)

Ph: 41512412, 9811156083

e-mail: peepee160@yahoo.co.in

e-mail: peepee160@gmail.com

www.peepeepub.com

Eighth Edition: 2025

ISBN: 978-81-9720-725-9

Special Thanks

I would like to convey my heartfelt thanks to all those, who had arranged or served me during my foreign (academic) trips.

S. No.	Countries	College	First Visit
1	**Georgia**	*i. Tbilisi*	Feb 2018
		ii. Batumi	Feb 2018
2	**Russia**	*iii. Nalchik*	Oct 2018
		iv. Cheboksary	Oct 2018
		v. Stavropol	Mar 2019
		vi. Kazan	Mar 2019
3	**Kyrgyzstan**	*vii. Jalalabad*	Dec 2018
		viii. Osh	May 2019
4	**Nepal**	*ix. Bishkek*	Dec 2022
		x. Bhairahawa	May 2019
		xi. Bharatpur	May 2019
		xii. Dharan	Sep 2019
5	**Ukraine**	*xiii. Vinnytsia*	Nov 2019
		xiv. Kiev	Nov 2019
6	**China**	*xv. Ningbo*	Oct 2018
		xvi. Nanchang	Nov 2018
		xvii. Nanning	Nov 2018
		xviii. Dali	Nov 2018
		xix. Fuzhou	June 2019
		xx. Guangzhou	June 2019
7	**Belarus**	*xxi. Minsk*	Jan 2020
8	**Kazakhastan**	*xxii. Almaty*	April 2023
		xxiii. Shymkent	Mar 2024
9	**Uzbekistan**	*xxiv. Fergana*	Feb 2024

Preface to Eighth Edition

For an author, there is nothing more pleasant view than to see a new edition of his book.

I feel very honoured to present the eighth and revised edition of this text.

In this edition, I have changed the presentation of the book. There were two reasons for this:

1. Nowadays, the exam pattern has changed. Few years back, most of the questions in the exam were one-liners but nowadays, the questions are clinical concept based.
2. Students always wished to have a concise theory book, which they can revise easily in the last few weeks of exam.

Based on these observations, I have kept two segments in the book.

Rapid Revision Notes are concise, to the point and MCQ yielding notes. Wherever needed, content has been arranged in the form of short tables for quick revision.

Clinical Questions are added at the end of each chapter to give an insight about the current pattern (of clinical questions) and trick/ concept to solve them.

As I always say, students are the best judge of an author's work. And I personally feel, there is always some room left for further improvement. So, I expect my dear students to share their valuable feedbacks regarding betterment of this text in subsequent editions.

Despite my best efforts, some errors must have crept in. I request dear readers to please forward the same to me.

Hope this title will serve its purpose.

04.10.2024

drkamalkv
Facebook, YouTube, Instagram: drkamalkvgroup
E-mail: drkamalkvgroup@gmail.com
Website: www.drkamalkvgroup.co.in
WhatsApp: 84 7000 4333

Preface to First Edition

Going through the MCQ banks of the previous years is equally important as knowing the detailed theoretical concepts for any subject.

During initial days of preparation, students can go through bulky MCQ banks. But the problem is that these titles are so vast, many find it very difficult to retain or revise.

This title plans to help you in this regard. It contains MCQ points of last 10 years of examinations. Important straightforward one-liners kind of MCQ has been selected and arranged in 2 parts (subject-wise and all subjects mix). Before MCQ points, important bits have been arranged in quick review format. Also, enough space has been provided for students to add up their notes.

Despite my best efforts, some errors must have crept in. I request dear readers to please forward the same to me.

Hope this title will serve its purpose.

drkamalkv

Acknowledgements

All thanks to almighty (for imparting me with this passion of writing books and teaching), to my parents (for imparting qualities of a good human being), my brothers & sister (for giving me some wonderful memories of childhood), my wife (for supporting me in all my endeavours), my daughters (for allowing me to use their share of time with my students) and my dear students (for accepting my all titles with equal enthusiasm and also, who made me academically strong, to an extent).

Thanks are due for everyone behind this project, from the publication house.

Special thanks to **Pawaninder Paul Vij** sir and **Anupam Vij** for accepting all my work, without any hesitancy or objection.

drkamalkv

Contents

CHAPTER 1

ANATOMY

RAPID REVISION NOTES

Upper limb muscles

Muscle	*Action*	*Nerve supply*
Trapezius	Elevates shoulder	Spinal accessory nerve
	Retracts scapula	
	Rotates scapula	
Serratus anterior	Protracts scapula (paralysis leads to winging of scapula)	Long thoracic nerve of bell
Pectoralis minor	Protracts scapula	Medial pectoral nerve
	Depresses shoulder	
Pectoralis major	Protracts scapula	Pectoral nerve
	Depresses shoulder	
Rhomboids	Retraction & medial rotation of scapula	Nerve to rhomboids
Levator scapula	Elevation & medial rotation of scapula	Dorsal scapular & C3, C4
Latissimus dorsi	Depressed shoulder	Thoracodorsal nerve
	Retracts scapula	
Deltoid	Flexion, abduction & rotation of shoulder	Axillary nerve
Biceps brachii	Flexion at elbow & shoulder	Musculo-cutaneous nerve
Coraco-brachialis	Flexion of shoulder	Musculo-cutaneous nerve
Teres major	Adduction & medial rotation	Subscapular nerve
Teres minor	Lateral rotation of shoulder	Axillary nerve
Triceps	Extension of elbow	Radial nerve
Brachialis	Flexion of elbow	Musculo-cutaneous nerve
Brachio-radialis	Flexion of elbow (midprone position)	Radial nerve
Pronator teres	Pronation at elbow	Median nerve
Pronator quadrates	Pronation at elbow	Anterior interosseous nerve (branch of median nerve)
Supinator	Supination	Radial nerve
Biceps brachii	Supination with elbow in flexion	Musculo-cutaneous
Brachio-radialis	Supination from pronation to mid-position	Radial
Lumbrical	Flexion at metacarpophalangeal & extension at interphalangeal joints	Median (1st & 2nd); ulnar (3rd & 4th)

Dorsal interossei	Abduction of MP of index, ring & middle finger	Ulnar nerve
Palmar interossei	Adduction of MP of thumb, index, ring & little finger	Ulnar nerve

JOINTS

- Temporomandibular joint: Condylar
- Shoulder & hip joint: Ball & socket
- 1st carpometacarpal & sternoclavicular joint: Saddle/ Sellar
- Wrist & metacarpophalangeal joint: Ellipsoid/ condyloid
- Superior & inferior radio-ulnar joint: Pivot
- Elbow, ankle & interphalangeal joint: Hinge
- Inferior tibio-fibular joint: Syndesmosis
- Symphysis pubis, Manubriosternal joint: Secondary cartilaginous/ symphysis
- Joint between epiphysis & diaphysis, 1st costochondral joint: Primary cartilaginous/ Synchondrosis
- Tooth in socket: Gomphosis
- Skull: Sutures

Nerves & their important branches

Nerve	*Branches*
Trigeminal nerve	Ophthalmic nerve Maxillary nerve Mandibular nerve (motor only)
Ophthalmic nerve	Lacrimal nerve Frontal nerve Nasociliary nerve
Maxillary nerve	Meningeal branch Anterior superior alveolar Middle superior alveolar Posterior superior alveolar Nasal
Mandibular nerve	Meningeal branch Deep temporal nerve Inferior alveolar nerve Auriculotemporal nerve Lingual nerve
Facial nerve	Chorda tympani Posterior auricular
Vagus nerve	Superior laryngeal nerve Recurrent laryngeal nerve Oesophageal Gastric Celiac Hepatic branches
Nervus intermedius	Sensory component of facial nerve
Suboccipital nerve	Ventral ramus of C1

CRANIAL NERVES

- Largest cranial nerve: V
- Longest course through a bony canal of skull: VII
- Longest intracranial course: IV
- Thinnest cranial nerve: IV
- Nerves having nuclei in midbrain:
  - III
  - IV
- Nerves having nuclei in pons:
  - V
  - VI
  - VII
  - VIII
- Nerves having nuclei in medulla:
  - IX
  - X
  - XI
  - XII
- Cranial nerve emerging from dorsal aspect of brain: IV
- Nerve MC involved in raised intra-cranial pressure: VI
- Nerve supply of platysma: VII
- Buccinator muscle is supplied by: VII
- Palatal muscles (except tensor palati) are supplied by: Pharyngeal plexus
- Lower motor neuron lesion of XII nerve results in deviation of tongue to: Same side

- Muscle of facial expression each supplied by: VII
- Glands supplied by VII nuclei:
  - o Submandibular gland
  - o Lacrimal gland
  - o Nasal gland
- REMEMBER: Facial nerve traverses the substance of parotid but DOES NOT supply it
- Ganglion related to facial nerve:
  - o Pterygopalatine palatine
  - o Geniculate ganglion
  - o Submandibular ganglion

DIAPHRAGMATIC OPENING

- Level of vena caval opening: T8
- Level of esophageal opening: T10
- Level of aortic opening: T12
- Caval opening is through: Central part
- Aortic opening is through: Osseo-aponeurotic opening (not a true opening)
- Esophageal opening is through: Muscular part of diaphragm
- Right phrenic nerve passes through: Vena caval opening
- Vagus nerve passes through: Esophageal opening
- Esophageal branch of left gastric artery passes through: Esophageal opening
- Azygous vein passes through: Aortic opening

CONDITIONS & SOURCE OF BLEEDING

- Duodenal ulcer: Gastroduodenal artery
- Extradural hemorrhage: Middle meningeal artery
- Tonsillectomy: Paratonsillar vein

Duct

Duct	*Description*
Duct of Bellini	Straight collecting tubules of kidney
Mullerian duct	Paramesonephric duct (Structure derived are fallopian tube, uterus, cervix & upper 2/3rd of vagina)
Wolffian duct	Mesonephric duct
Gartner duct	Remnant of mesonephric duct in females
Duct of Wirsung	Pancreatic duct
Duct of Santorini	Accessory pancreatic duct
Stensen duct	Duct of parotid gland
Wharton's duct	Duct of submandibular gland
Duct of Rivinus	Duct of sublingual glands

DUCTS

- Stensen duct: Parotid duct
- Pecquet's duct: Thoracic duct
- Remnant of mesonephric duct/ wolffian: Gartners duct

Membranes

Membrane	*Location*
Spiral membrane/ basilar membrane	Cochlea
Bowman's membrane	Anterior layer of cornea
Descemet's membrane	Posterior layer of cornea
Bruch's membrane	Basal membrane of choroid
Scarpa's membrane	Part of tympanic membrane

MEMBRANES

- Shrapnell membrane: Pars flaccida (tympanic membrane)
- Henle's membrane: Root sheath of hair (Outer layer of cells)
- Huxley membrane: Root sheath of hair (Inner layer of cells)

CANALS

- Schlemm canal: Canal at corneoscleral junction
- Haversian canal: Central vascular channels in bones around which lamellae are arranged concentrically

CELLS

- Gitter cells: Microglial (brain)
- Hofbauer cells: Ellipsoidal cells in chorionic villi of placenta
- JG cells: Smooth muscle cells (of afferent arteriole of kidney)
- Ito cells: Stellate cells in liver
- Muller's canal: Neuroglial cells in retina
- Glomus cells: Presents in carotid bodies

DIAPHRAGM

- Oral cavity diaphragm: Mylohyoid
- Urogenital diaphragm:
  - o Deep transverse perinei
  - o Sphincter urethrae
  - o Perineal membrane

FASCIA

- Buck's fascia: Deep fascia of penis
- Denonvilliers fascia: Fascia separating prostate & rectum
- Pelvic fascia: Hypogastric sheath

TRIANGLE

- Koch's triangle: Part of fibrous skeleton of heart; Bounded by:
  - o Tendon of todaro
  - o Tricuspid valve &
  - o Margin of coronary sinus opening
- Triangle of auscultation: Part of back, not covered by muscles so respiratory sounds are best heard; Bounded by:
  - o Trapezius (medially)
  - o Scapula (laterally) &
  - o Latissimus dorsi (inferiorly)
- Hesselbach's triangle:
  - o Rectus abdominis (medially)
  - o Inferior epigastric artery (laterally) &
  - o Inguinal ligament (inferiorly)
- MacEwen's triangle: Triangular depression posterior to the external acoustic meatus:
  - o External acoustic meatus (postero-superior)
  - o Supramastoid crest &
  - o Tangent to posterior border of external acoustic meatus

LENGTHS

- Male urethra: 18-20 cms
- Ureter, esophagus: 10 inches
- Spinal cord, vas deferens, thoracic duct: 18 inches/ 45 cm

NAMED FORAMEN

- Foramen of Winslow: Between greater & lesser sac
- Foramen of Morgagni: Opening in diaphragm

ARTERIES

- Formed by union of 2 vertebral arteries: Basilar A.
- Inferior vesical artery is a branch of: Anterior division of internal iliac artery
- Uterine A. is a branch of: Anterior division of internal iliac A.
- Inferior thyroid A. is a branch of: Thyrocervical trunk
- Ascending pharyngeal A. is a branch of: External carotid A.
- Internal pudendal A. is a branch of: Anterior division of: Internal iliac A.
- Left gastro-epiploic A. is a branch of: Splenic A.
- Splenic A. is a branch of: Coeliac trunk
- Cystic A. is a branch of: Right hepatic A.
- Cilio-retinal A. is a branch of: Choroidal A.
- Middle meningeal A. is a branch of: Maxillary A.
- Anterior spinal A. is a branch of: Vertebral A.

- Ophthalmic A. is a branch of: Internal carotid A.

EMBRYOLOGY

- Oogonia & germ cell are derived from: Yolk sac
- 1st polar body is formed during: Oogenesis
- 1st polar body is extruded: At the time of ovulation
- Y chromosome is: Acrocentric
- Sperms are stored in: Epididymis
- Length of human sperm: 50-60 microns

Sutures & conditions associated with their closure

- Dolichocephaly / Scaphocephaly [Closure of sagittal suture (anteroposterior widening)]
- Brachycephaly [Closure of coronal suture(transverse suture)]
- Oxycephaly/ Acrocephaly/ Turricephaly [All sutures are closed]

Structures derived from neural crest

- Pia mater
- Dental papillae
- Adrenal medulla
- Schwann
- Melanoblasts
- Dorsal root ganglia
- Autonomic ganglia
- Cells belonging to APUD series
- Bones and connective tissues of craniofacial structures
- Cells of truncoconal; cushions of heart

Structures derived from Pharyngeal pouches:

- 1st: Middle ear, Eustachian tube
- 2nd: Tonsil
- 3rd: Upper - Inferior parathyroid; Lower - Thymus
- 4th: Upper - Superior parathyroid
- 5th: Ultimobranchial body
- 4th + 5th forms caudal pharyngeal complex which forms superior parathyroid & parafollicular cells of thyroid

Structures derived from Pharyngeal clefts:

- 1st: External auditory canal
- 2nd, 3rd, 4th: Cervical sinus

Fetal structures & adult remnants

- The extra hepatic portion of umbilical vein: The round ligament of the liver (ligamentum teres hepatic), which lies in the free edge of the falciform ligament
- The intrahepatic portion (ductus venosus): Ligamentum venosus
- Closure of ductus arteriosus: Ligamentum arteriosum
- Closure of distal part of Umbilical arteries: Medial umbilical ligament

Must know facts

- Just prior to ovulation, the primary oocyte enters and completes 1st meiotic division
- During first 24 weeks, there is only fetal hemoglobin; after which adult type Hb appears, at term, 75-80 percent Hb is of fetal type, it is completely replaced by 4 months of age
- Order of development of paranasal sinuses: Maxillary – Ethmoid – Frontal - Sphenoid
- Occurrence of acute sinusitis and carcinoma in paranasal sinuses: Maxillary – Ethmoid – Frontal - Sphenoid

FETAL STRUCTURES & ADULT REMNANT

- Meckel's diverticulum: Remnant of vitelline duct
- Ligamentum venosum: Remnant of ductus venosus
- Ligamentum arteriosum: Remnant of ductus arteriosus
- Median umbilical ligament: Remnant of urachus
- Medial umbilical ligaments: Remnant of 2 umbilical arteries

DERIVATIVE OF GERM LAYERS

- Trigone of bladder: Mesoderm

- Somites: Paraxial mesoderm
- Epithelial lining of biliary tract: Endoderm
- Tympanic membrane: All the 3 germ layers
- Derivatives of neural crest:
  - Neurons of:
    - Dorsal root
    - Sensory &
    - Autonomic/ sympathetic ganglia
  - Schwann cells
  - Melanocytes
  - Mesenchyme of dental papillae etc.

Aortic arches & their derivatives

1st, 2nd & 5th (Most)	*Disappears*
3rd	Common Carotid artery & proximal Internal Carotid artery
4th (Left)	Arch of Aorta & Left Subclavian artery
4th (Right)	Proximal Right Subclavian artery & Brachiocephalic artery
6th	Right & Left Pulmonary arteries & Ductus Arteriosus (left only)

EMBRYOLOGY OF CVS

- Sinus venosus forms: Smooth part of right atrium, coronary sinus & oblique vein of left atrium
- Persistence of 4th aortic arch leads to: Double aortic arch

EMBRYOLOGY OF GENITO-URINARY TRACT

- Collecting duct develops from: Ureteric bud
- Epithelium of ureter develops from: Mesonephros
- Uterus/ appendix testes develops from: Mullerian duct/ paramesonephric duct
- Ovary develops from: Genital ridge
- Scrotum develops from: Genital swelling
- Clitoris develops from: Genital tubercle

PHARYNGEAL ARCH DERIVATIVES

- Meckel's cartilage develops from: 1st pharyngeal arch
- Sphenomandibular ligament develops from: 1st pharyngeal arch
- Stapes develops from: 2nd pharyngeal arch
- Stylohyoid ligament develops from: 2nd pharyngeal arch
- Greater cornua of hyoid develops from: 3rd pharyngeal arch
- Posterior belly of digastric develops from: 2nd pharyngeal arch
- Anterior belly of digastric develops from: 1st pharyngeal arch
- Platysma develops from: 2nd pharyngeal arch

NERVE SUPPLY OF PHARYNGEAL ARCHES

- 3rd arch: Glossopharyngeal nerve
- 6th arch: Recurrent laryngeal nerve

PHARYNGEAL POUCH & DERIVATIVES

- Palatine tonsil develops from: 2nd pharyngeal pouch
- Inferior parathyroid gland & thymus develop from: 3rd pharyngeal pouch
- Superior parathyroid gland & ultimobranchial body develop from: 4th pharyngeal pouch
- Parafollicular cells are derived from: Ultimobranchial body

EAR

- Nerve supply of pinna: Vagus & auriculotemporal nerve
- Tympanic plexus is formed by: Tympanic branch of glossopharyngeal nerve
- Second smallest muscle in body: Stapedius
- Smallest muscle in body: Erector pili

TONGUE

- Muscle of tongue develops from: Occipital myotomes

- Muscles of tongue are: Both smooth & skeletal muscles
- Safety muscle of tongue: Genioglossus
- Pain of Ca base of tongue is referred to the ear through: Glossopharyngeal nerve
- Circumvallate papillae of tongue are supplied by: Glossopharyngeal nerve
- Anterior 2/3rd of tongue develops from:
    - o Lingual swellings &
    - o Tuberculum impar
- Taste sensation from anterior 2/3rd of tongue is by: Chorda tympani (facial)
- Posterior 1/3rd of tongue develops from: Hypobranchial eminence

TONSIL

- Endodermal structure
- Main nerve supply is through: Glossopharyngeal nerve
- Lymphatic drainage: Jugulodigastric nodes

EPITHELIUM

- Mesothelium of pleura, peritoneum & pericardium is lined by: Simple squamous epithelium
- Nasal cavity, nasal air sinuses, nasopharynx, larynx, trachea & bronchi (EXCEPT true vocal cords) are lined by: Ciliated pseudo-stratified columnar epithelium
- True vocal cords, cornea, tonsil are lined by: Non keratinized stratified squamous epithelium
- Epithelium with extra reserve of cell membrane: Transitional epithelium
- Calyces, ureter, ureterovesical junction & urinary bladder have: Transitional epithelium

HISTOLOGY

- Function of gap junctions: Exchange between cells
- Gustatory system has: Sensory type of neuro-epithelium
- Intercalated disc is present in: Cardiac muscle
- Nucleus in cardiac muscle: Central
- Reticuloendothelial cells of liver are: Kupffer cells
- Space of Disse & space of Mall are seen in: Liver
- Intrinsic factor (Castle) is secreted by: Parietal/ oxyntic cells
- Chief/ peptic/ zymogen cells lines the: Body of the gland (secrete pepsinogen)
- Paneth cells (intestine) are rich in: Rough ER

Important cells

- Gitter cells: Microglia
- Dieter cells: Outer hair cells of organ of Corti
- Hofbauer's cells: Ellipsoidal cells in chorionic villi of placenta
- Juxtaglomerular cells: Smooth muscle cells of afferent arteriole
- Ito cells: Stellate cells in liver
- Langerhans cells: Antigen presenting epithelial dendritic cells
- Glomus cells: Present in carotid bodies

EPITHELIUM

- Simple squamous: Alveoli of lungs, mesothelium of pleura, peritoneum & pericardium, endothelium of heart & blood vessels
- Simple cuboidal: Lining of thyroid follicles, germinal epithelium of ovary
- Simple columnar: Lining of stomach, intestines, gall bladder
- Simple columnar ciliated: Fallopian tubes, uterus, osseous part of Eustachian tube
- Keratinized stratified squamous: Epidermis of skin, external ear, external nose
- Non keratinized stratified: Esophagus, tongue, true vocal cords, cornea, tonsil
- Transitional: Calyces, ureter, urinary bladder, male urethra

Muscles supplied by

Nerve	*Muscles supplied*
Median nerve	Flexor carpi radialis Pronator teres Pronator quadratus Flexor digitorum profundus Flexor pollicis longus Palmaris longus Lumbricals of index & middle fingers Abductor pollicis longus
Radial nerve	Brachioradialis Extensor carpi radialis Triceps Anconeus Supinator Extensor carpi ulnaris Extensor digitorum Extensor digiti minimi Extensor pollicis longus Extensor indicis Abductor pollicis brevis
Ulnar nerve	Flexor carpi ulnaris Lumbricals of ring & little fingers Interossei Flexor digiti minimi Opponens digiti minimi
Musculocutaneous nerve	Biceps brachii Brachialis coracobrachialis

UPPER LIMB

- Nerve arising from the trunks of brachial plexus:
  - o Suprascapular nerve
  - o Subclavius nerve
- Musculocutaneous nerve arises from: Lateral cord
- Subscapular nerve arises from: Posterior cord
- Shoulder joint is weakest: Inferiorly
- Flexion at shoulder joint is carried out by:
  - o Clavicular head of pectoralis major
  - o Anterior fibres of deltoid
- Suprascapular nerve supplies:
  - o Supraspinatus &
  - o Infraspinatus
- Function of levator scapulae: Elevation of scapula
- Erb's point is: Union of C5 & C6
- Erb's palsy involves: Upper trunk of brachial plexus
- Klumpke's paralysis is: Injury to lower trunk of brachial plexus
- Hypothenar area (medial third of palm) is supplied by: Ulnar nerve
- Palmar & dorsal interossei are supplied by: Ulnar nerve
- Adductor pollicis (adduction of thumb) is supplied by: Ulnar nerve
- Froment sign/ Book test is done for: Ulnar nerve injury
- Thenar eminence is supplied by: Median nerve
- Lunate dislocation may injure: Median nerve
- Ape thumb deformity is seen in: Median nerve injury
- Lower subscapular nerve supplies: Teres major (adducts & medially rotates the arm)
- Abduction & lateral rotation of the arm is done by:
  - o Supraspinatus &
  - o Infraspinatus (supplied by suprascapular nerve)
- Teres minor & deltoid are supplied by: Axillary nerve
- Musculocutaneous nerve supplies:
  - o Brachialis
  - o Biceps &
  - o Coracobrachialis (BBC)
- Flexors of forearm are:
  - o Biceps
  - o Brachialis
  - o Brachioradialis (3B)

- Muscles attached to greater tubercle of humerus:
  - o Supraspinatus
  - o Infraspinatus &
  - o Teres minor
- Muscle originating from coracoid process: Short head of biceps, coracobrachialis
- Abductors of shoulder joint:
  - o Supraspinatus (initiator; 0-15 degree)
  - o Deltoid (15 to 90 degree)
  - o Serratus anterior (beyond 90 degree)
  - o Trapezius (beyond 90 degree)
- Rotator cuff muscle includes:
  - o Supraspinatus
  - o Infraspinatus
  - o Teres minor &
  - o Subscapularis
- Dropped shoulder is seen in: Paralysis of deltoid

Spaces related to upper limb

i. *Upper triangular space:*
  - Medial boundary: Teres minor
  - Lateral boundary: Long head of triceps
  - Inferior boundary: Teres major
  - Contents: Circumflex scapular artery

ii. *Lower triangular space:*
  - Medial boundary: Long head of triceps
  - Lateral boundary: Medial border of humerus
  - Superior boundary: Teres major
  - Contents: Radial nerve and profunda brachi vessels

iii. *Anatomical snuff box/ radial fossa:*
  - Anterior boundary: Abductor pollicis longus and extensor pollicis Brevis
  - Posterior boundary: Extensor pollicis longus
  - Floor: Scaphoid, trapezium, radial artery
  - Roof: Origin of cephalic vein, dorsal cutaneous branch of radial nerve
  - Significance: Tenderness is suggestive of Scaphoid fracture

De Quervain's Stenosing Tenosynovitis

- Localized pain over radial styloid process
- Finkelstein's test is positive

Axial arteries of limbs

- Axial artery of upper limb: C7 intersegmental artery
- Axial artery of lower limb: L5 intersegmental artery

Infection of hand & their spread to spaces

- Thumb and index finger infection spread to Thenar space
- Middle and ring fingers infection spread to Mid-palmar space
- Little finger infection spreads to Forman space of parona

Effects of nerve injury

Nerve injured	*Effects*
Femoral nerve	Weakened hip flexion Loss of extension of knee joint Sensory loss on medial side of lower part of leg & medial border of foot
Obturator nerve	Loss of adduction at hip Instability in standing & walking
Sciatic nerve	Weakened hip extension Weakness of knee flexion Weakness of rotation of leg on thigh

LOWER LIMB

- Nerve of medial/ adductor compartment of thigh: Obturator nerve
- Gluteus maximus is supplied by: Inferior gluteal nerve
- Gluteus minimus, G. medius & tensor fascia lata are supplied by: Superior gluteal nerve
- Actions of Sartorius: Lateral rotation & abduction at hip; flexion at knee
- Quadratus femoris, Superior & inferior gemelli action: Lateral rotation

- Abductors of the hip: Gluteus medius & gluteus minimus
- Extensor of the knee joint: Quadricep femoris
- Function of iliofemoral ligament/ ligament of Bigelow: Prevents hyperextension at the hip
- Posterior dislocation of femur is prevented by: Anterior cruciate ligament
- Posterior dislocation of the tibia is prevented by: Posterior cruciate ligament
- Inversion & eversion occur at: Subtalar joint
- Root value of pudendal nerve: S2, S3, S4
- Root value of obturator nerve: L2, L3, L4

Fascial compartment of thigh & their nerve-artery

- Anterior: Femoral artery & Femoral nerve
- Medial: Profunda femoris artery & Obturator nerve
- Posterior: Branches of profunda femoris artery & Sciatic nerve

Fascial compartment of leg & their nerve-artery

- Anterior: Anterior tibial artery & Deep peroneal nerve
- Lateral: Branches of peroneal artery & Superficial peroneal nerve
- Posterior: Posterior tibial artery & Tibial nerve

Contents of the adductor canal

- Terminal part of femoral artery
- Femoral vein
- Saphenous nerve
- Nerve to vastus medialis
- Terminal part of obturator nerve
- Deep lymph vessels

Must know facts

- Nutrient artery to the tibia is the largest nutrient artery in the body
- Housemaid's knee- Prepatellar bursitis
- Clergyman's knee- Infrapatellar bursitis

THORAX

- Blood supply of breast is via:
  - o Internal thoracic artery
  - o Intercostal artery etc.
- Azygos vein passes through: Aortic opening
- Superior epigastric vessels & lymphatic passes through: Foramen of Morgagni
- Bochdalek's hernia occurs through: Posterolateral part of diaphragm
- Morgagni hernia occurs: Anteriorly (usually right side)

Bronchopulmonary segments

- It is an anatomic, functional and surgical unit of the lung
- As it is separated from rest of the lungs by a connective tissue septum, it can be separated surgically without affecting other segments
- It has a segmental bronchus, a segmental artery, lymph vessels and autonomic nerves
- There are 10 segments on each side

Esophagus

- It is 10 inches/25 cm long
- Constrictions of esophagus: 15 cm (Cricopharynx); 25 cm (Aortic arch); 27 cm (Left bronchus); 40 cm (Diaphragmatic entry)
- Cricopharynx is the narrowest region of gastrointestinal tract
- Esophagus shown three indentation on radiographic study; from above downwards they are: Aortic arch; Left bronchus; Left atrium
- Blood supply of esophagus: Upper third - Inferior thyroid artery; Middle third - Branches from descending thoracic aorta; Lower third - Left gastric artery

Diaphragmatic hiatus

- Esophageal hiatus transmits: Esophagus, anterior and posterior vagal trunks
- Aortic hiatus transmits: Aorta, thoracic duct, Azygos vein

Arterial supply of heart

- Right Coronary artery (Main branches are Posterior Descending & Marginal artery) supplies:
  - o Right atrium & ventricle
  - o Posterior 1/3rd of interventricular septum
  - o SA node & AV node
- Left Coronary artery (Main branches are Left Anterior Descending & Circumflex artery) supplies:
  - o Anterior 2/3rd of interventricular septum
  - o SA node (in 40% cases)
  - o Anterior part of right & left ventricle
  - o Lateral wall of left ventricle

Venous drainage

- 10% drains into heart chambers through venae cordis minimis
- 90% drains through Coronary Sinus into right atrium via Great, Small & Middle cardiac veins (GSM)

ESOPHAGUS

- Esophagus pierces diaphragm at a distance of: 15 inches (from incisor)
- Length of esophagus: 25 cm
- Esophagus commences at: Lower end of cricoid
- Epithelium of esophagus: Stratified squamous non-keratinized

THORACIC DUCT

- Thoracic duct crosses from right to left at the level of: T4
- Thoracic duct passes through: Aortic opening of diaphragm
- Thoracic duct is also known as: Pecquet's duct
- Thoracic duct commences in the abdomen as an elongated lymph sac of the: Cisterna chyli

HEART

- Inferior surface of the heart is formed by: Both ventricles
- Base of heart is formed by: Both atrium
- Part of heart lying close to esophagus: Left atrium
- Trabeculae carnea is present in: Right ventricle
- Right coronary artery arises from: Anterior aortic cusp
- In right dominance, posterior interventricular artery originates from: Right coronary artery
- SA node & AV node is supplied by: Right coronary artery
- Middle cardiac vein follows: Posterior interventricular artery
- SVC & IVC open into: Right atrium
- Coronary sinus drains into: Right atrium

LUNG

- Smallest physiological unit of lung is: Lobule
- Sequestered segments are supplied by: Systemic circulation

Branches of

Artery	*Main branches*
Coeliac artery	Left gastric artery Splenic artery (largest) Common hepatic artery Gastroduodenal artery Right gastric artery
Splenic artery	Branches to pancreas Branches to spleen Short gastric artery Left gastroepiploic artery
Inferior mesenteric artery	Left colic artery Sigmoid artery Superior rectal artery
Superior mesenteric artery	Middle colic artery Right colic artery Inferior pancreatico-duodenal artery Ilio-colic artery Appendicular artery Jejunal & ileal arteries

ABDOMEN

- Brunner's gland is present in: Duodenum
- Length of ureter is: 25 cm
- Superior suprarenal artery is a branch of: Inferior phrenic artery
- Middle suprarenal artery is a branch of: Abdominal artery
- Arrangement of structures at hilum of kidney (VAP):
  - o Vein
  - o Artery &
  - o Pelvis (anterior to posterior)

Length of:

- Duodenum: 1 foot
- Jejunum: 8 feet
- Ileum: 12 feet

Liver

- Liver is divided into right and left lobes by the attachment of the peritoneum of the falciform ligament.
- The right lobe is further divided into a quadrate lobe and caudate lobe, by gallbladder, fissure for the ligamentum teres, the inferior vena cava and the fissure for ligamentum venosum.

Tributaries of left renal vein

- Left gonadal vein
- Left suprarenal vein
- Left inferior phrenic vein

Coverings of kidney from inside outwards

- Fibrous capsule
- Perirenal fat
- Renal fascia (fascia of Gerota)
- Pararenal fat (Fascia of Zuckerkandl is the posterior layer of renal fascia)

The renal hilum transmits following structures from front to backwards

- Renal vein
- Two branches of the renal artery
- Ureter
- Third branch of the renal artery

Ureter

- 10 inches/25 cm long
- Has three constrictions in its course: Where the renal pelvis joins the ureter; Where it crosses the pelvic brim; Where it enters the bladder wall

Renal transplantation

- Iliac fossa is the preferred site for transplanted kidney

Prostate

- Prostatic urethra is the widest and the most dilatable part of urethra.
- Lobes of prostate: Anterior lobe; Median / middle lobe (enlarged in BPH); Posterior lobe (most common site of malignancy); Right and left lateral lobes

Superficial fascia is divided into

- Camper's fascia: Superficial fatty layer
- Scarpa's fascia: Deep membranous layer

Constituents of spermatic cord

- Ductus deferens
- Testicular and cremasteric arteries and artery of the ducts deferens
- Pampiniform plexus of veins
- Lymph vessels from testis
- Plexus of sympathetic nerves around the artery to the ductus deferens
- Remains of processus vaginalis

Coverings of the spermatic cord

- External spermatic fascia: Derived from external oblique aponeurosis
- Cremasteric fascia: Derived from internal oblique aponeurosis
- Internal spermatic fascia: Derived from fascia transversalis

Blood supply of the stomach

- Right gastric artery (Hepatic artery) supplies: Lower right part of the stomach
- Short gastric artery (Splenic artery) supplies: Fundus
- Left gastric artery (Celiac artery) supplies: Lower third of esophagus, upper right part of the stomach
- Left gastroepiploic artery (Splenic artery) supplies: Upper part of greater curvature
- Right gastroepiploic artery (Gastroduodenal artery) supplies: Lower part of greater curvature

HEAD & NECK

- Axillary sheath is the continuation of: Prevertebral fascia
- Thalamic nuclei for hearing (lateral lemniscus): Medial geniculate body
- Genu of internal capsule contains fibres:
    - Ascending: Sensory fibres (from thalamus to brain)
    - Descending: Corticonuclear
- Retrolentiform part of internal capsule contains: Optic radiation
- Sublentiform part of internal capsule contains: Auditory radiation
- Left middle cerebral artery blockage results in:
    - Right sided hemiplegia
    - Sensory deficits (face & arm)
- Right middle cerebral artery blockage results in:
    - Left side hemiplegia
    - Sensory deficits (face & arm)
- Right posterior cerebral artery blockade results in: Left sided visual field defect
- Medial medullary syndrome is due to occlusion of: Vertebral artery
- Lateral medullary syndrome is due to occlusion of: Posterior inferior cerebellar artery

Layers of SCALP

- S: Skin
- C: Connective tissue
- A: Aponeurosis
- L: Loose areolar tissue
- P: Pericranium

Branches of external carotid artery

- **Anterior:** Superior thyroid, Lingual, Facial
- **Posterior:** Occipital, Posterior auricular
- **Medial:** Ascending pharyngeal
- **Terminal:** Maxillary, Superficial temporal

Sensory innervation of tongue [General sensation (GS); Taste sensation (TS)]

- Anterior 2/ 3rd (including circumvallate papillae for taste sensation): Lingual nerve (GS); Chorda tympani branch of facial nerve (TS)
- Posterior 1/ 3rd (except circumvallate papillae for taste sensation): Glossopharyngeal nerve for GS & TS

Carotid sheath contains

- Carotid arteries (within the sheath common carotid divides into external and internal carotids)
- Internal jugular vein
- Vagus nerve

Ocular muscles (Nerve supply & Function)

- Superior rectus: Oculomotor nerve; Moves eyeball upward and medially
- Inferior rectus: Oculomotor nerve; Moves eyeball downwards and medially
- Medial rectus: Oculomotor nerve; moves eyeball medially
- Lateral rectus: Abducens Moves eyeball laterally
- Superior oblique: Trochlear; Moves eyeball downwards and laterally
- Inferior oblique: Oculomotor nerve; Moves eyeball upwards and laterally
- Orbicularis oculi: Facial nerve; Closes eyeball and dilates lacrimal sac
- Levator Palpebrae Superioris: Oculomotor nerve; Raises upper lid and sympathetic supply

- Sphincter Pupillae: Parasympathetic supply; Constricts pupil by Oculomotor nerve
- Dilator pupillae: Sympathetic supply; Dilates pupil
- Ciliary muscle: Parasympathetic supply by Oculomotor nerve; controls shape of eye, helps in accommodation

Must know facts

- Only cranial nerve to arise from the dorsal aspect of the brain stem is Trochlear nerve
- Facial vein communicates with the cavernous sinus through the superior and inferior ophthalmic veins
- Stensen's duct- Parotid gland
- Wharton's duct- Submandibular gland

Tracts & modality carried

Tract	*Fibres of*
Posterior column	Light touch Vibration
Lateral spinothalamic tract	Crude touch Pressure Temperature
Corticospinal tract	Motor fibres
Rubrospinal tract **Cerebello spinal tract** **Vestibulospinal tract**	Position sense

BRAIN & SPINAL CORD

Lesion of visual pathway

- Optic nerve: Blindness in that eye
- Crossing fibres of optic chiasma: Bitemporal hemianopia
- Lateral parts of chiasma: Binasal hemianopia
- Optic tract/ lateral geniculate body: Contralateral homonymous hemianopia
- Meyer's loop of optic radiation: Contralateral superior Quadrantic anopia
- Vascular lesion of occipital lobe: Contralateral homonymous hemianopia with macula sparing

Blood-brain barrier is absent at

- Pituitary
- Area postrema
- Organum vasculosum of lamina terminalis
- Subfornical organ
- Ventral part of median eminence of hypothalamus
- Anterior pituitary
- Pineal gland

CRANIAL NERVES

- Artery crossing optic nerve: Ophthalmic artery
- Cranial nerve having longest intracranial course: Trochlear
- Cranial nerves 3 & 4 have their nuclei in: Midbrain
- Cranial nerves 9, 10, 11, 12 have their nuclei in: Medulla
- Cranial nerve emerging from the dorsal aspect of brain: Trochlear
- MC nerve involved in intracranial pressure: Cranial nerve 6
- Common nucleus for cranial nerves 9, 10 & 11: Nucleus ambiguus
- Muscles supplied by facial nerve:
  - o Platysma
  - o Muscles of facial expression
  - o Buccinator etc.
- Glands supplied by facial nerve:
  - o Submandibular
  - o Lacrimal
  - o Nasal glands
- Gustatory sensation to soft palate is carried by: Facial nerve
- Ganglion related to facial nerve:
  - o Pterygopalatine ganglion
  - o Geniculate ganglion etc.

- Arterial supply to facial nerve: Ascending pharyngeal artery
- All palatal muscles (except tensor palati) are supplied by: Accessory nerve through pharyngeal plexus
- Spasmodic torticollis is due to: Irritation of cranial part of accessory nerve
- Right hypoglossal nerve palsy will deviate the tongue to: Right side
- Paralysis of 3, 4 & 6 cranial nerve indicates lesion of: Cavernous sinus (these nerve lies in lateral wall of cavernous sinus)

FORAMINA

- Contents of optic canal:
  - o Optic nerve &
  - o Ophthalmic artery
- Contents of foramen rotundum: Maxillary division of cranial nerve V
- Contents of foramen ovale (MALE):
  - o Mandibular division of cranial nerve V
  - o Accessory meningeal artery etc.
  - o Lesser petrosal nerve
  - o Emissary vein
- Content of foramen spinosum:
  - o Middle meningeal artery
  - o Meningeal branch of the mandibular nerve etc.
- Contents of foramen magnum:
  - o Accessory nerve
  - o Vertebral & spinal arteries (NOT spinal cord) etc.
- Contents of jugular foramen:
  - o 9, 10 & 11 cranial nerves
  - o Internal jugular vein
  - o Inferior petrosal sinus
- Contents of internal auditory meatus:
  - o 7 & 8 cranial nerve
  - o Labyrinthine artery
- Content of Dorello's canal: Cranial nerve 6

Cranial nerve & functions

- Olfactory (Sensory): Perceives smell
- Optic (Sensory): Vision
- Oculomotor (Motor): Supplies levator palpebrae superioris, superior rectus, medial rectus, inferior rectus, inferior oblique, supplies sphincter pupillae and ciliary muscle with parasympathetic fibres
- Trochlear (Motor): Supplies superior oblique
- Trigeminal (Mixed): Supplies sensory fibres to the skin of the scalp, face, mouth, teeth, nasal cavity and paranasal sinuses; supplies motor fibres to the muscles of mastication, tensor veli palatini and tensor tympani
- Abducent (Motor): Supplies lateral rectus
- Facial (Mixed): Supplies motor fibres to the muscles of face, scalp with auricle, buccinator, platysma, stapedius, stylohyoid and posterior belly of digastric; gives sensory supply to anterior 2/3rd of tongue, floor of mouth and the palate; gives parasympathetic secretomotor fibres to the submandibular and sublingual salivary glands, lacrimal glands and the glands of the nose and palate
- Vestibulocochlear (Sensory): Position and movement of head; hearing
- Glossopharyngeal (Mixed): Supplies stylopharyngeus muscle; supplies parasympathetic secretomotor fibres to the parotid gland, sensory and taste fibres to the posterior third of tongue and pharynx
- Vagus (Mixed): Supplies constrictor muscles of pharynx and intrinsic muscles of larynx involuntary muscles of trachea and bronchi, heart, alimentary tract from pharynx to splenic flexure of colon, liver and pancreas; Afferent fibres from the abdominal structures, taste from epiglottis and valleculae
- Spinal accessory (Motor): Supplies sternocleidomastoid and trapezius
- Hypoglossal (Motor): Supplies muscles of tongue, except palatoglossus

Cranial foramen with the structures passing through them

- Carotid canal: Internal carotid artery

- Foramen rotundum: Maxillary nerve
- Foramen lacerum: Internal carotid artery, nerve of pterygoid canal
- Jugular foramen: Inferior petrosal sinus, 9th, 10th, 11th cranial nerves, internal jugular vein
- Stylomastoid foramen: Facial nerve
- Foramen magnum: Medulla, tonsils of cerebellum, meninges.
  - o Through subarachnoid space - Spinal accessory nerve, vertebral artery, posterior spinal artery, anterior spinal artery
  - o Anterior part - Ligament of dens, membrana tectoria
- Optic canal: Optic nerve
- Superior orbital fissure: Superior ophthalmic vein, lacrimal, frontal, Trochlear, Oculomotor, nasociliary, abducens nerves
- Hypoglossal canal: Hypoglossal nerve
- Internal acoustic meatus: Vestibulocochlear and facial nerve
- Foramen spinosum: Middle meningeal artery, nervous spinosus, posterior trunk of middle meningeal artery
- Foramen ovale: Mandibular nerve, Accessory meningeal artery, Lesser petrosal nerve, vein connecting cavernous sinus with the pterygoid plexus of veins

CEREBROSPINAL FLUID

- CSF is principally secreted by: Choroid plexus
- Choroid plexus is absent in: Anterior horn of lateral ventricle
- Total volume of CSF: 150 ml
- pH of CSF: 7.33
- Main factor controlling CSF pressure: Rate of CSF absorption
- Neutrophils in CSF: Are normally absent

LARYNX

- Cartilages of larynx: 3 paired & 3 unpaired
- Sensory innervation above the level of vocal cords is by: Internal laryngeal nerve
- Sensory innervation of larynx below the level of vocal cords: Recurrent laryngeal nerve
- Nerve supply of cricothyroid: External laryngeal nerve
- Abductor of vocal cords: Posterior crico-arytenoid
- Tensor of vocal cords: Cricothyroid

TEMPOROMANDIBULAR JOINT

- Depressor: Lateral pterygoid
- Protrusion: Pterygoids (both medial and lateral)
- Retraction: Posterior fibres of temporalis

Location of

Nucleus	*Location*
Red nucleus	Midbrain
Reticular activating system	Brainstem
Substantia nigra	Midbrain
Nucleus ambiguous	Medulla
Nucleus gracilis	Nucleus of dorsal column
Nucleus cuneatus	Medulla
Spiral ganglion	Cochlea
Dentate nucleus	Cerebellum
Nucleus fastigii	Cerebellum
Acoustic pathway (passes through)	Medial geniculate body
Optic radiation (passes through)	Lateral geniculate body
Edinger Westphal nucleus	3rd nerve

BRAIN

- Primary auditory area is in: Superior part of the temporal gyrus
- Primary visual area is in: Occipital lobe
- Broca's area is in: Inferior frontal gyrus
- Loss of tactile localization & 2 point discrimination occurs in damage to: Somatosensory area 1
- Functions of limbic system:
  - o Emotions

- o Memory &
- o Higher functions

EYE

- Extorters of eyeball: Both Inferior's
- Intorters of eye: Both Superior's
- Action of superior oblique: Abduction, Intorsion & depression
- Nerve supply of superior oblique: Cranial nerve 4
- Muscle attached to posterior tarsal margin: Muller's muscle

DRAINING LYMPH NODES

- Clitoris & glans penis: Cloquet node/ Rosenmuller node/ deep inguinal
- Labium majus: Superficial inguinal node
- Testis: Pre-aortic & para-aortic nodes
- Tip of tongue: Submental nodes
- Spongiform urethra: Deep inguinal nodes (mainly)
- Lymphatics are not present in: Brain, choroid, internal ear, cornea

VEINS

- Great cerebral vein (of Galen) is formed by the union of: Internal cerebral veins
- Great cerebral vein drains into: Straight sinus
- Portal vein is formed by: Union of splenic vein & superior mesenteric vein (behind neck of pancreas)
- Normal portal pressure is: 5-10 mm Hg

EXCEPTS IN ANATOMY

- All intrinsic muscle of larynx are supplied by recurrent laryngeal nerve except: Cricothyroid (external laryngeal nerve)
- All muscles of tongue are supplied by hypoglossal nerve except: Palatoglossus (pharyngeal plexus)
- All muscles of pharynx are supplied by pharyngeal plexus except: Stylopharyngeus (Glossopharyngeal nerve)
- All muscles of the soft palate are supplied by pharyngeal plexus except: Tensor palati (nerve to medial pterygoid)

JOINTS

- Sutures are seen in: Skull
- Joint between diaphysis & epiphysis is: Primary cartilaginous (synchondrosis)
- Symphysis pubis is: Secondary cartilaginous (symphysis)
- Inferior tibiofibular joint is: Syndesmosis
- Elbow joint is: Hinge joint
- Temporomandibular joint is: Condyloid joint
- Wrist joint is: Ellipsoid joint
- First carpometacarpal joint is: Saddle joint

EPIPHYSES

- Head of femur is: Pressure epiphysis
- Tubercles of humerus, mastoid process is: Traction epiphysis
- Coracoid process of scapula is: Atavistic epiphysis

SESAMOID BONES

- Sesamoid bones develop in: Muscle tendons
- Sesamoid bones are devoid of: Periosteum
- Fabella is present in: Lateral head of gastrocnemius

Sesamoid bones (in the tendons of)

- Quadriceps femoris (Patella-largest sesamoid bone)
- Peroneus longus
- Tibialis anterior
- Tibialis posterior
- Lateral head of gastrocnemius

Peculiarities of sesamoid bones

- Ossify at birth
- Devoid of periosteum
- Absence of haversian system

MISCELLANEOUS

Spinal nerves

- Cervical: 8
- Thoracic:12
- Lumbar: 5
- Sacral: 5
- Coccygeal:1
- Total: 31

Vertebral levels & bony landmarks

- C7: Most prominent spinosus process at the base of neck
- T3: Level of the spine of scapula
- T7: Level of lower angle of scapula
- T12: Floating rib
- L4: Level of iliac crests
- S2: Level of posterior superior iliac spine

Structure & their levels in body

- Xiphoid process: T9
- Celiac trunk: T12 L1
- Spleen: 10th rib
- Superior mesenteric artery: L1
- Stomach pylorus: L1
- Spinal cord ends (adults): L1, L2
- Spinal cord ends (Children): L3
- Pancreas: L1, L2
- Inferior mesenteric artery: L3
- Umbilicus: L3, L4
- Highest point of iliac crest: L4
- Transtubercular plane: L5

Anatomy of heart

Area	*Formed by*
Anterior surface (sternocostal surface)	Right ventricle (mainly), partly be left ventricle & left auricle
Apex	Left ventricle
Base (posterior surface)	Left atrium receiving 4 pulmonary veins, some part of right Atrium
Inferior surface/ border (diaphragmatic surface)	Right ventricle plus some part of left ventricle
Left heart border	Left ventricle mainly, left atrial appendages, aortic knuckle, pulmonary artery
Right heart border	Superior vena cava, right atrium, inferior vena cava

CLINICAL QUESTIONS

1. **A young male was operated in the area of right submandibular gland and accidentally right hypoglossal nerve was injured. What will be the clinical finding in that patient?**

   A. Deviation of the tongue toward left side when the patient was told to protrude the tongue

   B. Deviation of the tongue toward right side when the patient was told to protrude the tongue

   C. Loss of general sensation over the anterior 2/3rd of the tongue

   D. Loss of taste sensation over the anterior 2/3rd of the tongue

   Clinical presentation is suggestive of lower motor type of hypoglossal nerve palsy.

   Following a lesion of the hypoglossal nucleus or nerve, there is atrophy of the muscles of the ipsilateral one-half of the tongue. This is a lower motor neuron lesion (the damaged neuron or axon directly innervates skeletal muscle). Upon closer examination, fasciculations (tiny, spontaneous contractions) can be seen. Both fasciculations and atrophy result from the loss of the normal innervation of the muscle by the lower motor neurons in the hypoglossal nucleus. Upon protrusion, the tongue will deviate toward the side of the lesion (i.e., same side). This is due to the unopposed action of the genioglossus muscle on the normally innervated side of the tongue (the genioglossus pulls the tongue forward).

   Answer: B i.e., Deviation of the tongue toward right side when the patient was told to protrude the tongue

2. **A 55 years old female has undergone mastectomy for carcinoma breast. After the surgery, she was unable to extend, adduct and internally rotate the arm. Nerve supply to which of the following muscle has been damaged:**

   A. Pectoralis major B. Teres minor

   C. Latissimus dorsi D. Lateral head of triceps

   Clinical presentation is suggestive of injury to thoracodorsal nerve.

   It supplies latissimus dorsi.

   Action of LD is extension, adduction and medial rotation of arm.

   The latissimus dorsi is a large, flat muscle on the back that stretches to the sides, behind the arm, and is partly covered by the trapezius on the back.

   Answer: C i.e., Latissimus dorsi

3. **Paralysis of 3rd, 4th and 6th cranial nerves with involvement of ophthalmic division of 5th cranial nerve suggest the possibility of lesion in:**

   A. Apex of the orbit B. Brainstem

   C. Base of the skull D. Cavernous sinus

   Clinical presentation is suggestive of cavernous sinus thrombosis.

   The cavernous sinus is part of the brain's dural venous sinus and contains multiple neuro-vasculatures. It is situated bilaterally to the sella turcica and extends from the superior orbital fissure anteriorly to the petrous part of the temporal bone posteriorly, and is about 1 cm wide and 2 cm long.

   Answer: D i.e., Cavernous sinus

4. **A child has recurrent abdominal pain and bilious vomiting. Condition was diagnosed by Barium follow through. Surgical procedures followed – Lad S band division, appendectomy and mesenteric widening. Diagnosis is:**

   A. Cecal volvulus B. Malrotation

   C. Acute appendicitis D. Duodenal web

   Clinical presentation is suggestive of malrotation.

   Malrotation is a birth defect link that occurs when the intestines do not correctly or completely rotate into their normal final position during development.

   Answer: B i.e., Malrotation

5. **A patient woke up from sleep with difficulty in extending the fingers. He can make a grip and hold the pen. Wrist extension was possible. No sensory disturbance was found. Site of injury:**

   A. Hand area in motor cortex

B. Lower part of brachial plexus

C. C8, T1

D. Posterior interosseous nerve

Clinical presentation is suggestive of finger drop due to posterior interosseous nerve palsy.

It is a purely motor nerve.

The posterior interosseous nerve (PIN) is a branch of the radial nerve, which comes off the posterior cord of the brachial plexus. The posterior interosseous nerve supplies motor innervation to the posterior forearm.

Answer: D i.e., Posterior interosseous nerve

6. **A patient is trying to make a fist, but can only partially flex index and middle finger. Which nerve is damaged most probably?**

A. Radial nerve

B. Median nerve

C. Ulnar nerve

D. Posterior interosseous nerve

Clinical presentation is suggestive of Benediction deformity, which is seen in median nerve palsy.

The hand of benediction, also known as benediction sign or preacher's hand, occurs as a result of prolonged compression or injury of the median nerve.

Answer: B i.e., Median nerve

7. **In a vehicular accident, the musculocutaneous nerve was completely severed, but still the person was able to weakly flex the elbow joint. Which of the following muscle is NOT responsible for this weak flexion?**

A. Brachioradialis

B. Flexor carpi radialis

C. Ulnar head of pronator teres

D. Flexor carpi ulnaris

Brachioradialis is a flexor of elbow and is supplied by radial nerve.

Muscles originating from medial epicondyle of humerus are weak flexors.

The common flexor tendon is the convergence of 5 muscles: pronator teres, flexor carpi radialis, palmaris longus, flexor digitorum superficialis, and flexor carpi ulnaris.

Answer: C i.e., Ulnar head of pronator teres

8. **After surgery on right side of neck, a person could NOT raise his arm above the head level and also could NOT shrug his shoulder. Which structure is paralyzed?**

A. Injury to axillary nerve

B. Paralysis of deltoid

C. Paralysis of trapezius muscle

D. Paralysis of latissimus dorsi

Clinical presentation is suggestive of injury to spinal accessory nerve resulting in paralysis of trapezius muscle.

The trapezius is a large paired trapezoid-shaped surface muscle that extends longitudinally from the occipital bone to the lower thoracic vertebrae.

Answer: C i.e., Paralysis of trapezius muscle

CHAPTER 2

PHYSIOLOGY

RAPID REVISION NOTES

Distribution of cardiac output

Brain	1/5th of cardiac output
Heart	5% of cardiac output
Kidney	1/4th of cardiac output
Liver	1500 ml/ min
Muscle	100-200 ml/ min

GENERAL PHYSIOLOGY

Normal values

- Normal blood volume: 5-5.5 liters (3 liters plasma + 2 liters of cell volume)
- Intracellular fluid - 55 percent
- Extracellular fluid - 45 percent
- Total plasma protein in blood is 6.4-8.3 gm/dl
- Normal albumin: globulin ratio is 1.8:1-2:1
- Na^+: 135-145 meq/l
- K^+: 3.5-5.5 meq/l
- Ca^{++}: 9-11 meq/l
- pH: 7.35-7.45
- PCO_2: 34-45 Hg
- PO_2: 85-100 mm Hg
- HCO_3^- 25-28 meq/l
- O_2 saturation: 92-96 percent
- Normal anion gap: 8-16 meq/l
- Normal glomerular filtration rate-125 ml
- Renal blood flow-1200 ml/min
- Renal threshold for glucose -180 mg/dl
- Tubular maximum for glucose- 320 mg/min

Half lives of proteins

- Albumin: 2-3 weeks
- Transferrin: 1 week
- Pre-albumin, retinol binding protein, Fibronectin: 2 days

Function of cell organelles

- Mitochondria: Production of energy
- Rough endoplasmic reticulum: Packaging of proteins
- Smooth endoplasmic reticulum: Lipid synthesis
- Ribosomes: Protein synthesis
- Golgi apparatus: Concentration of proteins and polysaccharides
- Centriole: Initiates the process of cell division

- Lysosome: Breaks down bacteria and debris from dead tissue cells
- Peroxisomes: Destroy harmful substances

Types of cell transport

- Passive diffusion(simple passive+ facilitated diffusions): Transport of a substance along the gradient, energy is not required
- Simple passive diffusion: Diffusion along the gradient, without the requirement of carrier. Not rate limiting. doesn't follow saturation kinetics
- Primary active transport: Transport against gradient. Energy is obtained by breakdown of ATP. Requires transport protein. Rate limiting and saturable
- Secondary active transport: Energy for transport is derived from sodium gradient. Transport against gradient requires transport protein. Rate limiting and saturable

Rheobase & chronaxie

- Rheobase: The least strength or current which excites the excitable tissue
- Chronaxie: Minimum time required to stimulate the excitable tissue when strength of the current used is double the rheobase

Reflexes/ Law's/ Rule's in physiology

- Cushing's reflex: The reflex that tends to restore the blood flow to medulla by causing rise in systemic arterial pressure, slowing of respiration and reflex bradycardia in case of raised intracranial pressure
- Bainbridge reflex: A true reflex rather than local response to stretch, causes receptor mediated increase in heart rate, is abolished by bilateral Vagotomy
- Starling's law: Within physiological limits, force of contraction is directly proportional to the initial length of the muscle fibres, provided conditions remain the same
- Bezold-Jarisch reflex: Is a coronary chemoreflex mediated by left ventricular stretch receptors that are C fibers endings, it causes a fall in systemic arterial pressure and heart rate and apnoea followed rapid breathing
- Bohr effect-effect of CO_2 in the affinity of Hemoglobin for O_2: Shift of oxygen hemoglobin dissociation curve by change in the blood in the blood CO_2, and hydrogen ions to enhance oxygenation of blood in lungs and to enhance release of oxygen from blood in the tissue
- Haldane effect: Binding of oxygen with hemoglobin tends to displace CO_2 from blood; Important in promoting carbon dioxide transport
- Hering-Breuer reflex: The stretch receptors in bronchi and bronchioles send inhibitory signals through vagi to inspiratory centre when the lung is overinflated
- Cushing's response: Onset of irregular respiration, bradycardia and final increased blood pressure with increasing intracranial tension due to brain stem compression
- Landsteiner's law: States that if an agglutinogen is present in the red cells of the blood, the corresponding agglutinin must be absent from the plasma, if the agglutinogen is absent, corresponding agglutinin must be present in the plasma
- Sham rage behavior: Physical and motor manifestation of anger seen in destruction of ventromedial hypothalamic nuclei and septal nuclei
- Muller's doctrine of specific nerve energies: When the nerve pathways from particular sense organs are stimulated, the sensation evoked is that for which the receptor is specialized no matter how or where along the pathway the activity is initiated
- Weber-Fechner law: Interpreted signal strength = Log x stimulus intensity + constant

Resting membrane potential

RBC	-7 mV
Smooth muscle	-50 mV
Nerve	-70 mV
Cardiac muscle	-90 mV

BASICS

- RMP of nerve fibre is: -70 mV
- RMP is due to: Potassium ions
- RMP is close to isoelectric potential of: Chloride ions

- Inhibitory post synaptic potential/ IPSP is due to: Chloride influx
- At synapse, nerve impulse flow is: Unidirectional

CELL MEMBRANE

- Main constituent of cell membrane is: Protein
- Fluidity of cell membrane is increased by: Polyunsaturated fatty acids
- RBC membrane has: Spectrin (maintains integrity) & glycophorin
- Basement membrane contains: Laminin, nidogen, type IV collagen etc.

CELL ORAGENELLES & FUNCTIONS

- Agranular endoplasmic reticulum: Synthesis of lipids
- Rough ER: Synthesis of proteins
- Microtubules: Cell shape & motility
- Peroxisomes: Catabolism of H_2O_2
- Mitochondria: Site of ATP synthesis

CELL ORGANELLES & MARKERS

- Mitochondria: Glutamic dehydrogenase
- Golgi bodies: Galactosyl transferase
- Plasma membrane: Adenylyl cyclase 5 nucleotidase

BODY FLUIDS

- Water constitutes about: 60% of body weight
- Sodium, chloride & bicarbonate ions are predominant in: Extracellular fluid
- Intracellular fluid is rich in: Potassium
- Endolymph is rich in: Potassium
- Measurement of total body water: Tritiated water, deuterium oxide
- Measurement of ECF: Inulin, mannitol
- Measurement of plasma volume: Evans blue, radiolabeled albumin
- Normal anion gap (cations - anions): 10-12 mmol/ L

Centre of reflexes

Reflex	*Centre*
Jaw jerk	Vth cranial nerve
Conjunctival & corneal	Afferent – Vth; efferent – VIIth
Anal, bulbocavernosus	S3, 4
Ankle	S1
Plantar	L5, S1
Knee	L3, 4
Cremaster	L1, 2
Triceps	C7, 8
Pronator	C6
Biceps, supinator	C5, 6

NERVE & MUSCLE PHYSIOLOGY

- Band which narrows during contraction: H band
- Active sites of actin are covered by: Tropomyosin
- Essential for smooth muscle contraction: Cellular calcium
- Order of susceptibility of nerve fibres to anaesthesia & pressure: Type C > type B > type A
- REMEMBER: Force of contraction of muscle is INDEPENDENT of amplitude of action potential

GOLGI TENDON ORGAN

- GTO detects: Muscle tension
- Impulses are transmitted by: Type Ib nerve fibres
- Golgi tendon reflex is: Bisynaptic

MUSCLE SPINDLE

- It is a receptor for: Myotatic/ stretch reflex
- Peripheral zone of muscle spindle has: Actin & myosin

CVS PHYSIOLOGY

- Resistance vessel: Arteriole
- Exchange vessel: Capillaries (maximum surface area)
- Capacitance vessel: Vein

- BP is calculated as: Cardiac output X peripheral resistance
- Small cuff, thick walled vessels & obesity will give a: High BP
- Ventricular end diastolic volume: Volume of blood in ventricular cavity at the end of atrial contraction (120 ml); determines preload
- Ejection fraction: Ratio of stroke volume to end diastolic volume (SD/ EDV); 50-70%
- Stroke volume: Volume of blood ejected with each heart beat (CO/ HR); 70-80 ml
- Cardiac index: Cardiac output/ Body surface area; 3.2 is the normal value

Volumes related to cardio-physiology

- Stroke volume: Volume of blood that is ejected by each ventricle with each beat. It is normally 70 ml
- Ventricular end diastolic volume: Volume of blood in the ventricle just prior to the onset of ventricular contraction. Normal 110-120 ml
- Ventricular end systolic volume: Volume of blood remaining in the ventricle at the end of ejection. Normally 40- 50 ml

REGIONAL BLOOD FLOW

- Blood flow is mainly controlled by: Arterioles
- Effect of CO_2 on brain vasculature: Vasodilation
- Effect of hypoxia in pulmonary circulation: Vasoconstriction
- Depolarization proceeds from: Endocardium to epicardium
- Speed of conduction is fastest in: Purkinje fibres

ELECTROCARDIOGRAM

- QRS complex is due to: Ventricular depolarization
- Duration of QRS complex: 0.08 – 0.10 sec
- 3rd heart sound is hear during: Ventricular filling phase
- Y wave in JVP is due to: Opening of AV valve & emptying of blood into ventricle

ECG (Parameters & coincident event)

- P wave (0.08): Atrial depolarization
- PR interval (0.12-0.20 sec): Atrial depolarization and conduction through AV node measured from beginning of QRS complex.
- QRS duration (0.08-0.10 sec): Ventricular depolarization and atrial repolarization
- T wave: Ventricular repolarization
- U wave: Slow repolarization of papillary muscles.

Life span

Cells	*Life span (days)*
Monocytes	1-3
Basophils	12-15
Platelets	9-11
Eosinophils	8-12
Lymphocytes	2-3
Neutrophils	2-4

HEMOGLOBIN

- Hb A: Alpha2, Beta2/ $\alpha 2\beta 2$
- Hb A2: Alpha2, Delta2/ $\alpha 2\delta 2$
- Hb F: Alpha2, Gamma2/ $\alpha 2\gamma 2$
- Bart's Hb: Gamma4/ $\gamma 4$

Hypoxia

Type of hypoxia	*Pathophysiology*	*Example*
Stagnant	Due to slow circulation	Circulatory shock, congestive heart failure
Histotoxic	Inability of cells to utilize available oxygen	Cyanide poisoning
Hypoxic	Due to inadequate gas exchange	High altitude, respiratory disease (COPD)
Anemic	Due to reduced oxygen carrying capacity	Anemia, CO poisoning

RESPIRATORY PHYSIOLOGY

- CO_2 is primarily transported in arterial blood as: Bicarbonate
- Normal value of pO_2: 80 mm Hg
- Arterial level of CO_2: 40 mm Hg
- During inspiration, intrapleural pressure becomes: More negative
- Total lung capacity: Volume of air contained in the lung at the end of maximal inspiration; 6 L (male); 4.7 L (female)
- Total lung capacity depends upon: Lung compliance
- Vital capacity: Amount of air that can be forced out of the lungs after maximal inspiration; 4.8 L (male); 3.6 L (female)
- Tidal volume: Amount of air breathed in or out during normal breathing; 500 ml (male); 390 ml (female)
- Functional residual capacity: Amount of air left in the lungs after normal expiration; 2.4L (male); 1.9 L (female)
- Physiologic dead volume: Anatomic dead space + alveolar dead space; 155 ml (male); 120 ml (female)
- At the apex of lung: V>Q (wasted ventilation)
- Volume of lung at the end of quite expiration, which can be expired with maximal effect: Expiratory reserve volume
- Minute alveolar ventilation is: 3.5 – 4.5 L
- Response to high altitude:
  - o Increased ventilation (earliest)
  - o Increased response to carotid bodies
  - o Respiratory alkalosis etc.
- Increased pulmonary capillary pressure results in: Pulmonary edema
- Pulmonary surfactant is secreted by: Type II pneumocytes
- Surfactant is: Dipalmitoyl phosphatidyl choline (DPPC)
- Surfactant production is accelerated by: Glucocorticoids
- Respiratory distress syndrome is due to: Deficiency of surfactant
- Nernst equation/ chloride shift: Bicarbonate diffuses into plasma & same quantity of chloride diffuses into RBC in venous circulation
- Bohr effect: Affinity of oxygen for hemoglobin decreases with fall in pH
- Heads reflex: Inflation of lungs induces more inflation
- Pneumotaxic centre is present in: Pons (dorsal)
- Shape of oxygen hemoglobin dissociation curve: Sigmoid
- Decrease in temperature shifts the curve to: Left
- Increase in affinity of oxygen for hemoglobin shifts the curve to: Left
- Increased pCO_2 shifts the curve to: Right
- Sickle cell hemoglobin presence shifts the curve to: Right
- Respiratory distress syndrome shifts the curve to: Right
- 2,3 DPG (increased in anemia) shift the curve to: Right
- MC type of hypoxia: Hypoxic hypoxia
- Hypoxia is defined as: Low pO_2

O_2 dissociation curve

- Shift to left: Increased pH, Decreased temperature, Fetal hemoglobin
- Shift to right: Decreased pH, Increased temperature, Increased 2,3, DPG

Respiratory capacities and volumes

- Tidal volume: Air that is taken in or given out during normal quiet respiration
- Inspiratory reserve volume: Air that can be taken in over and above the tidal volume
- Expiratory reserve volume: Maximum volume of air that can be expired over and above the tidal volume
- Residual volume: Volume of air that remains in the lungs after forceful expiration
- Inspiratory capacity: Maximum volume of air that can be inspired after normal tidal expiration (IC=IRV+TV)
- Vital capacity: Maximum volume of air that can be expired after deepest possible inspiration (VC=IRV +TV+ERV)

- Total lung capacity: Sum of vital capacity and residual volume

GASTROINTESTINAL TRACT

- Site of absorption of iron: Duodenum
- Intrinsic factor is secreted by: Oxyntic/ parietal cells
- HCl is secreted by: Oxyntic/ parietal cells
- Gastrin is secreted by: G cells of stomach, duodenum etc.
- Actions of gastrin:
  - o Stimulates secretion of gastric juice
  - o Increases gastric motility etc.
- Actions of secretin:
  - o Stimulates secretion of watery, alkaline & pancreatic secretions, Inhibit gastric secretion
  - o Causes contraction of pyloric sphincter
- Most potent stimulator of secretion of secretin is: Acidic chyme
- Action of cholecystokinin: Stimulates contraction of gallbladder
- CCK-PZ secretion is stimulated by: Proteins
- Gastric secretion is stimulated by:
  - o Gastrin
  - o Histamine etc.
- Pacemaker of small intestine is in: Second part of duodenum
- Gastric phase of gastric secretion is mediated by: Hormones
- Intestinal motility is stimulated by:
  - o Distension
  - o Acetylcholine etc.
- Fat is maximally absorbed in: Jejunum
- Calcium is maximally absorbed in: Ileum
- Electrolytes are absorbed in: Colon
- Effect of dietary fibres (e.g. pectin):
  - o Increases bulk of stool
  - o Increases metabolism of sugar in GIT
- Largest reserve of energy in body: Fat
- Gastric lipase helps in digestion of: Fats
- Indicator of malabsorption: Fat in stool (> 6 gms/ day)

Gastric acid secretion

- Excitatory: Acetylcholine, Gastrin, Histamine
- Inhibitory: Enterogastric reflex, Enterogastrone, Somatostatin

Hepatic cells

- Ito cells are fat containing lipocytes in the space of Disse of the liver
- Kupffer cells are phagocytic cells, part of monocyte and macrophage cells

Half life

Substance	*Half life*
Albumin	20-26 days
Fibrinogen	100 hours
Factor VIII	8 hours
Heparin	60-90 minutes

ENDOCRINOLOGY

- Insulin increases:
  - o Glycogen synthesis
  - o Fat synthesis
  - o Protein synthesis etc.
- Insulin is a: Hypoglycemic hormone
- Insulin is secreted by: Beta cells of pancreas
- In fetus, secretion of insulin begins by: 3 months
- Insulin secretion is inhibited by: Epinephrine
- Delta cells of pancreas secrete: Somatostatin
- Hormones acting on intracellular nuclear receptors:
  - o Steroids
  - o Thyroid hormones
  - o Vitamin D etc.
- cAMP mediates action of:

  - o ADH
  - o PTH etc.
- cGMP mediates action of: NO (cellular signalling molecule)
- Insulin acts through: Tyrosine kinase activity
- Hormones belonging to steroid receptor family:
  - o Vitamin D3
  - o Thyroid
- Effects of parathormone:
  - o Stimulates osteoclastic activity
  - o Augments absorption of calcium from the gut
- Effects of calcitonin:
  - o Opposite to that of PTH
  - o Lowers serum calcium
  - o Acts by decreasing osteoclasis (bone resorption)
- PTH-rP/ PTH related protein is: Hypercalcemic factor
- PTH-rP secretion is stimulated by: Low calcium levels
- Feature of PTH-rP: Important hormonal mediator of cancer associated hypercalcemia
- Active form of calcium: Ionized form
- A decrease in concentration of free calcium ions in plasma results in:
  - o Increased neuromuscular irritability & tetani
  - o Chvostek's sign etc.
- ECG finding of hypocalcemia: Lengthening of the QT interval
- ACTH & TSH are secreted by: Anterior pituitary gland
- Vasopressin & oxytocin are secreted by: Posterior pituitary gland

Hormone Receptors

- Cell membrane receptors:
  - o cAMP pathway: Adrenaline, Calcitonin, Glucagon, TSH, FSH, LH, ACTH, PTH
  - o IP3-DAG: Vasopressin, Oxytocin
  - o Tyrosine- kinase: Insulin, Growth hormone
- Cytoplasmic receptors: Steroids (Glucocorticoids, Mineralocorticoids), Estrogen, Progesterone
- Nuclear receptors: Thyroxine

Zones of adrenal cortex & hormones secreted (GFR)

- Zona **G**lomerulosa: Aldosterone
- Zona **F**asciculate: Cortisol
- Zona **R**eticularis: Androgens

Hormones & their site of action

Hormone	*Site of action*
Atrial natriuretic peptide	Collecting duct
Antidiuretic hormone	Medullary collecting duct
Aldosterone	Cortical collecting duct & distal tubules
Angiotensin II	Constricts afferent arterioles, helps to reduce GFR

EXCRETORY SYSTEM

- Action of renin: Converts angiotensinogen to angiotensin I
- Factors stimulating renin secretion:
  - o Low BP
  - o Hyponatremia etc.
- Major part of glomerular filtrate is absorbed in: PCT
- Substances completely reabsorbed in PCT:
  - o Glucose
  - o Potassium
  - o Amino acid
- In presence of vasopressin, maximum reabsorption of eater takes place in: PCT
- Substances partially reabsorbed in PCT:
  - o Sodium,
  - o Bicarbonate
  - o Water
  - o Chloride
- Glucose transport occurs with: Sodium

- Macula densa is: Epithelial lining of distal tubule
- Tubuloglomerular feedback is mediated by sensing: Sodium chloride in densa
- Loop of Henle does not handle: Urea
- Filtration fraction is calculated as: GFR/ RPF; 20%
- GFR (inulin clearance) is: 125 ml/ min
- Normal creatinine level: 0.6-1.2 mg%
- Urea clearance: 88 ml/ min

Juxtaglomerular apparatus

- Macula densa: Epithelial cells of the initial part of distal tubule, lying in the angle between afferent and efferent arteriole of the glomerulus
- Juxtaglomerular cells/ Granular cells: Smooth muscle cells of afferent and efferent arterioles containing dark granules, coming in contact with macula densa

REPRODUCTIVE SYSTEM

- Functions of LH:
  - o Stimulates ovulation
  - o Maintains corpus luteum
- FSH receptors are present in: Granulosa cells
- Hormonal status in menopause:
  - o Decreased estrogen
  - o Raised FSH & LH
- Spermatozoa acquire motility in: Epididymis
- Capacitation occurs in: Female genital tract (fallopian tube)
- In female genital tract, sperm don't survive more than: 48 hours
- Testosterone is produced from: Pregnenolone
- Testosterone is produced by: Leydig cells
- Blood testis barrier is formed by: Sertoli cells
- Inhibin is secreted by: Sertoli cells
- Most useful physiologic marker of thyroid hormone action: TSH
- Hormones increased in stressful conditions:
  - o Adrenaline
  - o Vasopressin
  - o Cortisol
  - o Glucagon
- Insulin is NOT increased in stressful conditions
- Melatonin is a: Pineal hormone
- In darkness: Activity of serotonin-N-acetyl transferase is increased

Hormones & their effects

- Prolactin: Promotes breast development in pregnancy & lactation
- FSH: Stimulates ovarian follicle growth in female & spermatogenesis in male
- LH: Stimulates ovulation & luteinization of ovarian follicles in female & testosterone secretion in male
- Estrogen: Responsible for maintenance of oogenesis, development of sex organs & secondary sexual characters in females at puberty
- Progesterone: Prepares the endometrium for implantation of the fertilized ovum & promotes the growth & development of the breast
- Testosterone: Responsible for maintenance of spermatogenesis, development of sex organs & secondary sexual characters in males at puberty
- Oxytocin: Uterine contraction during labour & promotes milk ejection during breast feeding

Electroencephalogram/ EEG

Alpha	Seen at rest with eyes closed & mind wandering Frequency 8-12/second Amplitude of 50 mV Most marked in parieto-occipital area
Beta	18-30/second Seen over frontal region
Theta	4-7/second Occurs in children Over hippocampus
Delta	<4/second Large, slow waves

NERVOUS SYSTEM

- Theta waves (4-7 Hz) are seen in: Hippocampus
- Delta waves (3-5 Hz) are seen in: Deep sleep
- Nightmares are seen in: REM sleep
- Helmholtz theory (of colour vision): There are 3 kinds of cones in retina, corresponding to 3 colours
- Protanomaly is: Defect in red cones
- Visible range of electromagnetic spectrum of human eye: 370-740 nm
- Function of amacrine cells: Regulates relative color & luminosity of photoreceptive input under changing light
- Most sensitive (pathway) for stimulus of colour contrast: Parvocellular pathway (from lateral geniculate body to visual cortex)
- Blobs of visual cortex are associated with: Colour processing
- Function of pacinian corpuscles: Senses rapidly adapting touch, pressure & vibration
- Region of CNS, which degenerate in Huntington's disease (GABAergic neurons): Caudate nucleus
- Cingulate gyri & amygdaloid nucleus are part of: Limbic system
- Wernickes aphasia is: Impaired comprehension of spoken & written language
- Broca's aphasia is concerned with: Word formation
- Broca's area is present in: Inferior frontal gyrus
- Nuclei of hypothalamus controlling thirst & water balance: Supraoptic nucleus
- Nuclei of hypothalamus controlling circadian rhythm: Suprachiasmatic nucleus
- Nuclei of hypothalamus controlling shivering: Postero-lateral hypothalamus
- Functions of hypothalamus:
  - o Food intake
  - o Hypophyseal control
  - o Non shivering thermogenesis (because of noradrenaline; mediated by beta 3 receptors)
- Hormone important for cold adaptation: Thyroxine (piloerection is NOT significant)
- Main excitatory neurotransmitter in CNS is: Glutamate
- Flight or fight response includes:
  - o Increased heart rate
  - o Increased BP
  - o Increased total peripheral resistance
- Functions of cerebellum:
  - o Coordinates & smoothens the action of different muscle groups
  - o Producing smooth & accurate movements
- Intention tremors are seen in: Lesions of cerebellum
- Function of basal nuclei/ basal ganglia: Planning & programming of movements
- Caudate nucleus & lentiform nuclei (corpus striatum) are a part of: Basal ganglia

Cells of nervous system

- Macroglia: CNS macrophages
- Astrocytes: Maintain blood-brain barrier. Repair and scar formation
- Oligodendrocytes: Formation of myelin in CNS
- Ependymal cells: Line the ventricular system

Route of CSF Flow

- Choroid plexus - Lateral ventricle - Foramen of Monro - Third ventricle - Aqueduct of Sylvius - Fourth ventricle - Foramina of Luschka and Magendie - Subarachnoid space - Venous outflow

Nuclei of Hypothalamus

- Lateral nucleus: Feeding centre
- Ventromedial nucleus: Satiety centre

Reflexes & root values

- Ankle: S1, S2
- Knee jerk: L3, 4
- Biceps reflex: C5, 6
- Triceps jerk: C7, 8

- Radial jerk: C6
- Plantar reflex: S1,S2
- Abdominal reflex: T7, T11
- Cremasteric reflex: L1

Receptors

- Free nerve endings: Detect touch and pressure
- Meissner's corpuscles: Detect movement of light touch
- Merkel's disc: Localizing touch sensations and determining texture
- Hair end organs: Detect the movement of objects on the surface of body
- Ruffini's end organs: Detect degree of joint movement
- Pacinian corpuscles: Detect tissue vibration, extremely rapid changes in mechanical state of tissue

Coagulation factors

Factor	*Remarks*
5, 10	Good for growth of hemophilus organism
5, 8	Unstable in stored blood
1, 2, 10	Both PTT & PT increased
2, 7, 10	PT
2, 7, 9, 10	Vitamin K dependent
2, 7, 8, 9, 10	Levels increased with oral contraceptives
1, 2, 5, 7, 9, 10	Produced in liver

MISCELLANEOUS

- Nitric oxide/ NO is also known as: EDRF/ endothelial derived relaxing factor
- Nitric oxide is produced from: Arginine (by NO synthetase)
- NO has half life of: 4 seconds (short $t_{1/2}$)
- NO acts as:
    - o Free radical
    - o Vasodilator
    - o Oxidizing agent
- Histamine is formed by: Decarboxylation of histidine
- Function of histamine: Mediates triple response
- Effects of release of Atrial natriuretic peptide/ ANP:
    - o Excretion of sodium & water (augments GFR)
    - o Inhibiting sodium reabsorption in PCT
    - o Arteriolar & venous dilatation (by antagonizing vasoconstrictors)
    - o Decreases BP
- ANP acts by: cGMP pathway
- Changes seen with exercise:
    - o Increased cardiac output
    - o Increased respiratory rate
    - o Blood flow to brain is unaltered
- Changes with aging:
    - o Vital capacity decreases
    - o Hematocrit remains the same

LAWS IN PHYSIOLOGY

- Weber Fechner law: Magnitude of sensation felt is proportionate to the log of the intensity of the stimulus
- Law of projection: No matter where a particular sensory pathway is stimulated along its course to the cortex, the conscious sensation produced is referred to the location of the receptor
- Phantom limb sensation is based on: Law of projection
- Receptor of hearing: Hair cells of organ of corti
- Receptors for linear acceleration: Hair cells of utricle & saccule
- Function of bradykinin: Stimulation of visceral smooth muscle
- Function of clathrin: Receptor mediated endocytosis
- Muscle spindle detects: Muscle length

Hemophilia

Type	*Deficient factor*
Hemophilia A	VIII
Hemophilia B	IX
Hemophilia C	XI
Parahemophilia	V
Pseudo-hemophilia	Vascular hemophilia, von-willebrand's disease

CLINICAL QUESTIONS

1. **A 25 years old female was watching TV for long hours keeping her right hand under the head. Later on, she experienced tingling sensation over her right upper limb. Most likely affected nerve fibers are:**

   A. Type A B. Type B

   C. Type C D. Sympathetic fibers

   Type A nerve fibers are most susceptible to pressure.

   Answer: A i.e., Type A

2. **A patient slept the whole night keeping his arm under his head. Next morning when he woke up, he had paresis and numbness in that upper limb. Which of the following physiological fact is true in relation to the clinical presentation?**

   A. A fibers are more prone to pressure than C fibers

   B. C fibers are more prone to pressure than A fibers

   C. A fibers are more prone to hypoxia than C fibers

   D. C fibers are more prone to hypoxia than A fibers

   ***A** fibers are most susceptible to **P**ressure.*

   ***B** fibers are most susceptible to **H**ypoxia.*

   C** fibers are most susceptible to **local anesthetics**. **(Mnemonic: ABC – pH of local anesthetic).

   Answer: A i.e., A fibers are more prone to pressure than C fibers

CHAPTER 3

BIOCHEMISTRY

RAPID REVISION NOTES

Amino acids/ AA and proteins

Amino acid	*Characteristic*
Glycine	Simplest AA
Proline, hydroxyl-proline, tryptophan, histidine	Hetero-cyclic AA
Tryptophan	Source of nicotinic acid & serotonin
Gelatin	Protein which is not an antigen
Branched chain AA	Lost in urine in Maple syrup urine disease
Tryptophan	Disturbed metabolism in Hartnup disease
Ornithine, arginine, citrulline, ammonia	Required for urea formation
Alanine, aspartic acid, glutamic acid	Glycogenic AA
Leucine	Ketogenic AA
Isoleucine, phenyl-alanine, tyrosine	Glucogenic plus ketogenic AA
Tyrosine	Precursor of thyroxine, dopa, dopamine, norepinephrine, melanin
Cystine, ornithine, lysine, arginine	Excreted in urine in cystinuria
Histidine	AA excreted in pregnancy
Histidine	Abundant in hemoglobin
Glutathione	Source of ammonia
Leucine, isoleucine, lysine, valine	Branched chain AA
Cystine, cysteine, methionine	Sulphur containing AA
Protamine	Antidote of heparin
Proteins	16% nitrogen

BASICS

Respiratory quotient

- Carbohydrates: 1
- Protein: 0.8
- Fat: 0.7

Cells & their fuel

- Muscle cells: Can utilize glucose, fatty acids and ketone bodies
- Brain: Can utilize ketone bodies and glucose
- Hepatocytes: Cannot utilize ketone bodies (As it lack the enzyme necessary to convert acetoacetate to acetoacety CoA)

Must know facts

- Ubiquitin: Eukaryotic protein for degradation of intracellular proteins
- Chaperones: Proteins which play a role in the assembly or proper folding of other proteins without themselves being components of the latter
- Shine-Dalgarno sequence: A polypurine sequence in bacterial mRNA, 7 nucleotides in front of initiation codon AUG. It is involved in binding of mRNA to ribosome, and hence initiation of protein synthesis
- HbS: Substitution of glutamate by valine in B chain in the 6th position

ENZYMES

- Enzyme activity is measured as: Micromoles/ min
- In competitive inhibition, Vmax is: Same (Km is increased)
- Coenzyme is: Non protein organic compounds
- Abzyme is: Antibody with catalytic activity
- Ribozymes are: RNA molecules with catalytic activity
- Km (Michaelis Menten) reflects: Affinity of enzymes to that substrate
- Fumarase belongs to: Lyase
- Tyrosinase belongs to: Oxidase
- Hexokinase belongs to: Transferase

Isoenzymes of Lactate dehydrogenase

- LDH1: Heart and RBC
- LDH2: Heart and RBC
- LDH3: Brain and kidney
- LDH4: Liver and skeletal muscle
- LDH5: Skeletal muscle and liver

Type of enzyme inhibition

- Uncompetitive inhibition: Inhibitor doesn't bind with enzyme, but only binds with the enzyme-substrate complex
- Competitive inhibition: Inhibitor competes with the substrate and binds to the active site of the enzyme but doesn't undergo any catalysis
- Non-competitive inhibition: The inhibitor has no structural resemblance with substrate and binds at a site other than the active site on the enzyme surface and thus impairs enzyme function
- Allosteric inhibition: The allosteric modulator binds to the allosteric site and regulates enzyme activity

Enzyme deficiencies diseases/ syndromes

- Acute Intermittent Porphyria: Uroporphyrinogen -1 synthase
- Congenital erythropoietic porphyria: Uroporphyrinogen -3 synthase
- Porphyria cutanea tarda: Uroporphyrinogen decarboxylase
- Erythropoietic porphyria: Ferrochelatase
- Crigler- Najjar: UDP- glucuronyl transferase
- Von-Gierke's: Glucose-6-phosphatase
- Pompe's: Acid maltase (Acid alpha glucosidase)
- Mc Ardle's: Muscle glycogen phosphorylase
- Niemann- Pick's: Sphingomyelinase
- Faber's: Ceramidase
- Gaucher's: Beta-glucosidase
- Krabbe's: Beta -galactosidase
- Tay-Sach's: Hexosaminidase –A
- Phenylketonuria: Phenylalanine hydroxylase
- Alkaptonuria: Homogentisate oxidase
- Albinism: Tyrosinase
- Metachromatic leukodystrophy: Arylsulfatase A
- Lesch-Nyhan syndrome: HGPRT
- Xeroderma pigmentosa: DNA exonuclease
- Maple syrup urine: Branched chain alpha-ketoacid dehydrogenase complex (BCKDC)
- MPS-1/Hurler's syndrome: Alpha-L- iduronidase
- MPS-2: **L-iduronate 2-sulfatase**

Commonly asked rate limiting steps

- Urea synthesis: Carbamoyl phosphate synthase I
- Glycolysis: Phosphofructokinase

- Bile acid synthesis: 7- alpha hydroxylase
- Cholesterol synthesis: HMG-CoA reductase

Commonly asked rate limiting enzymes

- Uric acid synthesis: Xanthine oxidase
- Denovo purine biosynthesis: PRPP synthetase
- Porphyrin synthesis: ALA synthetase
- Fatty acid synthesis: Acetyl CoA carboxylase

DNA

- Bases in DNA:
    - o Adenine (A)
    - o Guanine (G)
    - o Cytosine (C) &
    - o Thymine (T)
- The double helix are bonded together by: Hydrogen bonds
- RNA differ from DNA in that:
    - o Deoxyribose sugar of DNA is replaced by a ribose moiety,
    - o Instead of thymine (T), Uracil (U) is present in RNA
- New synthesized strand is made in: 5' → 3' direction
- Cistron: Smallest fundamental unit coding for DNA synthesis
- Okazaki fragments: DNA fragments with RNA head
- Okazaki fragments are formed during: Replication
- Microsatellite sequence: Short sequence repeat DNA
- Proteins binding to DNA contains: Zinc
- Protein synthesis occurs mainly in: Ribosomes
- Function of helicase: Unwinding of DNA helix
- Fidelity enzyme in protein synthesis is: Amino acyl t RNA synthetase
- AMBER codon is: Termination codon
- Function of chaperones: Protein folding
- Transposons: Jumping genes

RNA

- Abnormal purine bases are present in: tRNA
- Highest % of modified bases are present in: tRNA
- Prokaryotic RNA is: 70S (30S & 50S)
- Normal role of micro-RNA: Gene regulation
- Splicing activity is a function of: Sn-RNA
- Sigma subunit of prokaryotic RNA polymerase: Specifically recognizes the promoter site

MITOCHONDRIAL DNA

- Mitochondrial DNA is: Closed & circular
- Diseases associated with mt-DNA:
    - o Mitochondrial encephalopathy with lactic acidosis & stroke like disorders/ MELAS
    - o Myoclonic epilepsy & ragged red fibres/ MERRF syndrome etc.

MEDICALLY IMPORTANT ENZYMES

- Reverse transcriptase: RNA dependent DNA polymerase
- Telomerase are expressed in:
    - o Germ cells
    - o Cancer cells
    - o Human pluripotent stem cells

GENETIC CODE

- Genetic code is:
    - o Unambiguous (Each codon specifies no more than 1 amino acid)
    - o Degenerate (More than one codon can specify a single amino acid)
- Non-sense codon: New codon is stop codon (usually non-functional)

DIAGNOSTIC TECHNIQUE

- Northern blot: RNA

- Microarray: RNA/ complimentary-DNA
- FISH/ fluorescence in situ hybridization: Rapid method of chromosome identification

POLYMERASE CHAIN REACTION

- PCR is: Enzymatic DNA amplification
- In PCR, oligonucleotides build copies of the DNA using a: Heat stable polymerase (Taq1)
- Substances required for PCR:
  - o Primers
  - o DNA polymerase
  - o Magnesium
- Advantage of PCR: Can be used to study mRNA as well as DNA

AMINO ACIDS

- Branched chain amino acid whose metabolism is abnormal in maple syrup urine disease/ MSUD:
  - o Valine
  - o Isoleucine
- Essential amino acids:
  - o Methionine
  - o Arginine
  - o Threonine
  - o Tryptophan
  - o Valine
  - o Isoleucine
  - o Leucine
  - o Phenylalanine
  - o Histidine
  - o Lysine
- Naturally occurring amino acids are: L isomers
- Most non-polar amino acid is: Leucine
- Amino acid containing indole ring: Tryptophan
- Melatonin is synthesized from: Tryptophan
- Ammonia is produced in kidney from: Glutamine
- Ammonia is detoxified in brain to: Glutamine
- Precursor of tyrosine: Phenylalanine
- Creatinine is synthesized from:
  - o Glycine
  - o Arginine
  - o Methionine
- Buffering action of blood is due to: Histidine

Phenylketonuria

- Autosomal recessive inheritance
- Deficiency of: Phenylalanine hydroxylase
- Cause of neurological signs & mental retardation: As brain cell are deprive of essential amino acids
- High phenylalanine concentration results in: Competitive inhibition of tyrosine leading to:
  - o Blonde hair
  - o Blue eyes
  - o Fair skin
- Accessory metabolic pathway leads to: Accumulation of phenylacetic acid and other metabolites leading to mousy odour
- Diagnosis: Provocative protein meal test; A plasma phenylalanine level >20 mg/dl; A normal plasma tyrosine level
- Screening tests: Guthrie's test ferric chloride solution- green colour; 2,4 dinitrophenol hydrazine - Yellow precipitate
- Treatment: Low phenylalanine levels, however it should not be completely eliminated; Tyrosine becomes essential, hence adequate intake should be ensured

Hartnup's disease

- Hereditary disorder of tryptophan metabolism
- Clinical symptoms include dermatitis, ataxia, and mental retardation
- Characterised by low plasma levels of tryptophan and their elevated urinary excretion

Essential amino acids (Mnemonic: MATTVILPhly)

- Methionine
- Arginine
- Threonine
- Tryptophan
- Valine
- Isoleucine
- Leucine
- Phenylalanine
- Lysine

Semi-essential amino acids

- Histidine
- Arginine

Protein structure (bonds & detection)

- Primary: Linear sequence of amino acids, consisting of peptide bonds; Edman's degeneration technique
- Secondary: Special structure of proteins, by twisting of polypeptide chains, consisting of alpha helix and beta pleated sheets (Hydrogen bonds); X-ray diffraction, crystallography and nuclear magnetic resonance
- Tertiary: Three dimensional structure of functional proteins (Disulfide bonds); X-ray diffraction, crystallography and nuclear magnetic resonance
- Quaternary: Three dimensional structure of functional proteins; Detected by X-ray diffraction, crystallography and nuclear magnetic resonance

Some important proteins & their functions

- Haptoglobin: Binds with free hemoglobin
- Ceruloplasmin: Transports copper
- Alpha 1 antitrypsin: Inhibitor of trypsin
- Alpha 1 lipoprotein: Transport of cholesterol and phospholipids

PROTEINS

- Quaternary structure of proteins is: Spatial relationship between individual polypeptide chains
- Secondary structure (alpha helix & beta sheet) are stabilized by: Hydrogen bonds
- SDS PAGE/sodium dodecyl sulfate polyacrylamide gel electrophoresis is used for separation & purification of individual proteins on: Basis of size
- SDS PAGE is used for determining: Molecular weight of a protein
- Ion exchange chromatography separates proteins on the basis of: Their charge
- Hemoglobin electrophoresis is done on the basis of: Charge

IMPORTANT TESTS

- Modified Koppanyi test: Barbiturates
- Guaiac test: Haematuria
- Rothera's test: Ketone bodies
- Gerhardt's test: Ketosis
- Molisch's test: Sugar (Colour test)
- Millon's test: Tyrosinosis
- Sulkowitch test: Urinary calcium
- Biuret test: Protein

VITAMINS

- Features of vitamin A deficiency:
  - Night blindness
  - Xerophthalmia
  - Follicular hyperkeratosis
- Vitamin which prevents lipid peroxidation: Vitamin E
- Vitamin needed for gamma carboxylation: Vitamin K
- Vitamin which is a post-translation modifier: Vitamin K

Vitamins as coenzymes

- Thiamine: TPP, TDP
- Riboflavin: FAD, FMN
- Niacin: NAD, NADP
- Pantothenic acid: CoA, Acyl carrier protein
- Pyridoxine: Pyridoxal phosphate
- Folic acid: Tetrahydrofolate

Markers for vitamin deficiencies

- B_1: RBC transketolase
- B_2: RBC glutathione peroxidase
- B_6: Urine xanthurenic acid
- Folic acid: Urine FIGLU
- B_{12}: Urine methylmalonic acid

VITAMIN DEFICIENCIES

- Wernicke's Korsakoff syndrome is associated with deficiency of: Thiamine (B1)
- Consumption of egg (containing avidin) may lead to deficiency of: Biotin
- Methyl malonic aciduria is seen in deficiency of: Vitamin B12/ extrinsic factor of castle
- Scurvy is seen in deficiency of: Vitamin C

ENZYMES RELATED TO VITAMINS

- Alpha-keto glutarate dehydrogenase is associated with: Thiamine (B1)
- Transketolase is associated with: Thiamine (B1)
- Pyruvate carboxylase is associated with: Biotin
- Aminotransferases is associated with: Pyridoxine

HAEMOGLOBIN

- 'Haem' in Haemoglobin lies in: Hydrophobic pockets
- 'Haem' in haemoglobin is bonded to: Histidine
- Iron in haemoglobin is present in: Ferrous state
- Iron in haemoglobin is held by: Polar bonds
- Alpha2, gamma2 is: Hb fetal

Carbohydrates

Sugar	*Osazones*	*Shape*
Glucose	Glucosazones	Needles & sheaves of corn
Sucrose	No osazone	-
Maltose	Maltosazones	Sunflower
Fructose	Fructosazones	Needles & sheaves of corn

GLYCOLYSIS

- Mature RBC lacks enzymes of: TCA cycle
- Cancer cells derives energy by: Glycolysis
- Anticoagulant added for estimating blood glucose (added to prevent glycolysis): Sodium fluoride
- Fluoride inhibits: Enolase
- Enzymes responsible for complete oxidation of glucose are present in: Mitochondria
- Substances which can prevent glycolysis:
  - o Potassium oxalate
  - o Sodium fluoride
- Glycolysis is regulated at:
  - o Hexokinase
  - o Phosphofructokinase
  - o Pyruvate kinase

Glycolysis

- Location: Cytosol
- Substrate level phosphorylation: Phosphoglycerate kinase, Pyruvate kinase
- Inhibitors:
  - o Fluoride: Enolase
  - o Oxamate: Glyceraldehyde-3-phosphate dehydrogenase
  - o Bromohydroxyacetone phosphate: Phosphate isomerase
- Irreversible steps: Hexokinase, Phosphofructokinase, Pyruvate kinase

Carbohydrates

Substance	*Features*
Glycogen	Animal starch
Glycogen	Mainly found in liver & muscle
Inulin	GFR measurement
Amylose	Linear bands present between glucose molecules
Galactose	Best absorbed sugar

Sucrose	Glucose + fructose
Maltose	Glucose + glucose
Maltose	End product of starch metabolism
Sucrose	Invert sugar

CITRIC ACID/ KREBS CYCLE

- First substrate of citric acid cycle is: Pyruvate
- Substrate level phosphorylation occurs in reaction catalyzed by enzyme: Succinyl-CoA-thiokinase
- Location: Mitochondria
- Substrate level phosphorylation: Succinate thiokinase
- Inhibitors:
  - Arsenite: Alpha ketoglutarate dehydrogenase
  - Malonate: Succinate dehydrogenase
  - Fluoroacetate/ Flurorocitrate: Aconitase
- Energy: 1 Acety1 CoA, 12 ATP
- 1 mole of glucose gives: 2 ATP anaerobically & 38 ATP aerobically

Uncouplers of electron transport chain are:

- 2,4 dinitrophenol
- Dinitrocresol
- Pentachlorophenol
- Trifluoro carbonyl
- Long chain free fatty acids
- Unconjugated bilirubin

GLUCONEOGENESIS

- Gluconeogenesis occurs from:
  - Glycerol
  - Alanine
  - Lactate
- Enzyme common to glycolysis & gluconeogenesis is: Phosphofructokinase
- Muscle cannot make use of glycogen as they lack: G-6-Phosphatase

HMP SHUNT

- HMP shunt is important as it produces: NADPH
- ATP produced in HMP shunt: No ATP is directly produced/ consumed

NADPH

- NADPH is produced in: HMP shunt
- NADPH is used for:
  - Fatty acid synthesis
  - Steroid synthesis etc.
- Important enzyme involved in NADPH synthesis: G6PD

ENERGY YIELD

- Stearic acid oxidation:New: 120; Old: 146 ATP
- HMP shunt: 0
- Kreb's cycle: New: 10 ATPS; Old: 12 ATP (per acetyl CoA)
- Aerobic glycolysis: New: 5/7; Old: 8 ATP (per glucose molecule)
- Anaerobic glycolysis: 2 ATP (per glucose molecule)

Mucopolysaccharides/ MPS

Sites	*MPS*
Connective tissue, cartilage, vitreous	Hyaluronic acid
Cartilage, vitreous	Chondroitin sulphate
Skin	Dermatan sulphate
Cornea	Keratan sulphate

GLYCOGEN STORAGE DISEASES

- Enzyme deficient in von-Gierke's disease: Glucose-6-phosphatase deficiency
- Enzyme deficient in Andersons disease: Branching enzyme
- Enzyme deficient in McArdle's disease: Muscle phosphorylase
- Lactic acid & hyperuricemia is a feature of: Von-Gierke's disease (GST-I)

- Muscles are not involved in: Von-Gierke's disease (GST-I)
- Hypoglycemia, non-responsive to epinephrine is a feature of: Von-Gierke's disease (GST-I)

Increase in blood glucose

Mechanism	*Hormone*
Lipolysis, glycogenolysis, neoglucogenesis	Glucagon
Glycogenolysis, decreasing insulin levels	Adrenaline
Lipolysis	Nor-adrenaline
Gluconeogenesis, decreased utilization of glucose	Cortisol

GALACTOSEMIA

- Most common (of the 3) enzyme deficient in galactosemia: GPUT/ Galactose-1-phosphate-uridyl transferase
- Cataract occurs because of the accumulation of: Galactilol
- Substance present in urine: Reducing sugars

ELECTRON TRANSPORT CHAIN

- Electron transport chain is located in: Inner mitochondrial membrane
- Internal respiration is: Exoergic & catabolic
- Mitochondrial membrane protein contain transporter of:
    - o NAD
    - o NADPH &
    - o ATP
- SGOT is an: Mitochondrial enzyme
- In electron transport chain, FADH gives: 1.5 ATP
- In electron transport chain, NADH gives: 2.5 ATP
- Cyanide inhibits:
    - o Cytochrome oxidase (inhibits electron flow)
    - o Complex IV
    - o Cellular oxidation
- Cytochrome oxidase is inhibited by:
    - o Cyanide
    - o Carbon monoxide
    - o Hydrogen sulphide
    - o Azide
- Uncoupler of oxidation & phosphorylation: Dinitrophenol

FATTY ACIDS

- Monosaturated fatty acids:
    - o Oleic acid
    - o Elaidic acid
- Essential fatty acids:
    - o Linoleic acid
    - o Linolenic acid
    - o Arachidonic acid
    - o Eicosapentaenoic acid
    - o Docosahexaenoic acid
- Most essential fatty acid is: Linoleic acid

Terms

Description	*Term*
When exposed to atmosphere, edible fats become auto-oxidated and give bad odour and become unfit for consumption	**Rancidity**
Process of alkali hydrolysis	**Saponification**

LIPIDS METABOLISM

Apolipoproteins

- Chylomicron: AI, A II, B 48
- VLDL: B100, CI, C II, C III, E
- LDL: B 100
- HDL: AI, AII, CI, C II, C III D, E.

Function of:

- Chylomicron: Transport exogenous triglycerides
- VLDL: Transports endogenous triglyceride
- LDL: Transports cholesterol to peripheral tissues
- HDL: Transports cholesterol from peripheral tissues to liver for degradation

CHOLESTEROL

- Rate limiting enzyme in cholesterol synthesis: HMG CoA reductase
- Bile acids are derived from: Cholesterol

Lipids

Lipid	*Features*
Linoleic acid	Definitely essential fatty acid
Arachidonic acid, linoleic acid, linolenic acid	Essential fatty acids
Keracin, cerebran, nervon, oxyneuron	Cerebrosides
Lecithin & sphingomyelin	Choline is a component
Lecithin, cephalin, sphingomyelin	Phospholipids
Cerebrosides, gangliosides	Glycolipids
Triglycerides	Storage form of lipids
Sulpholipids	Abundant in brain
Lipoproteins	Rhodopsin, thromboplastin
Hydnocarpic acid, chaulmoogric acid	Cyclic acid

FATTY ACID SYNTHESIS

- Synthesis of fatty acid occurs in: Cytosol
- Reducing equivalents for fatty acid synthesis are provided by: NADPH
- Rate limiting step in fatty acid synthesis: Acetyl CoA carboxylase (contains biotin)
- Fatty acid synthetase contains: Acyl carrier protein & pantothenic acid
- Beta oxidation of fatty acids produces: Propionyl CoA
- ATP produced by beta oxidation of palmitic acid: 129

KETOSIS

- Ketone bodies are formed in: Liver
- Ketone bodies are product of: Fatty acids metabolism
- Ketone bodies are normally produced from: Acetyl CoA
- Normal excretion of ketone bodies is: 1 mg/ day
- Ketone bodies are utilized by conversion of acetoacetate to: Acetoacetyl CoA
- Important feature of starvation: Ketone body formation without glycosuria

LIPOPROTEINS

- Activator of LCAT: ApoA
- Activator of lipoprotein lipase: ApoC-II
- Apoprotein associated with HDL: ApoA-1
- Apoprotein associated with LDL: B100
- Most atherogenic lipoprotein: LDL
- Lipoprotein with highest cholesterol content: LDL
- Lipoprotein with highest triglyceride content: Chylomicrons
- Apoproteins associated with chylomicrons: ApoA, ApoB, ApoC & ApoE
- Lipoprotein which reverses cholesterol transport: HDL
- Chylomicrons have least: Electrophoretic mobility

AMINO ACID METABOLIC DEFECTS

- Phenylketonuria/ PKU is due to deficiency of: Phenylalanine hydroxylase
- Mousy/ musty odour of urine is present in: PKU
- Alkaptonuria is due to deficiency of: Homogentisate oxidase
- Arthritis & urine turns black in: Alkaptonuria
- Maple syrup urine is due to deficiency of: Branched chain alpha ketoacid dehydrogenase

UREA CYCLE

- First 2 reactions of urea cycle occurs in: Mitochondria
- Source of ammonia in urine is: Glutamine

ENZYMES & INHIBITORS

- Aconitase: Fluoroacetate
- Succinate dehydrogenase: Malonate
- Enolase: Fluoride

NUCLEOTIDE METABOLISM

- Nucleoside: Pentose + N-base
- Nucleotide: Nucleoside + phosphate
- Nucleic acid: Polymerization of nucleotides

CLINICAL QUESTIONS

1. **A 40 years old woman presented with progressive palmoplantar pigmentation. X-ray spine shows calcification of intervertebral discs. On adding Benedict's reagent to urine, it gives greenish brown precipitate and blue-black supernatant fluid. Most likely diagnosis:**

A. Phenylketonuria

B. Alkaptonuria

C. Tyrosinosis type II

D. Argininosuccinic aciduria

Clinical presentation is suggestive of alkaptonuria.

By the 3rd or 4th decade of life, patient with alkaptonuria may develop ochronosis (deposition of alkaptone bodies in intervertebral discs, cartilages of nose, pinna of ear).

Diagnosis of alkaptonuria is suggested by blackish discoloration of urine, a positive Benedict's test, silver nitrate reduction and detection of elevated homogentisic acid by GC/ MS (Gas Chromatography/ Mass spectrometry).

Answer: B i.e., Alkaptonuria

2. **A 6 years old patient presented with fatigue on normal outdoor activity. In blood there was raised triglycerides, increased cholesterol, fatty acid and lactate. Blood sugar was 60 mg/ dL. USG shows enlarged liver and kidney. Liver biopsy showed increased glycogen. Most likely diagnosis:**

A. Von-Gierke's disease B. Pompe's disease

C. Cori's disease D. McArdle's disease

Clinical presentation is suggestive of Von-Gierke's disease.

In Von-Gierke's disease, there is fasting hypoglycemia that does not respond to stimulation by adrenaline.

There is hyperlipidemia, lactic acidosis and ketosis.

Glycogen gets deposited in liver and massive liver enlargement can lead to cirrhosis.

Answer: A i.e., Von-Gierke's disease

3. **A patient had normal blood glucose level as estimated by Glucose-Oxidase Peroxidase method. Urine examination showed a positive Benedict's test. Most likely condition:**

A. Fructosuria

B. Galactosemia

C. Denaturation of glucose

D. Faulty tests

Clinical presentation is suggestive of Fructosuria.

Fructosuria is a benign metabolic defect due to deficiency of fructokinase.

There is no abnormality other than excretion of fructose in urine.

Urine gives positive Benedict's and Seliwanoff's tests.

Answer: A i.e., Fructosuria

4. **A child was found to have hypoglycemia, hepatomegaly and accumulation of highly branched glycogen called limit dextrin. Most likely diagnosis:**

A. Cori's disease B. Von-Gierke's disease

C. Anderson's disease D. McArdle's disease

Clinical presentation is suggestive of Cori's disease.

Cori's disease/ Limit dextrinosis is characterized by accumulation of highly branched dextrin, fasting hypoglycemia, hepatomegaly & myopathy.

Answer: A i.e., Cori's disease

5. **An infant present with hepatosplenomegaly, hypoglycemia, hyperuricemia and lactic acidosis. Liver biopsy shows normal structured glycogen deposition. Which enzyme is deficient:**

A. Debranching enzyme B. Branching enzyme

C. Glucose-6-phosphatase D. Muscle phosphorylase

Clinical presentation is suggestive of Von-Gierke's disease.

Findings are suggestive of Von-Gierke's disease, which occurs because of deficiency of the enzyme Glucose-6-phosphatase.

Answer: C i.e., Glucose-6-phosphatase

6. **A person on a fat-free, carbohydrate-rich diet continues to grow obese. Which of the following lipoprotein is likely to be elevated in his blood?**

A. Chylomicrons B. VLDL

C. LDL D. HDL

Clinical presentation is suggestive of elevated VLDL levels.

The lipid abnormalities in patients who are obese include elevated serum triglyceride, VLDL, apolipoprotein B, and non-HDL-C levels.

The increase in serum triglycerides is due to increased hepatic production of VLDL particles and a decrease in the clearance of triglyceride rich lipoproteins.

Carbohydrate rich diet results in more production of Acetyl CoA, which leads to synthesis of fats in the body.

Since these fats are endogenous fats, they are transported in VLDL.

Answer: B i.e., VLDL

7. **A person was diagnosed with isolated increase in LDL. His father and brother had the same disease with increased cholesterol. Most likely diagnosis:**

A. Familial type III hyperlipoproteinemia

B. Abetalipoproteinemia

C. Familial lipoprotein lipase deficiency type I

D. LDL receptor defect

Clinical presentation is suggestive of LDL receptor mutation.

In type IIA hyperlipoproteinemia (Primary Familial Hypercholesterolemia), there is elevation of LDL.

The cause is LDL receptor defect.

Receptor deficiency in liver and peripheral tissues will result in the elevation of LDL levels in plasma, leading to hypercholesterolemia.

Answer: D i.e., LDL receptor defect

8. **A 48 years old lady presented with bone pain and hepatosplenomegaly. On examination of biopsy specimen from spleen, crumpled tissue paper appearance is seen. Which product is likely to have accumulated:**

A. Glucocerebroside B. Sphingomyelin

C. Sulfatide D. Ganglioside

Clinical presentation is suggestive of Gaucher's disease.

In Gaucher's disease, there is beta-glucosidase deficiency leading to accumulation of glucocerebroside.

There is hepatosplenomegaly, erosion of bone and moderate anemia.

Gaucher cells have the appearance of signet rings with 'wrinkled tissue paper' because the nucleus is pushed to the periphery of the cells.

Answer: A i.e., Glucocerebroside

9. **A 7 years old boy presented with severe abdominal pain. On examination, he has xanthomas. Blood drawn for work up has milky appearance of plasma. Which lipoprotein is increased:**

A. Chylomicron

B. Chylomicron remnants

C. LDL

D. HDL

Clinical presentation is suggestive of increased chylomicron levels.

Lipoprotein fraction elevated in a patient with type I hyperlipoproteinemia is chylomicron.

Plasma after 24 hours shows creamy layer over clear plasma.

Clinical features are eruptive xanthoma, hepatosplenomegaly and pain in abdomen.

Answer: A i.e., Chylomicron

10. **In a person, LDL is highly elevated but the level of LDL receptors is normal. What could be the cause:**

A. Phosphorylation of LDL receptors

B. ApoB100 mutation

C. Lipoprotein lipase deficiency

D. Cholesterol acyl CoA transferase deficiency

Clinical presentation is suggestive of ApoB100 mutation.

A mutation in apoB-100 that inhibits its binding to the LDL receptor is another genetic cause of elevations in LDL-cholesterol.

This is also known as familial defective Apo B100 (Autosomal Dominant hypercholesterolemia).

There is a mutation in the gene encoding Apo B100, specifically at the LDL-receptor binding domain of Apo B100.

Answer: B i.e., ApoB100 mutation

11. **If in a person, total cholesterol: 300 mg/dL, HDL: 25 mg/ dL and triglyceride: 150 mg/ dl. What would be the value of LDL?**

A. 245 mg/ dL B. 125 mg/ dL

C. 95 mg/ dL D. 55 mg/ dL

LDL cholesterol = Total cholesterol – HDL cholesterol – 1/5 (Triglycerides)

LDL cholesterol = 300-25-1/5(150) = 300-25-30 = 245

Answer: A i.e., 245 mg/ dL

12. **A 10 years old child with aggressive behavior and poor concentration is brought with presenting complaints of joint pain and reduced urinary output. Mother gives history of self-mutilation behavior stating that he tends to mutilate his fingers. Enzyme deficiency in such a case:**

A. HGPRTase B. Adenosine deaminase

C. APRTase D. Acid maltase

Clinical presentation is suggestive of Lesch-Nyhan syndrome.

Lesch-Nyhan syndrome is characterized by self-mutilation, mental retardation, excessive uric and nephrolithiasis. Gout develops in later life.

There is deficiency of hypoxanthine guanine phosphoribosyl transferase/ HGPRTAse.

Answer: A i.e., HGPRTase

13. **A four years old child diagnosed with Duchenne muscular dystrophy, an X-linked recessive disorder. Genetic analysis shows that the patient's gene for the muscle protein dystrophin contains a mutation in its promoter region. Most likely effect of this mutation:**

A. Tailing of dystrophin mRNA will be defective

B. Capping of dystrophin mRNA will be defective

C. Termination of dystrophin transcription will be deficient

D. Initiation of dystrophin transcription will be deficient

Duchenne muscular dystrophy/ DMD is a degenerative disease of muscle affecting only male children.

The gene is in the middle of the short arm of X-chromosome.

This gene produces a protein called dystrophin with 3700 amino acids.

In DMD patients, the gene for dystrophin is mutated.

These mutations affect the normal transcription of dystrophin.

Answer: D i.e., Initiation of dystrophin transcription will be deficient

14. **A lady presented with fatigue and tingling sensation in both hands and legs. On examination, she is found to have a fissured red tongue, lesions at angle of mouth with a decreased RBC glutathione reductase activity. Likely vitamin deficiency:**

A. Riboflavin B. Thiamine

C. Vitamin B_{12} D. Vitamin B_6

Clinical presentation is suggestive of riboflavin deficiency.

Manifestations of riboflavin (vitamin B_2) deficiency include glossitis, magenta colored tongue, cheilosis (redness and shiny appearance of lips), angular stomatitis (lesions at muco-cutaneous junction at corners of mouth) and circum-corneal vascularization.

Proliferation of the bulbar conjunctival capillaries is the earliest sign of riboflavin deficiency.

Glutathione reductase (RBC) is an FAD (Flavin adenine dinucleotide) requiring enzyme, which is the marker for vitamin B_2 deficiency.

Answer: A i.e., Riboflavin

15. A child was weaned from breast milk on the fifth day and was given sugar cane juice. The child developed hypoglycemia and hepatomegaly. Biochemical examination showed hypophosphatasia and reducing substances in urine. Likely enzyme deficiency:

A. Aldolase B B. Fructokinase

C. Glucose-6-phosphatase D. Beta-galactosidase

Clinical presentation is suggestive of deficiency of aldolase-B.

In hereditary fructose intolerance, the defect is in aldolase-B, hence fructose-1-phosphate cannot be metabolized. This is seen when sucrose (containing fructose) is introduced in the diet of the infants, usually around 6 months of age. Accumulation of fructose-1-phosphate will inhibit glycogen phosphorylase.

This leads to accumulation of glycogen in liver and associated hypoglycemia.

Fructose is also excreted in urine when urine gives positive Benedict's test.

Answer: A i.e., Aldolase B

16. A 28 years old female presented with obstructive jaundice. Which of the following type of reaction will be seen in Van Der Bergh test:

A. Direct positive B. Indirect positive

C. Both positive D. Biphasic

In obstructive jaundice, Van Der Bergy reaction will be direct positive.

Van Der Bergh reaction is direct positive in conjugated hyperbilirubinemia.

Obstructive jaundice causes conjugated hyper-bilirubinemia.

Answer: A i.e., Direct positive

17. In lead poisoning, there is inhibition of some of the enzymes of the heme biosynthetic pathway. This is reflected by the raised urinary levels of:

A. Uroporphyrinogen III

B. Ferrochelatase

C. Porphyrobilinogen

D. Delta-Amino Levulinic Acid

Clinical presentation is suggestive of raised urinary levels of delta-amino-levulinic acid.

Lead inhibits heme synthesis.

Basophilic stippling of red cells is seen in peripheral blood and bone marrow smears.

This is due to agglutination of ribosomes.

Globin synthesis is adversely affected.

Lead particularly inhibits ferrochelatase/ Heme synthase and ALA-dehydratase/ PBG synthase, though activity of ALA synthase is increased.

Answer: D i.e., Delta-Amino Levulinic Acid

18. 10 years old boy presented with muscle weakness and fatigue with increased lead in blood. Which of the following enzyme production in liver is increased?

A. Ferrochelatase B. PBG deaminase

C. Heme oxygenase D. ALA synthase

Clinical presentation is suggestive of increased production of ALA synthase.

Porphyria can result from lead poisoning (acquired porphyria).

Most of the paints contain lead more than the permitted levels.

Children suck painted toys; and they get the poison.

The toxic effect of lead is due to inhibition of ferrochelatase.

So, there is decreased level of heme with consequent increased activity of ALA synthase.

Answer: D i.e., ALA synthase

19. A 4 years old boy of first-degree consanguineous couple presented with complaints of backache and bilateral knee pain. All blood investigations were normal. Urine routine microscopy is normal. However, on keeping urine outside for sometimes, it turned black. Which of the enzyme is likely to be deficient in such a patient?

A. Xanthine oxidase

B. Homogentisate oxidase

C. Tyrosinase

D. Fumaryl-acetoacetate hydroxylase

Clinical presentation is suggestive of deficiency of Homogentisate oxidase.

The patient is suffering from alkaptonuria, which is because of deficiency of homogentisate oxidase.

Urine becomes dark on exposure to air.

Answer: B i.e., Homogentisate oxidase

20. **Young male presented with pain in calves during excessive exercise without any other symptom or sign. His blood lactate levels did not increase after exercise. His blood glucose levels were found to be normal. Muscle biopsy shows increased glycogen. The enzyme deficient is:**

A. Debranching enzyme

B. Muscle phosphorylase

C. Glucose-6-phosphorylase

D. Muscle phosphofructokinase

Clinical presentation is suggestive of deficiency of muscle phosphorylase.

In type V glycogen storage disease (McArdle's disease), there is exercise intolerance, accumulation of glycogen in muscles and myoglobinuria.

This occurs because of deficiency of the enzyme muscle phosphorylase (skeletal muscles).

Answer: B i.e., Muscle phosphorylase

21. **A man complaint of diarrhoea with dairy products. He must avoid all EXCEPT:**

A. Condensed milk B. Skimmed milk

C. Yogurt D. Ice cream

Clinical presentation is suggestive of lactose intolerance.

The person is suffering from lactose intolerance, which is because of deficiency of the enzyme lactase.

In this condition, lactose accumulates in the gut.

Irritant diarrhoea and flatulence are seen.

If milk is withdrawn completely, diarrhoea will be limited.

Curd is an effective treatment, because the lactobacilli present in the curd contains the enzyme lactase.

Lactase is abundantly seen in yeast, which could also be used for treatment.

Answer: C i.e., Yogurt

22. **Patient presents with inability to convert pyruvate to Acetyl coA. Treatment of this condition is with the supplementation of:**

A. Thiamine B. Biotin

C. Free fatty acids D. Vitamin B6

Pyruvate to Acetyl CoA conversion is catalyzed by pyruvate dehydrogenase.

The co-enzyme form of the enzyme pyruvate dehydrogenase is TPP (thiamine pyrophosphate).

This enzyme is used in oxidative decarboxylation of alpha keto acids, e.g., pyruvate dehydrogenase catalyzes the breakdown of pyruvate to acetyl CoA, and carbon dioxide.

Answer: A i.e., Thiamine

23. **After a fatty meal, in a patient with lipoprotein lipase deficiency, which of the following will be raised?**

A. HDL B. LDL

C. IDL D. Chylomicrons

Clinical presentation is suggestive of raised levels of chylomicrons.

The dietary triglycerides are transported by chylomicrons.

The lipoprotein molecules are broken down by the lipoprotein lipase present on the capillary wall.

Lipoprotein lipase hydrolyzes triglycerides present in chylomicrons into fatty acids and glycerol.

Answer: D i.e., Chylomicrons

24. **A patient presented with mental retardation and cherry red spots on the retina. Most likely condition:**

A. Krabbe's disease B. Tay Sach's disease

C. Gaucher's disease D. McArdle's disease

Clinical presentation is indicative of Tay Sach's disease.

Patient presents with mental retardation and cherry red spot in the macula.

There is progressive deterioration and the patient dies by the age of 3-4 years.

Answer: B i.e., Tay Sach's disease

25. A Mediterranean person was taking primaquine and he developed hemolytic anemia. It was found that he was having G-6-PD deficiency. Which of the pathway is associated with this clinical syndrome?

A. Kreb's cycle B. HMP pathway

C. Glycolysis D. Gluconeogenesis

The affected pathway in G-6PD deficiency associated hemolysis is HMP shunt.

The first step catalyzed by glucose-6-phosphate dehydrogenase (G-6-PD) is the rate-limiting step in the HMP pathway.

NADPH generated as a result of HMP pathway is essential to maintain transparency of the eye lens, to prevent met-hemoglobinemia and to maintain erythrocyte membrane integrity.

Deficiency of G-6PD leads to drug-induced hemolytic anemia.

The deficiency is manifested only when exposed to certain drugs or toxins, e.g., intake of anti-malarial drugs like primaquine.

Primaquine stimulates peroxide formation inside RBC.

In G-6PD deficient cells, the level of NADPH is low; hence further production of peroxides will lead to cell lysis.

Answer: B i.e., HMP shunt

CHAPTER 4

PATHOLOGY

RAPID REVISION NOTES

Some terms

Description	*Term*
Gangrene developing when there is sudden vascular obstruction (intussusceptions, strangulated hernia)	**Moist gangrene**
Gangrene developing when there is gradual narrowing of arteries	**Dry gangrene**
Massive necrosis with superadded putrefaction	**Gangrene**
Deposition of calcium salts under skin, muscles, tendons etc.	**Calcinosis**
Complete absence of development	**Agenesis**
Defective embryologic development	**Dysgenesis**
Necrosis and loosening of tissue	**Necrolysis**
Physiological death of cells due to changes with development	**Necrobiosis**
Death of a cell surrounded by living cells	**Necrosis**
Intracellular hyaline is seen in mesenchyme (seen in striated muscles)	**Zenker's degeneration**
Reversible changes in epithelium due to chronic inflammation or irritation	**Dysplasia**
Change of one type of tissue into another type	**Metaplasia**
Increase in size of cells	**Hypertrophy**
Increase in number of cells	**Hyperplasia**

GENERAL PATHOLOGY

- Dystrophic calcification occurs in: Dying tissues
- Calcium level in dystrophic calcification is: Normal
- Red infarct (venous occlusion, seen in organ with dual blood supply) is seen in:
  - o Brain
  - o Gut etc.
- Most common type of necrosis is: Coagulative necrosis
- Features of irreversible injury:
  - o Flocculent, amorphous densities in mitochondria
  - o Swelling & disruption of lysosomes etc.
- Features of apoptosis:
  - o Condensation of nuclear chromatin followed by fragmentation
  - o Formation of cytoplasmic/ membrane blebs
  - o Cytoplasmic chromophilia etc.
- Phagocytosis is inhibited by: bcl2
- Examples of autoimmune diseases:
  - o SLE
  - o Graves' disease
  - o Myasthenia gravis etc.

- Chronic venous congestion of liver is known as: Nutmeg liver
- Gamma Gandy bodies are seen in: Chronic venous congestion of spleen
- Leukotrienes (LTC4, LTD4, LTE4) causes: Vasoconstriction
- LTB4 causes: Adhesion of WBC
- Prostacyclin inhibits: Platelet aggregation
- C5a is: Important mediator of chemotaxis
- Wound contraction is mediated by: Fibroblast
- Epithelioid & multi-nucleated giant cells are derived from: Monocyte-macrophages
- ARDS/ diffuse alveolar damage is also known as: Shock lung
- Lines of Zahn are seen in: Thrombus
- Chicken fat clot is: Post mortem thrombus
- Heart failure cells are seen in: Lungs
- Cells first involved in tissue injury are: Neutrophils
- Procoagulant states:
  - o Protein C & protein S deficiency
  - o Factor V/ Leiden mutation etc.
- Hyperviscosity is seen in:
  - o Multiple myeloma
  - o Cryoglobulinemia etc.

Stains & tissue stained

- Alcian blue stains: Acid mucin, mast cells
- Masson Fontana stains: Melanin
- Masson's trichrome stains: Collagen

Giant cells & associated diseases

- Langhan's: Tuberculosis, Sarcoidosis
- Aschoff: Rheumatic heart disease
- Touton: Xanthomas
- Warthin-Finkeldey: Measles

Intracellular accumulations & stains used

- Fat: Sudan 4, Oil red O
- Glycogen: PAS, Best carmine
- Iron: Prussian blue
- Amyloid: Congo red, crystal violet, methyl green, Thioflavin, toluidine blue DMAB nitrite

Pathological calcification

- Dystrophic calcification: Deposition occurs in non-viable or dying tissue despite normal serum calcium levels
- Metastatic calcification: Deposition occurs in normal tissues due to hypercalcemia

Amyloid proteins

- AL: Primary amyloidosis
- AA: Secondary amyloidosis
- Beta-2 microglobulin: Hemodialysis associated amyloidosis
- Beta-2 amyloid protein: Alzheimer's disease
- Transthyretin: Hereditary amyloidosis, senile amyloidosis

Exudative effusion

- Protein: More than 3 gm percent; Mostly fibrinogen
- Specific gravity: < 1.018
- pH: >7.3
- LDH: Increased
- Effusion LDH/ serum LDH: <0.6
- Effusion protein/ serum protein: <0.5

Transudative effusion

- Protein: <3 gm percent; Mostly albumin
- Specific gravity: <1.015
- pH: >7.3
- LDH: Decreased
- Effusion LDH/ serum LDH: <0.6
- Effusion protein/ serum protein: <0.5

Virchow's triad

- Endothelial injury
- Abnormal blood flow
- Hypercoagulability

Skin markers (of internal malignancy)

- Acanthosis nigricans
- Lentigines
- Café-au-lait
- Nevi
- Pemphigoid
- Dermatophytosis
- Erythema gyratum repens

Carcinoma & their genetic associations

- RET proto oncogene: Medullary carcinoma thyroid, papillary carcinoma
- Rb gene (13q14): Retinoblastoma
- BRCA1: Ca breast (females), Ca ovary
- APC gene: Familial adenomatous polyposis coli
- Chromosome 3: Renal cell carcinoma
- 11p13: Wilm's tumor
- Xp2l: Duchenne muscular dystrophy
- APP gene: Alzheimer's disease

Cytochemical features of malignancy

- CML: Decreased leucocyte alkaline phosphatase
- Accelerated and blastic phases of CML: Increased leucocyte alkaline phosphatase
- Lymphoblasts of ALL: Negative for sudan black B, myeloperoxidase, ASD

Chloroacetate esterase

- Myeloblasts of AML: Positive for Suden black B, myeloperoxidase, ASD-chloroacetate esterase
- Hairy cell leukemia: Tartrate resistant acid phosphatase

Psammoma bodies are associated with

- Papillary carcinoma thyroid
- Serous cystadenocarcinoma ovary
- Meningioma

Histopathological characteristics

- H-X bodies, Birbeck granules: Langerhans cell Histiocytosis
- Flexner-Wintersteiner rosettes, Homer-Wright rosette, Fleurette: Retinoblastoma
- Neurofibrillary tangles, Senile/ neuritic plaques, Amyloid angiopathy: Alzheimer's disease
- Lewy bodies: Parkinson's disease
- Henderson- Peterson bodies: Molluscum contagiosum
- Russell bodies: Multiple myeloma
- Halberstaedter- Prowazeke bodies: Chlamydia trachomatis
- Dohle bodies: Severe inflammatory disease or sepsis

IMMUNITY

- Major histocompatibility complex/ MHC/ Human leucocyte complex/ HLA complex is located on: Chromosome 6
- Cells which are a part of innate immunity: Natural killer cells
- NK cells are expressed on: CD16, CD56
- NK kills: Infected cells & cancer cells
- Killing by NK cells is: MHC independent (not dependent of foreign antigen presentation)

TRANSLOCATIONS

- t(8;14): Burkitt's lymphoma
- t(9;22): CML
- t(11;22): Ewing's sarcoma

TUMOUR MARKERS

- Endodermal sinus tumours: AFP/ alpha Fetoprotein
- Yolk sac tumours: AFP
- Pancreatic neuroendocrine tumours: Gastrin
- Ca cervix: Keratin

HYPERSENSITIVITY REACTIONS

- PK/ Prausnitz reaction: Type I
- Casoni's test: Type I
- Asthma. Hay fever, atopy etc.: Type I (IgE mediated)
- Contact dermatitis: Type IV (delayed hypersensitivity)
- Schick's test: Type III (Immune complex mediated)
- Serum sickness: Type III
- Arthus reaction: Type III
- Immune thrombocytopenic purpura/ ITP: Type II (IgM/ IgG mediated)
- Immune hemolytic anemia: Type II
- Blood transfusion reactions: Type II
- Good pastures syndrome: Type II
- Graves' disease: Type II

COLLAGEN

- Most abundant collagen of human body: Type I
- Basal lamina has: Type IV collagen

Conditions & pathologic features

Condition	*Pathologic features*
Human papilloma virus infection	Koilocytes
Burkitt's lymphoma	Starry sky appearance
Cystic glandular hyperplasia	Swiss cheese endometrium
Lupus nephritis	Sub-endothelial immune deposit
Focal glomerulonephritis/ GN	Flea bitten kidney
Membrano-proliferative GN	Tram track appearance
Rapidly progressive GN	Epithelial crescents
Lipid nephrosis	Fusion of foot processes of podocytes
Chronic active hepatitis	Piecemeal necrosis & bridging necrosis
Typhoid	Erythro-phagocytosis
Focal amyloidosis	Sago spleen
Diffuse amyloidosis	Lardaceous spleen
Alcoholic hepatitis	Mallory hyaline
Chronic pyelonephritis	Thyroidisation of kidney
Chronic gastritis	Intestinalisation of stomach
Pneumonia	Grey & red hepatisation of lung
SLE	Lumpy bumpy basement membrane
Chronic venous congestion/ CVC liver	Nutmeg liver

AMYLOIDOSIS

- Amyloid protein associated with primary amyloidosis/ myeloma: AL
- Amyloid protein associated with secondary amyloidosis (TB, RA): AA
- Amyloid protein associated with cardiac amyloidosis: ATTR
- MC site of amyloidosis: Kidney (followed by liver)
- Thyroid Ca showing amyloid stroma is Medullary thyroid Ca/ MTC
- Best diagnostic method for amyloidosis: Rectal biopsy
- Congo red stain in ordinary light gives: Pink colour
- Congo red stain in polarizing light gives: Yellow green birefringence

GENETICS

- Homocystinuria is: Autosomal recessive/ AR
- Von Willebrand's disease is: Autosomal dominant/ AD
- Retinoblastoma is: Autosomal dominant/ AD
- Familial hypercholesterolemia is: Autosomal dominant/ AD
- Achondroplasia is: Autosomal dominant/ AD
- Hereditary spherocytosis is: Autosomal dominant/ AD
- Chromosome 4 is involved in: Huntington's chorea
- Chromosome 7 is involved in: Cystic fibrosis
- Gene for major histocompatibility is located on chromosome: 6

- Gene for folate carrier protein is located on chromosome: 21
- Short arm of chromosome is designated as: p
- Long arm of chromosome is designated as: q
- Genes regulating morphogenesis: Homeobox genes (HOX)
- APC gene is located on chromosome: 5
- BRCA1 gene is located on chromosome: 17

IMMUNOGLOBULINS

- First antibody to be synthesized after primary immunization: IgM
- First antibody to be synthesized after exposure to new antigen: IgM
- First antibody to be synthesized by fetus: IgM
- Antibody which fixes complement: IgM
- Only immunoglobulin that crosses placenta: IgG
- Immunoglobulin found in mucous secretions (saliva, tears, colostrum etc.): IgA/ secretory antibody
- Immunoglobulin elevated in atopic diseases (asthma, hay fever etc.): IgE
- Immunoglobulin mediating reaginic hypersensitivity: IgE

INTERFERONS

- IFN produced by leucocytes: IFN-alpha
- IFN produced by fibroblasts: IFN-beta
- IFN produced by T lymphocytes and NK cells: IFN-gamma

COMPLEMENT COMPONENTS

- Opsonization: C3b
- Chemotaxis: C5a

TUMOUR SUPPRESSOR GENE

- VHL is a tumour suppressor gene for: Von Hippel Lindau disease
- Rb is a tumour suppressor gene for:
  - o Retinoblastoma
  - o Osteosarcoma
- BRCA is a tumour suppressor gene for: Hereditary breast carcinoma

TRISOMIES

- Trisomy 21: Downs syndrome
- Trisomy 18: Edwards syndrome
- Trisomy 13: Patau's syndrome

VASCULAR SYSTEM PATHOLOGY

- Medium sized vessel arteritis includes:
  - o Polyarteritis nodosa/ PAN
  - o Kawasaki disease
- ESR is markedly elevated (over 100 mm/ hour, Westergren method) in: Temporal arteritis
- Pathological feature of malignant hypertension: Fibrinoid necrosis
- Hyaline arteriosclerosis is seen in: Benign hypertension
- Pseudoaneurysm/ false aneurysm: Haematoma, as a result of injury
- MC cause of abdominal aneurysms: Atherosclerosis
- MC cause of aneurysm: Atherosclerosis
- Luetic/ syphilitic aneurysm involves: Ascending aorta
- Tree bark calcification is seen in: Syphilis

CARDIAC PATHOLOGY

- Aschoff bodies are a feature of: Rheumatic heart disease
- Anitschkow cells/ caterpillar cells are seen in: Rheumatic heart disease
- Valve least commonly used in RHD: Tricuspid valve
- MC cause of mitral stenosis: Rheumatic fever
- MC cause of myocarditis: Viral (Coxsackie virus B)
- MC primary cardiac tumours: Myxoma
- Libman Sacks endocarditis is seen in: SLE
- Dressler's syndrome is: Autoimmune

Acute Rheumatic Fever

- Affects all the three layers of heart
- The stenotic mitral value appears like button-hole or fish mouth
- MacCallum's patch – Rough portion of endocardium of left atrium
- Characteristic distribution of erythema marginatum in rheumatic heart disease is bathing suit distribution
- Bread and butter pericarditis

Must know facts

- Tree barking of aortic intima – Syphilitic aortitis
- Most common site of coronary atherosclerosis – left anterior descending branch
- Vegetations of NBTE are sterile, nondestructive, small, singly or multiple along the lines of closure of the leaflets or cusps

Blood transfusion

- Stored at 4 degrees centigrade
- Those who have received HBIG- should not donate for 6 months
- Those who have received Rabies vaccine- should not donate for 1 year

MYOCARDIAL INFARCTION

- MC involved artery in MI: Left anterior descending artery/ LAD
- Earliest change seen in MI: Waviness of fibres
- Change noticed within 1-3 days of MI:
    - o Coagulation necrosis
    - o Neutrophilic infiltration
- Change seen around 1 week after MI: Granulation tissue
- Scarring in MI is complete by: 3 months
- Troponin T: Marker of MI

RESPIRATORY PATHOLOGY

- Charcot layden crystals are seen in: Asthma
- Curschmann spirals are seen in: Asthma
- Reid index is used for: Chronic bronchitis
- Alpha1 antitrypsin deficiency is associated with: Panacinar emphysema
- Important cause of emphysema: Smoking
- Non caseating granulomas with bilateral hilar lymphadenopathy is a feature of: Sarcoidosis
- Test used for sarcoidosis: Kveim's test
- Features of sarcoidosis:
    - o End stage lung disease
    - o Epithelioid cells with no caseation
    - o Does NOT involve brain
- Condition which may mimic sarcoidosis: Beryllium inhalation
- Egg shell pattern is seen in: Silicosis
- Intense fibrosis is a pathological feature of: Mesothelioma
- Particle size dangerous for pneumoconiosis: 1-5 micrometer

Reids index

- Thickness of mucous gland layer/ Thickness of wall between the epithelium and cartilage
- Normal ratio = 0.14 to 0.36
- Increased in chronic bronchitis

Pathological conditions

Description	*Entity*
Multiple discrete, laminated calcareous bodies seen in tumours from meninges, choroid plexus, ovary	**Psammoma bodies**
Alcoholic liver disease, Indian childhood cirrhosis, Wilson disease	**Mallory bodies**
Nuclear remnants in RBC; seen after spleen atrophy and folate deficiency after splenectomy	**Howell jolly bodies**
End product of degraded haemoglobin; seen in in chemical poisoning, drug intoxication	**Heinz bodies**
Iron containing granules in RBC precursors in haemolytic anaemia	**Pappenheimer cells**
Seen in CML	**Auer rods**

GIT PATHOLOGY

- Squamous cell esophageal Ca is related to:
    - o Alcohol
    - o Smoking
    - o Chronic achalasia
    - o Plummer vinson syndrome
    - o Tylosis etc.
- Virus causing esophagitis:
    - o HSV1 & 2
    - o Varicella zoster
    - o CMV etc.
- GIST/ gastrointestinal stromal tumours are expressed on:
    - o CD117 &
    - o CD34
- Gardner's syndrome:
    - o Rectal & colonic polyposis
    - o Skin cysts
    - o Osteomas
    - o Dentigerous cysts etc.
- Peutz Jeghers syndrome:
    - o Hamartomatous polyps of GIT &
    - o Mucocutaneous pigmentation
- Von recklinghausen's disease:
    - o Generalized neurofibromatosis
    - o Café au lait pigmentation
- Genetic predisposition for celiac disease:
    - o HLA B8
    - o DR3 &
    - o DQ2
- Typhoid ulcers are:
    - o Longitudinal
    - o Ulceration of peyer's patches
    - o Stricture is RARE

INFLAMMATORY BOWEL DISEASE

- Pipe stem colon is seen in: Ulcerative colitis
- Skip lesions is seen in: Crohn's disease
- Transmural inflammation is seen in: Crohn's disease
- Pseudopolyps are seen in: Ulcerative colitis
- MC site of involvement in Crohn's disease: Ileum

Crohn's disease

- Bowel region: Ileum, Colon
- Distribution: Skip lesion
- Stricture: Yes
- Wall appearance: Thick
- Inflammation: Transmural
- Pseudopolyps: Moderate
- Ulcers: Deep, knife like
- Lymphoid reaction, Fibrosis, Serositis: Marked
- Granulomas: Yes (35%)
- Fistulae/ Sinuses: Yes
- Perianal fistula: Yes (in colonic disease)
- Fat/ vitamin malabsorption: Yes
- Malignant potential: With colonic involvement
- Recurrence after surgery: Common
- Toxic megacolon: No

LIVER

- Mallory bodies are composed of: Eosinophilic intracytoplasmic inclusions
- Mallory bodies are seen in:
    - o Primary biliary cirrhosis
    - o Alcoholism etc.
- Mallory hyaline is ABSENT in:
    - o Secondary biliary cirrhosis
    - o Hepatitis etc.
- Acute infection of HBV:
    - o HBsAg +
    - o IgM anti-HBc +

- MC cause of post transfusion hepatitis: HCV
- HCV causes: Chronic hepatitis
- MC cause of sporadic cases of hepatitis in adults: HEV
- Hepatitis having worst prognosis in pregnancy: HEV
- MC route of spread of HEV: Feco-oral
- Angiosarcoma of liver is associated with:
  - Vinyl chloride
  - Aflatoxin etc.

Centrilobular necrosis is associated with

- Chronic venous congestion
- Hemorrhagic shock
- Carbon tetrachloride
- Halothane
- Acetaminophen
- Rifampicin

Amyloidosis of the spleen

- Sago spleen: Deposit mostly limited to splenic follicles
- Lardaceous spleen: Amyloid spares the follicle and involves the walls of the splenic sinuses and connective tissue framework of the red pulp

Mallory bodies are associated with

- Alcoholic liver disease
- Primary biliary cirrhosis
- Wilson's disease
- Chronic cholestatic syndromes
- Hepatocellular carcinoma

Hepatitis markers

- HbsAg: Acute or chronic HBV infection
- Anti- HBs: Immunity against HBV
- IgM Anti-HBc-high titre: Acute HBV infection
- IgM Anti-HBc-low titre/ absent: Chronic HBV infection
- IgG Anti-HBc: Past exposure to HBV
- HBV DNA: Continued infectious state
- HBeAg: Continued infectious state, Acute or chronic HBV infection
- Anti-HBe: Convalescence

RENAL PATHOLOGY

- Renomegaly is seen in:
  - Diabetic nephropathy
  - Amyloidosis
  - Polycystic kidney disease etc.
- Contracted kidney is seen in:
  - Chronic glomerulonephritis
  - Chronic pyelonephritis etc.
- Flea bitten kidney is seen in:
  - Malignant hypertension
  - Acute post streptococcal glomerulonephritis etc.

Urinary casts

- Hyaline casts: Normal
- RBC casts: Glomerular injury
- WBC casts: Interstitial nephritis/ pyelonephritis
- Broad granular casts: Chronic renal failure
- Pigmented muddy brown granular casts: Tubular necrosis

Electron microscopic features of glomerulonephritis

- Type I MPGN: Subendothelial & mesangial deposition of IgG & C3
- Type II MPGN: Dense deposit disease, deposits within basement membrane, deposition of C3
- PSGN:
  Immunofluorescence microscopy shows diffuse granular deposition of IgG and C3, giving rise to starry sky appearance

Must know facts

- Hyaline arteriosclerosis is seen in benign nephrosclerosis
- Fibrinoid necrosis and hyperplastic arteriosclerosis is seen in malignant hypertension

GLOMERULOPATHIES

- MC cause of nephrotic syndrome in children: Lipoid nephrosis/ Minimal change disease
- Anti-GBM antibodies are seen in: Goodpasture's syndrome
- Diffuse involvement is seen in: Post-streptococcal glomerulonephritis/ PSGN
- Sub-epithelial humps are seen in: PSGN
- FSGN having worst prognosis: Collapsing variety
- Sub-epithelial spikes (with M spike) is a feature of: Membranous GN
- Tram track appearance: Membranoproliferative GN
- Crescents (epithelial cells + fibrin + macrophage) are seen in: Rapidly progressive GN
- Alport's syndrome:
  - o Hereditary nephritis
  - o Nerve deafness &
  - o Eye disorders
- Lung involvement in Wegner's granulomatosis is: Bilateral nodular cavitary infiltrates (showing necrotizing granulomatous vasculitis)
- Renal biopsy in Wegner's granulomatosis is that of: Pauci-immune necrotizing & crescentic GN
- Bilateral renal cell Ca may be seen in: Von Hippel Lindau disease
- Kimmelstiel Wilson disease is seen in: Diabetic nephropathy
- Finnish type of nephritic syndrome is due to: Mutation of nephrin
- MC gene defect in steroid resistant nephritic syndrome is: NPHS2
- Michaelis Gutmann bodies are seen in: Malakoplakia
- Salt losing nephritis is seen in: Interstitial nephritis

THYROID

- Thyroid Ca which spreads by lymphatics: Papillary Ca thyroid
- Psammoma bodies are seen in: Papillary Ca thyroid
- Orphan annie eyed nuclei are seen in: Papillary Ca thyroid
- Hurthle cell Ca is a variant of: Follicular Ca thyroid
- Tumour arising from parafollicular/ C cells: Medullary Ca thyroid
- Thyroid tumour which secretes calcitonin: Medullary Ca thyroid
- Thyroid Ca associated with MEN-II: Medullary Ca thyroid
- RET proto-oncogene is involved in: Medullary Ca thyroid

Differential diagnosis microcytic hypochromic anemia

Serum values	*Iron deficiency anemia*	*Beta-thala-ssemia*	*Anemic of chronic diseases*	*Sidero-blastic anemia*
Iron	Low	Normal	Low	High
TIBC	High	Normal	Low	Normal
Ferritin	Low	Normal	High	High
HBA2	Low	High	Normal	Low

HAEMATOLOGY

- Bite cells are seen in: G6PD deficiency
- Helmet cells are seen in:
  - o Hemolytic uremic syndrome
  - o Coombs positive
- Schistocytes are seen in: Acquired spherocytosis
- Ring sideroblasts (iron granules in mitochondria around the nucleus) are seen in: Sideroblastic anemia
- 'Tear drop' poikilocytes are seen in:
  - o Myeloid metaplasia &
  - o Myelofibrosis
- Post splenectomy changes include:
  - o Howell jolly bodies
  - o Heinz bodies etc.
- Burr cells are seen in: Uremia

- Acanthocytes are seen in: Abetalipoproteinemia
- Macropolycytes are seen in: Megaloblastic anemia
- Hypersegmented neutrophils are seen in: Megaloblastic anemia
- Spur cells are seen in: Chronic liver disease

Peripheral smear features

- Basophilic stippling: Iron deficiency anemia, Lead poisoning, Thalassemia, Sideroblastic anemia
- Heinz bodies: Glucose- 6-phosphate deficiency, Thalassemia
- Acanthocytes: Abetalipoproteinemia
- Spiculated RBC: Pyruvate kinase deficiency
- Burr cells: HUS, Uremia

Pentad of thrombocytopenic purpura (TTP)

- Thrombocytopenia
- Fever
- Microangiopathic hemolytic anemia
- Transient neurological deficits
- Renal failure

Myelofibrosis

- Marked splenomegaly (tear drop cells)
- Peripheral blood shows leukoerythroblastic anemia
- In bone marrow dysplastic megakaryocytes are characteristically seen
- Characteristic dry tap

Peripheral smears & conditions

Findings	***Condition***
Starry sky appearance in lymph node biopsy	**Burkitt's lymphoma**
Increased eosinophils	**Eosinophilic leukaemia**
Large lymphocytes with prominent nucleolus	**Pro-lymphocytic leukaemia**
Increased small lymphocytes, rare blasts, auto-immune haemolytic anaemia present	**CLL (B-cell)**
All series of cells seen, myeloblasts greater than 10, increased basophils, eosinophils, thrombocytes	**CML**
Iron granules in mitochondria around the nucleus	**Ring sideroblasts**
Neutropenia, hairy cells, splenomegaly	**Hairy cell leukemia**
Megakaryocytosis in bone marrow	**Idiopathic thrombocytopenic purpura, myeloid metaplasia, polycythemia vera**
Polychromasia & spherocytosis	**Warm antibody AIHLA (auto-immune hemolytic anemia)**
Giant platelets, microcytic anemia, tear drop poikilocytes, leuko-erythroblastic picture	**Myeloid metaplasia & myelofibrosis**
Increased RBC, platelets, leukocytes, splenomegaly	**Polycythemia vera**
Ring sideroblast	**Sideroblastic anemia**
Anisocytosis, poikilocytosis, fragmented RBCs, neutrophil lobes increased, platelets normal, absolute reticulocyte count low	**Pernicious anemia & folate deficiency anemia**
Pancytopenia present, platelets maximum affected and last to recover	**Aplastic anemia**
Negative coombs test	**Hereditary spherocytosis**
Schistocytes present, Coombs test positive	**Acquired spherocytosis**
Tactoids & sickling	**Sickle cell anemia**
Decreased osmosis, microcytic hypochromic anemia, increased HbF & HbA2	**Thalassemia major**
Spur cells	**Cirrhosis**
Burr cells	**Uremia**

Must know facts

- Most sensitive and specific test for diagnosis of iron deficiency is –Serum ferritin level
- Thrombocytopenia indicates platelet count below 1 lac/ cu mm

- Wiskott-aldrich syndrome shows – small platelets
- Crumbling brick wall appearance seen in Hailey- Hailey disease
- Mycosis fungoides is a: T-cell lymphoproliferative disorder
- von Willebrand's factor can be assayed by: Ristocetin aggregation test

SICKLE CELL ANEMIA

- SCA is due to replacement of: Glutamate by valine
- SCA is due to: Structurally abnormal hemoglobin

HEREDITARY SPHEROCYTOSIS

- HS is due to: Spectrin deficiency
- Basically HS is a: Cell membrane defect
- Proteins defective in HS:
  - o Ankyrin
  - o Paladin
  - o Anion transport protein

APLASTIC ANEMIA

- Causes:
  - o Drugs (chloramphenicol)
  - o Viruses etc.
- Feature ABSENT in aplastic anemia: Splenomegaly
- Most effective treatment of aplastic anemia: Bone marrow transplant

LEUKEMIA

- Conditions associated with AML:
  - o Down syndrome
  - o Bloom syndrome etc.
- Features of AML:
  - o Chloroma
  - o Auer rods
  - o Positive non-specific esterase etc.
- AML subtype which is NOT positive for non-specific esterase: M6
- AML with gum infiltration: M4
- DIC is associated with: APML
- t(15;17) is seen in: APML
- Basophilic leukocytosis occurs in: CML
- B cell neoplasms include:
  - o Hairy cell leukemia
  - o Mantle cell lymphoma etc.

MULTIPLE MYELOMA

- Russel bodies & Flame cells are seen
- Bence Jones proteins are: Light chains
- Urea level in MM are: Raised

HAIRY CELL LEUKEMIA

- HCL is a: B cell neoplasm
- Associated feature: Splenomegaly
- Cells are: TRAP (tartrate resistant phosphatase) positive
- DOC for HCL: Cladribine

LYMPHOMA

- Malignant cells of Hodgkin's disease are: Reed Sternberg cells/ RS
- RS cells are positive for:
  - o CD15 &
  - o CD30
- Subtype of Hodgkin's disease, which is NOT positive for CD15 & CD30: Lymphocytic predominant
- Lacunar cells are seen in: Nodular sclerosis type of lymphoma
- Hilar lymphadenopathy is a feature of: Nodular sclerosis type
- MC type of Hodgkin's lymphoma: Nodular sclerosing
- MC site of extranodal non-Hodgkin's lymphoma: Stomach
- Starry sky appearance is seen in: Burkitt's lymphoma

ANTIPHOSPHOLIPID ANTIBODY SYNDROME

- Features of APAS:
  - o Arterial/ venous thrombosis (NOT bleeding)
  - o Recurrent fetal loss (2nd trimester abortions)
- Lab findings of APAS:
  - o Prolonged APTT
  - o Normal PT

NERVOUS SYSTEM PATHOLOGY

- Macrophage of brain: Microglia
- Complex granular corpuscles are produced by: Microglia
- CSF findings in pyogenic meningitis:
  - o Increased protein
  - o Decreased sugar
- Features of tubercular meningitis:
  - o Increased protein
  - o Decreased sugar
  - o Increased lymphocytes

CNS TUMOURS

- MC primary brain tumour: Glioma
- MC brain tumour in adults: Astrocytoma
- MC type of glial tumours: Astrocytoma
- MC posterior fossa tumour in children: Cerebellar astrocytoma
- Pseudo-rosette are seen in: Neuroblastoma
- Enamel like structure is found in: Craniopharyngioma
- Glial fibrillary proteins are seen in: Astrocytoma

Histopathological pentad of Alzheimer's disease

- Neuritic plaques
- Neurofibrillary tangles
- Granulo-vacuolar degeneration
- Amyloid angiopathy
- Gliosis

Neurotransmitters depletion & neurological diseases

- Alzheimer's: Decreased Acetylcholine
- Parkinson's disease: Dopamine <Acetylcholine
- Schizophrenia: Dopamine> Acetylcholine
- Huntington's disease: Loss of GABA-ergic and Cholinergic neurons

BERRY ANEURYSM

- MC cause of subarachnoid hemorrhage: Berry aneurysm
- MC site of Berry aneurysm: Anterior circle of Willis

'BODIES' & CONDITIONS

- Hirano bodies & neurofibrillary tangle are seen in: Alzheimer's disease
- Pick bodies are seen in: Picks disease
- Lewy bodies are seen in: Parkinsonism

ONCOLOGY

- MC bilateral breast tumour: Lobular Ca
- BRCA1 gene is located on: Chromosome 17
- MC tumours of ovary: Primary epithelial tumours (cystadenoma, clear cell Ca etc.)
- Call Exner bodies are seen in: Granulosa cell tumour
- Reinke's crystal are seen in: Hilus cell tumour
- Schiller Duval bodies: Endodermal sinus tumour
- Conditions associated with germ cell tumours/ GCT of testes:
  - o Cryptorchidism
  - o Testicular feminization syndrome
- Klinefelter's syndrome is associated with: Mediastinal GCT
- Seminoma corresponds to: Dysgerminoma of ovary

HIV

- Window period: Time period between infection & detection of antibodies against HIV

- Hallmark of HIV:
  - o Profound immunodeficiency
  - o Quantitative & qualitative deficiency of helper or inducer T cells
- AIDS related neoplasm:
  - o Kaposi sarcoma
  - o B cell non-Hodgkin's lymphoma
  - o Primary lymphoma of brain
- Kaposi sarcoma arises from: Cells lining lymph vessels or blood vessels
- Kaposi sarcoma is associated with:
  - o HIV
  - o Immunosuppression/ organ transplants

Familial syndromes associated with Phaeochromocytoma & extra-adrenal paraganglioma

- Multiple endocrine neoplasia (MEN) type-2A: Phaeochromocytoma, Medullary carcinoma of thyroid, Parathyroid hyperplasia
- MEN type-2B: Phaeochromocytoma, Medullary carcinoma of thyroid, Marfanoid habitus
- Neurofibromatosis (NF) type-I: Phaeochromocytoma, Neurofibromatosis, Café-au-lait spots, Optic nerve glioma
- Von-Hippel Lindau: Phaeochromocytoma, Paraganglioma, Renal cell carcinoma, Haemangioblastoma, Pancreatic endocrine neoplasm

Down's syndrome

- Muscle hypotonia
- Oblique eye fissures with epicanthic skin folds on the inner corner of the eyes
- Flat nasal bridge
- Excessive space between large toe and second toe
- Single palmar fold (Simian crease)
- Protruding tongue
- Short neck
- White spots on the iris known as Brushfield spots
- Single flexion furrow of the fifth finger
- Higher number of ulnar loop dermatoglyphics

Autosomal dominant disorders

- Huntington disease
- Familial hypercholesterolemia
- Familial adenomatous polyposis
- Von Hippel Lindau syndrome
- MEN type 1 and 2
- Retinoblastoma
- Spherocytosis
- Antithrombin III and factor V Leiden
- von Willebrand's disease
- Polycystic kidney disease
- Achondroplasia
- Marfan's syndrome
- Amyloidosis

Autosomal recessive disorders

- Cystic fibrosis
- Galactosemia
- Alpha-1 antitrypsin deficiency
- Ataxia telangiectasia
- Alkaptonuria
- Phenylketonuria
- Alpha and beta Thalassemia
- Sickle cell disease
- Hereditary spherocytosis
- Wilson's disease
- Hemochromatosis
- Gaucher's disease
- Niemann- Pick disease
- Tay-Sachs disease
- MPS I-VII
- Glycogen storage disorders I-VIII
- Congenital adrenal hyperplasia

X Linked dominant disorders

- Vitamin D resistant rickets
- Orofacial digital syndrome
- Incontinentia pigmenti

Mitochondrial disorders

- Kearns-Sayre syndrome
- MELAS
- Leber's hereditary optic neuropathy
- Myoclonic epilepsy

Traits inherited along Y chromosome

- Male infertility
- Gonadoblastoma

Chromosomal breakage disorders

- Fanconi's syndrome
- Bloom's syndrome
- Ataxia – telangiectasia

Mutations

- Silent mutation: Codon containing the changed base codes for the same amino acid
- Missense mutation: Codon containing the changed base codes for a different amino acid, this mistaken codon may be acceptable, partially acceptable or unacceptable to functioning of that protein molecule
- Nonsense mutation: Codon containing the changed base becomes the termination codon

Prion diseases

- Kuru
- Creutzfeldt-Jakob disease
- Fatal familial insomnia
- Madcow disease

Must know facts

- Regular Trisomy 21 is found in 94 percent cases of Down's syndrome
- Fragile X syndrome is the second most common cause of mental retardation after Down's syndrome in males
- Achondroplasia: Most common disproportionate dwarfism; Trident hand (index and ring finger are divergent)
- Ataxia telangiectasia: Autosomal recessive; Basic defect in abnormal sensitivity to X-ray and certain radiomimetic chemicals which leads to chromosome and chromatid breakage
- G6 PD deficiency is X-linked recessive transmission
- Marfan's syndrome is associated with mutation in fibrillin protein
- Hamartomas: Excessive and focal overgrowth of cells and tissues native to the organ in which it occurs
- Choristoma / heterotropia: Microscopically normal cells or tissues that are present in abnormal locations

Stain

Stain	*Used for*
Schiller's iodine	**Cervix (carcinoma)**
Von kossa stain, Alizarin stain, Haematoxylin Eosin stain	**Calcium**
Leishman stain, Giemsa stain, Delafield's stain	**Microfilaria in blood**
JSB stain, Giemsa stain, Leishman stain	**Malarial parasite**
PAS positive granules	**Whipple's disease**
Sudan black, Osmic acid, Nile blue sulphate	**Fat**
Lugol's iodine, Congo red, PAS (periodic acid schiff), Van Gieson stain, UV light	**Amyloid**
Alcohol, Best carmine, PAS	**Glycogen**

CLINICAL QUESTIONS

1. **A 60 years old female has history of 8 blood transfusions in past 2 years. Her Hb: 6.0 g/ dL, TLC: 5800, platelets: 3.4 lakhs, MCV: 60, RBC: 2.1 lakhs/ mm^3. She is having hypochromic microcytic anemia. Which investigation is NOT needed?**

A. Evaluation of pulmonary hemosiderosis

B. Urinary hemosiderin

C. Bone marrow examination

D. Gastrointestinal endoscopy

Clinical presentation is suggestive of deficiency of iron (normal MCV is 77-93 fl).

So, evaluation of pulmonary hemosiderosis is not needed.

Hemosiderosis is an iron-storage disorder in which there is excessive accumulation of iron in parenchymal cells with eventual tissue damage and functional insufficiency of organs such as liver, pancreas, heart and pituitary gland.

Answer: A i.e., Evaluation of pulmonary hemosiderosis

2. **During autopsy of a patient died due to suspected myocardial infarction, the heart tissue was stained with triphenyl-tetrazolium chloride dye. What would be the color of viable myocardium?**

A. Blue B. White

C. Red D. Dark brown

Color of viable myocardium will be red, when stained with triphenyl-tetrazolium chloride stain.

Early myocardial infarcts (3-6 hours) can be detected by histochemical staining for dehydrogenases on unfixed slice of the heart.

This consists of immersing a slice of unfixed heart in the solution of triphenyl-tetrazolium chloride (TTC) which imparts red colour to the normal heart muscle, while the area of infarcted muscle fails to stain due to lack of dehydrogenases.

Answer: C i.e., Red

3. **A 19 years old female with short stature, widespread nipples and primary amenorrhea, would likely to have which karyotype:**

A. 47, XX+18 B. 46, XXY

C. 47, XXY D. 45X

Clinical findings are suggestive of Turner's syndrome.

The karyotype is 45XO.

It is an example of monosomy (45, XO) most often due to loss of X chromosome in paternal meiosis.

Answer: D i.e., 45X

4. **In a 30 years old female patient with polyarthritis, testing reveals nucleolar pattern of ANA staining. What is the likely course of this patient?**

A. Malar rash, alopecia and renal failure

B. Sclerodactyly, esophageal dysmotility and Raynaud's phenomenon

C. Sjogren syndrome

D. Painful genital and oral blisters and ulcers

Clinical presentation is suggestive of CREST syndrome.

*CREST syndrome is characterized by **C**alcinosis, **R**aynaud's phenomenon, **E**sophageal hypomotility, **S**clerodactyly and **T**elangiectasia.*

CREST syndrome is one of the two types of scleroderma.

Answer: B. i.e., Sclerodactyly, esophageal dysmotility and Raynaud's phenomenon

5. **A 28 years old female presents with recurrent abortions and pain in the calves. She is most likely suffering from a deficiency of which of the following?**

A. Protein C B. Thrombin

C. Factor XIII D. Plasmin

Clinical presentation is suggestive of deficiency of protein C.

Deficiency of both protein C and S are autosomal dominant disorders having either reduced amount of protein C or S, or both, or their functional defect.

Clinically, both the conditions are associated with lifelong risk of thrombosis of deep leg veins (which present as calf pain).

Answer: A i.e., Protein C

6. **A 17 years old boy presented with TLC of 138 × 10^9/L with 80% blasts on the peripheral smear. Chest X-ray demonstrated a large mediastinal mass. Immunotyping of this patient blasts would likely demonstrate:**

A. No surface antigens (null phenotype)

B. An immature T cell phenotype (Tdt/ CD3/ CD7 positive)

C. Myeloid markers, such as CD13, Cd33 and CD15

D. B cell markers such as CD19, CD20 and CD22

Clinical presentation is suggestive of precursor T-cell lymphoblastic leukemia/ lymphoma/ ETP-ALL.

Immunotyping will demonstrate an immature T-cell phenotype (Tdt/ D3/ CD7 positive).

Since the precursor T-cells differentiates in the thymus, this tumour often presents as mediastinal mass and pleural effusion and progresses rapidly to develop leukemia in the blood and bone marrow.

On immunophenotyping, TdT (terminal deoxynucleotidyl transferase) is expressed by the nuclei of pre-T stages of differentiation of lymphoid cells.

Answer: B i.e., An immature T cell phenotype (Tdt/ CD3/ CD7 positive)

7. **A 55 years male presented with dry mouth and rheumatoid arthritis with high titer of anti SS-A and anti SS-B antibodies, diagnosed as a case of minor salivary gland tumour. The earliest histological finding is:**

A. Endothelial cells　B. Basophils

C. Lymphocyte　D. Eosinophils

Clinical presentation is suggestive of Sjogren's syndrome.

Sjogren's syndrome is characterized by the triad of dry eyes (keratoconjunctivitis sicca), dry mouth (xerostomia), and rheumatoid arthritis.

The combination of the former two symptoms is called as sicca syndrome.

In early stage, the lacrimal and salivary glands show periductal infiltration by lymphocytes and plasma cells, which at times may form lymphoid follicles (pseudo-lymphoma).

Answer: C i.e., Lymphocyte

8. **An undifferentiated malignant tumour on immuno-histochemical stain shows cytoplasmic positivity of most of the tumour cells for cytokeratin. Most probable diagnosis of the tumour is:**

A. Sarcoma　B. Lymphoma

C. Carcinoma　D. Malignant melanoma

Presentation is suggestive of carcinoma.

Immuno-stains for epithelial tumours (carcinomas) include pankeratin (fractions; high and low molecular weight keratins), epithelial membrane antigen (EMA), carcinoembryonic antigen (CEA) and neuron specific enolase (NSE).

Answer: C i.e., Carcinoma

9. **A 15 years old girl presented with weakness for 2 months. On examination, she had pallor and icterus. Spleen was palpable. Lab examination showed decreased MCV, increased MCHC and reticulocytosis. Osmotic fragility test is positive. Coomb's test is negative. Most likely diagnosis:**

A. Iron deficiency anemia

B. Auto-immune hemolytic anemia

C. G-6-PD deficiency

D. Hereditary spherocytosis

Clinical presentation is suggestive of hereditary spherocytosis.

Clinical features of hereditary spherocytosis include anemia (manifests as weakness and icterus), splenomegaly (a constant feature), jaundice and pigment gallstones.

Laboratory findings include reticulocytosis (usually 5-20%), MCV is usually normal or slightly decreased but MCHC is increased.

Osmotic fragility is increased (spheroidal nature of red cells make them lyse more readily in solutions of low salt concentration).

Direct Coomb's test (antiglobulin) is negative so as to distinguish this condition from acquired spherocytosis of AIHA (autoimmune hemolytic anemia), in which it is positive.

Answer: D i.e., Hereditary spherocytosis

10. A 2 years old child presents with scattered lesions in the skull. Biopsy revealed Langerhans cells. The most commonly associated marker with this condition would be:

A. CD1a B. CD57

C. CD3 D. CD68

Clinical presentation is suggestive of Langerhans cell histiocytosis.

Demonstration of common antigens on these Langerhans cells can be done by immune-histochemical stains for S-100 protein, CD1a and HLA-DR.

Answer: A i.e., CD1a

11. One sided kidney is normal whereas the other side kidney is contracted with scar formation. Most likely diagnosis:

A. Chronic pyelonephritis

B. Polycystic kidney disease

C. Renal artery stenosis

D. Tuberculosis of kidney

Presentation is suggestive of chronic pyelonephritis.

In chronic pyelonephritis, the kidney shows characteristic appearance.

The kidneys are usually small and contracted (weighing less than 100 gram) showing unequal reduction, which distinguishes it from other forms of contracted kidney.

The surface of the kidney is irregularly scarred; the capsule can be stripped off with difficulty due to adherence to scars.

Answer: A i.e., Chronic pyelonephritis

12. Patient with cirrhosis is HBsAg positive and has increased level of alpha fetoprotein. Most likely diagnosis:

A. Submassive hepatic necrosis

B. Hepatocellular carcinoma

C. Massive hepatic necrosis

D. Normal

Clinical presentation is suggestive of hepatocellular carcinoma.

Genesis of hepatocellular carcinoma/ HCC is linked to prolonged infection with HBV.

Cirrhosis of all etiologic types is more commonly associated with HCC but the most frequent association is with macronodular post-necrotic cirrhosis.

Laboratory findings of HCC yield nonspecific results like anemia, markedly elevated serum alkaline phosphatase as found in cirrhosis, and high serum alpha-fetoprotein (AFP). Elevated AFP level is quite specific; very high levels of AFP (above 500 ng/ ml) are observed in 70-80% cases of HCC, but lacks sensitivity since AFP is also found elevated in yolk sac tumour, cirrhosis, chronic hepatitis, massive liver necrosis and normal pregnancy.

Answer: B i.e., Hepatocellular carcinoma

13. A 35 years old male presented with history of bleeding. Peripheral smear shows platelet count: 50,000/ mm^3, leukocytosis, decreased neutrophils, normal lymphocytes, blast: 20%. t(8;21) is positive. Band forms, myelocyte and metamyelocytes were also seen. Most likely diagnosis:

A. CLL

B. CML

C. AML

D. Myelodysplastic syndrome

Clinical presentation is suggestive of AML.

Acute myeloblastic leukemia has bleeding manifestations (due to thrombocytopenia; causing spontaneous bruises, petechiae, bleeding from gums etc.).

The platelet count is usually moderately to severely reduced (below 50,000/ microL).

The total WBC count ranges from subnormal to markedly elevated values (leukocytosis).

Majority of leucocytes in the peripheral blood are blasts and there is often neutropenia due to marrow infiltration by leukemic cells.

A few important examples of chromosomal mutations in AML are translocations {(t8;21)(q22q22)} and {(t15;17)(q22;q12)} and inversions {inv(16)(p13;q22)}.

WHO classification for AML has revised and lowered the cut off percentage of marrow blasts to 20% (from 30% in the FAB classification) for making a diagnosis of AML.

Answer: C i.e., AML

14. A 40 years old man presented with painless hematuria. Bimanual examination revealed a ballotable mass over the right flank. Subsequently right nephrectomy was done and the mass was seen to be composed of cells with clear cytoplasm. Areas of hemorrhage and necrosis were frequent. Cytogenetic analysis would show:

A. Abnormality of chromosome 1

B. Abnormality of chromosome 3

C. Abnormality of chromosome 11

D. Abnormality of chromosome 17

Clinical presentation is suggestive of RCC.

The classical clinical evidence for diagnosis of renal cell carcinoma (RCC) is the triad of gross hematuria, flank pain and abdominal mass.

Clear cell type is the most common variety of RCC, histology of which shows clear cytoplasm (due to glycogen and lipid).

There is homozygous loss of VHL (Von-Hippel-Lindau) gene on chromosome 3 in clear cell type.

Answer: B i.e., Abnormality of chromosome 3

15. A lady with abdominal mass was investigated. On surgery, she was found to have bilateral ovarian masses with smooth surface. On microscopy, they revealed mucin secreting cells with signet ring shape. Most likely diagnosis:

A. Dysgerminoma

B. Krukenberg tumour

C. Mucinous adenocarcinoma of the ovaries

D. Dermoid cyst

Clinical presentation is suggestive of Krukenberg tumour.

Krukenberg tumours forms moderately large, rounded or kidney-shaped, firm, multinodular masses in both ovaries. Microscopically, it is characterised by the presence of mucin-filled signet ring cells which may lie singly or in clusters.

Answer: B i.e., Krukenberg tumour

16. A 45 years old patient presented with history of fever, night sweats and weight loss. On X-ray a mass in the apical lobe of lung is seen. On histopathology, it was found to have caseous necrosis. What is the likely underlying process involved?

A. Enzymatic degeneration

B. Hypersensitivity reaction with modified macrophages, lymphocytes and giant cells

C. Acute decrease in blood supply

D. Decreased supply of growth factors

Clinical presentation is suggestive of tuberculosis.

Some macrophages, unable to destroy tubercle bacilli, fuse together and form multinucleated giant cells.

Around the mass or cluster of epithelioid cells and a few giant cells, a zone of lymphocytes and plasma cells is formed which is further surrounded by fibroblasts.

The lesion at this stage is called hard tubercle due to the absence of central necrosis.

Within 10-14 days, the centre of the cellular mass begins to undergo caseation necrosis, characterised by cheesy appearance of high lipid content.

Answer: B i.e., Hypersensitivity reaction with modified macrophages, lymphocytes and giant cells

17. A patient presented with arthritis, hepatosplenomegaly, hyperpigmentation and raised serum ferritin levels. Most likely diagnosis:

A. Pseudogout

B. Hemochromatosis

C. Rheumatoid arthritis

D. Osteoarthritis

Clinical presentation is suggestive of hemochromatosis.

Hemochromatosis is characterised by a triad of features – micronodular pigment cirrhosis, diabetes mellitus and skin pigmentation.

On the basis of last two features, the disease also has come to be termed as 'bronze diabetes.'

In hemochromatosis, iron absorption goes up to 4 mg/ day or more (normally around 1 -1.5 mg/ day), as evidenced by elevated serum iron (normal about 125 mg/ dl) and increased serum transferrin saturation (normal 30%).

The serum ferritin is raised in iron overload states (normal 30-250 ng/ ml).

Answer: B i.e., Hemochromatosis

18. A 50 years old lady, who was obese and hypertensive, came with complaints of bleeding and abdominal pain, is diagnosed to have endometrial carcinoma. Which gene is mutated?

A. JAK2 B. PTEN

C. TET D. CFTR

Endometrial hyperplasia is a forerunner of endometrioid cancer is supported by mutated PTEN gene (located on chromosome 10) seen in 20% cases of complex hyperplasia, while it is seen in 40-80% cases of endometrioid carcinoma.

Other gene mutations in these cases are hMLH, K-RAS and beta-catenin oncogenes.

Answer: B i.e., PTEN

19. A female patient presented with diarrhea and abdominal pain. Small intestinal biopsy shows villous atrophy and crypt hyperplasia. Most likely diagnosis:

A. Celiac sprue

B. Tropical sprue

C. Whipple's disease

D. Hirschsprung's disease

Clinical presentation is suggestive of Celiac sprue.

Celiac sprue is the most important cause of malabsorption syndrome/ MAS occurring in temperate climates.

Clinical features of MAS include steatorrhoea (pale, bulky, foul-smelling stools), chronic diarrhoea, abdominal distension etc.

In Celiac sprue, there may be partial villous atrophy which is replacement of normal villous pattern by convolutions, or subtotal villous atrophy characterised by flat mucosal surface.

Epithelial cells show compensatory hyperplasia, suggesting a turnover of these cells.

Lamina propria shows increased number of plasma cells and lymphocytes.

Answer: A i.e., Celiac sprue

20. A 40 years old hypertensive male was admitted to the hospital with sudden onset of headache and altered sensorium. On examination, his blood pressure was observed to be 220/ 110 mm Hg and the patient died four hours later. Most likely pathological findings in his kidneys:

A. Small kidney with granular surface

B. Small kidney with petechial hemorrhages

C. Large kidney with waxy appearance

D. Large kidney with granular surface

Clinical presentation is suggestive of malignant nephrosclerosis.

Malignant nephrosclerosis is the form of renal disease that occurs in malignant or accelerated hypertension.

Blood pressure is around 200/ 140 mm Hg or higher. Headache, dizziness and impaired vision are commonly found. Azotaemia (high blood urea nitrogen/ BUN and serum creatinine) and uraemia develop soon if malignant hypertension is not treated aggressively.

In a case of malignant hypertension superimposed on pre-existing benign nephrosclerosis, grossly, the kidneys are small in size, shrunken and reduced in weight and have finely granular surface.

Answer: A i.e., Small kidney with granular surface

21. A 40 years male has hemoglobin 10 gm%, MCV: 65 fL, RDW: 16% and platelet count: 4.5 lakhs/ microL. What additional finding could be seen in such a patient?

A. Low serum transferrin

B. Raised iron binding capacity

C. Increased HbA_2

D. Increased serum copper

Clinical presentation is suggestive of iron deficiency anemia/ IDA.

Features of iron deficiency anemia include a fall in haemoglobin concentration, diminished MCV (normal is 77-93 fl), increased red cell distribution width (normal up to 14.5% in males), platelet count is usually normal (1.5-4 lakhs/ microL) but may be slightly to moderately elevated in patients who have recent bleeding and total iron binding capacity/ TIBC is high (normal 250-450 microgram/ dl).

Answer: B i.e., Raised iron binding capacity

22. Arterial biopsy of elderly male shows fragmentation of elastic lamina, lymphocyte infiltration and giant cells. Most likely diagnosis:

A. Temporal arteritis B. Takayasu disease

C. Polyarteritis nodosa D. Kawasaki disease

Clinical presentation is suggestive of temporal arteritis.

Histologically in temporal (giant cell) arteritis, the internal elastic lamina of artery is fragmented, non-specific inflammatory cell infiltrate consisting of neutrophils, lymphocytes and eosinophils is found throughout the arterial wall and giant cells of foreign body or Langhan's are found (in two-third of cases).

Answer: A i.e., Temporal arteritis

23. A 55 years old, chronic smoker underwent mass resection from bronchus. Most useful immuno-histochemical marker to make a proper diagnosis would be:

A. Cytokeratin

B. Vimentin

C. Desmin

D. Leucocyte common antigen

Clinical presentation is suggestive of bronchial carcinoma.

Immuno-stains for epithelial tumours (carcinomas) include pankeratin (fractions; high and low molecular weight keratins), epithelial membrane antigen (EMA), carcinoembryonic antigen (CEA) and neuron specific enolase (NSE).

Answer: A i.e., Cytokeratin

24. Kinky hair disease/ Menkes disease is a disorder where an affected child has peculiar white stubby hair, growth is retarded, brain degeneration is seen and dies by the age of 2 years. Mrs. 'X' is hesitant about having children because her 2 sisters had sons who died from Kinky hair disease. Her mother's brother also died of the same condition. Possible mode of inheritance:

A. X-linked recessive B. X-linked dominant

C. Autosomal recessive D. Autosomal dominant

Presentation is suggestive of X-linked recessive inheritance.

X-linked genetic disorders are conditions caused by a non-working gene on the X chromosome and manifest in males.

Females that have a non-working gene present on one of their X chromosomes are carriers for that disorder.

Carrier females usually do not display symptoms because females have two X chromosomes and only one carries the non-working gene.

However, since males have one X chromosome, inherited from the mother, if a male inherits an X chromosome harbouring a non-working gene, he will develop the disease (in question, it's mentioned that all the males died because of the disease).

Female carriers of an X-linked disorder have a 50% chance to have a son affected with the disease and a 50% chance of an unaffected son.

There is a 50% chance with each pregnancy to have asymptomatic "carrier" daughter like themselves, and a 50% chance to have a non-carrier daughter.

If a male with an X-linked disorder is able to reproduce, he will pass the non-working gene to all of his daughters who will be carriers.

A male cannot pass an X-linked gene to his sons because males always pass their Y chromosome instead of their X chromosome to male offspring.

Answer: A i.e., X-linked recessive

25. A 30 years old lady presents with an erythematous butterfly rash on her cheeks. Which antibody should be assayed initially for her suspected condition?

A. Anti-ds DNA

B. Anti-Ro

C. Anti-centromere

D. Anti-mitochondrial

Clinical presentation is suggestive of SLE.

Cutaneous lesions (erythematous eruptions) in systemic lupus erythematosus / SLE include butterfly area on nose and cheek. Antibodies to double-stranded DNA (anti-dsDNA) is the most specific antibodies for SLE, especially in high titres, and is present in 70% cases.

Answer: A i.e., Anti-Ds DNA

26. A child is born with a single functional copy of a tumour suppressor gene. At the age of 5 years, the remaining normal allele is lost through mutation. As a result, the ability to control the transition from G-1 to S phase of the cell cycle is lost. This mechanism can result in which neoplasm:

A. Retinoblastoma

B. Breast carcinoma

C. Adenocarcinoma of colon

D. Cerebral astrocytoma

Presentation is suggestive of retinoblastoma.

Retinoblastoma (RB) gene has been identified as 14 band on the long arm of chromosome 13 (13q 14) and is a 'cancer suppressor' or 'anti-oncogenic' gene.

Deletion or inactivation of both the normal alleles of this protective gene by two mutations (Knudson's two hit hypothesis, 1971) results in occurrence of retinoblastoma.

Answer: A i.e., Retinoblastoma

27. A patient presented with anemia. Peripheral smear of a patient showed feature of thalassemia. Family history is also positive. Investigation needed to establish the diagnosis would be:

A. ESR estimation

B. Blood spherocyte estimation

C. Bone marrow aspiration

D. Hemoglobin electrophoresis

Hemoglobin electrophoresis is confirmatory for the diagnosis of thalassemia and shows increased amounts of HbF, increased amount of HbA_2, and almost complete absence or presence of variable amounts of HbA.

The increased level of HbA_2 has not been found in any other hemoglobin abnormality except beta-thalassemia.

Answer: D i.e., Hemoglobin electrophoresis

28. A 45 years old female presented with painless supraclavicular lymphadenopathy. Biopsy revealed binucleated eosinophilic owl eye appearance with floating lymphocytes in empty space, which was CD15 and CD30 positive. Most likely diagnosis:

A. Lymphocyte predominant Hodgkin disease/HD

B. Nodular sclerosis Hodgkin disease/HD

C. Mixed cellularity Hodgkin disease/HD

D. Lymphocytic depleted Hodgkin disease/HD

Clinical presentation is suggestive of NS type of HD

Nodular sclerosis is the most frequent type of HD, seen more commonly in women than in men.

It is characterised by bands of collagen and lacunar type Reid Sternberg/ RS cells (there is distinctive pericellular halo; cells appear lacunar due to the shrinkage of cytoplasm in formalin-fixed tissue).

The nodules between the fibrous septa consist predominantly of lymphocytes and macrophages. RS cells are CD15+ and CD30+.

Answer: B i.e., Nodular sclerosis Hodgkin lymphoma

29. A renal biopsy from a 56 years old woman with progressive renal failure for the past 3 years shows glomerular and vascular deposition of pink amorphous material. It shows apple green birefringence under polarized light after Congo red staining. These deposits are positive for lambda light chains. Diagnosis:

A. Rheumatoid arthritis

B. Tuberculosis

C. Systemic lupus erythematosus

D. Multiple myeloma

Clinical presentation is suggestive of multiple myeloma (plasma cell dyscrasia).

In multiple myeloma, renal failure occurs in about 25% of patients, while renal pathology occurs in 50% of cases. Causes of renal failure in myeloma are hypercalcemia, glomerular deposits of amyloid, hyperuricemia and infiltration of the kidney by myeloma cells.

Amyloid deposition occurs primarily in the glomeruli.

Amyloid tissue when, stained with Congo red stain and viewed in polarized light, the amyloid tissue characteristically shows apple-green birefringence due to cross-beta-pleated sheet configuration of amyloid fibril.

Answer: D i.e., Multiple myeloma

30. A 20 years old female is diagnosed with granulosa cell tumor of the ovary. Which biomarker would be most useful for follow-up of patient?

A. CA 19-9

B. CA-50

C. Inhibin

D. Neuron specific enolase

Granulosa-cell tumors produce inhibin.

Since serum inhibin levels reflect the size of the tumor, measurements of inhibin can be used as a marker for primary as well as recurrent disease.

Answer: C i.e., Inhibin

31. A 50 years old male presented with skin rash and glomerulonephritis. What could be the next investigation:

A. c-ANCA B. HBsAg

C. Anti-HBs D. Anti-HCV

Clinical presentation is suggestive of Wegener's granulomatosis.

Focal or diffuse necrotizing glomerulonephritis is one of the essential features of clinicopathologic triad of Wegener's granulomatosis.

There can be involvement of skin as well.

The serum of these patient shows c-ANCA positivity.

Answer: A. i.e., c-ANCA

32. A 50 years old patient presented with a lesion in the midline involving the sacrum. It is found to be osteolytic. Most likely diagnosis:

A. Metastatic B. Chordoma

C. Osteosarcoma D. Chondrosarcoma

Clinical presentation is suggestive of chordoma.

Chordoma is a slow growing malignant tumour arising from remnants of notochord.

Notochord is the primitive axial skeleton which subsequently develops into spine.

Chordomas thus occur in the axial skeleton, particularly sacrum and coccyx (50%), spheno-occipital region (35%) and less often in the spine (15%).

Radiographically, the tumour usually appears as an osteolytic lesion.

Answer: B i.e., Chordoma

33. There are electron dense deposits in the region of hyalinosis and sclerosis with diffuse loss of foot process seen in electron microscopy suggest the diagnosis of:

A. Minimal change disease

B. Membranous glomerulonephritis

C. Membrano-proliferative glomerulonephritis

D. Focal segmental glomerulosclerosis

Presentation is suggestive of FSGS

Electron microscopy of focal segmental glomerulo-sclerosis (focal sclerosis/ focal hyalinosis) shows diffuse loss of foot processes as seen in minimal change disease, but, in addition, there are electron-dense deposits in the region of hyalinosis and sclerosis which are believed to be immune complexes.

Answer: D i.e., Focal segmental glomerulosclerosis

34. A 20 years old patient presented with a small firm nodular swelling in wrist joint for 2 years. Swelling was mobile only in one direction. Biopsy of nodule performed showed presence of spindle cells with Verocay bodies. Most likely diagnosis:

A. Lipoma B. Schwannoma

C. Neurilemmoma D. Neuroma

Clinical presentation is suggestive of Schwannoma.

Characteristic Verocay bodies may be seen in schwannoma.

These consist of parallel columns of elongated nuclei on either side of a homogenous acellular material.

Answer: C i.e., Schwannoma

Chapter 5

MICROBIOLOGY

RAPID REVISION NOTES

Basis for typing

Technique for typing	*Bacteria*
Voges-proskauer test & haemolytic activity	**Vibrio cholera**
Carbohydrate (Lancefield classification)	**Streptococci**
Bacteriophage	**Diphtheria**
Structural formula of H & O antigen	**Salmonella**
Antigenic nature of capsular polysaccharide (specific soluble substance)	**Pneumococci**
Lactose fermentation	**Enterobacteriaceae**
Reduction of nitrates & fermentation of glycerol	**Yersinia**
Sugar reaction	**Neisseria**

PROKARYOTE & EUKARYOTE

- In prokaryotes, nuclear membrane, nucleolus, cytoplasmic organelles & sterols are absent (present in eukaryotes)
- In prokaryotes, DNA, muramic acid (cell wall) & DAPA (in cell wall) is present
- Eukaryotic cell membrane/cell wall contains carbohydrate, lecithin & cholesterol (but muramic acid, DAPA & triglycerides are absent)
- Eukaryotes include fungi, protozoa, slime moulds

Bacteria

- Sterols absent
- They are prokaryotes; nucleus and cytoplasm not well developed
- Divide by binary fission
- Do not show true branching EXCEPT actinomycetes

STERILIZATION & DISINFECTION

- Ridel Walker test: Phenol is taken as the standard & measuring phenol coefficient of the disinfectant
- Savlon is a combination of: Cetrimide + Chlorhexidine (hibitane)
- All disposable items like endotracheal tube, breathing circuits, face masks, reservoir bags, adaptors, airways are best sterilized by: Ethylene oxide gas (all are heat sensitive)
- Laryngoscopic blades, Magill's forceps & stylets and spinal/ epidural sets for reuse: Autoclaved

- Removal of slough from wound: Eusol solution, hydrogen peroxide
- For cleaning infected wounds: Iodophors, acriflavine, savlon, hydrogen peroxide
- For hand wash: Chloroxylenol, chlorobutane, savlon, spirit, iodophors
- Bladder wash is done by: 0.1% potassium permanganate (Candy's lotion), Solution of acetic acid & silver nitrate

2% Glutaraldehyde

- 2nd Agent of choice for all disposable items like endotracheal tube, breathing circuits, face masks, reservoir bags, adaptors, airways (after ethylene oxide gas)
- Fibre optic scopes/ endoscopes

Resistance

- Prion & spores are most resistant to sterilization
- Coxiella burnetti is relatively heat resistant & survives in the holder method of pasteurization
- Clostridium botulinum spores are most heat resistant organism & requires 120 degree Celsius for 4 minutes or 100 degree Celsius for 330 minutes for their killing

Indicators

- Moist heat efficacy is shown by bacillus stearothermophilus
- Bacillus stearothermophilus is the most heat resistant organism known & because of this property, it is the biological indicator for testing autoclaves (plasma sterilization control), saturated steam & automatic steris sterilizer
- Bacillus subtilis is the biological indicator for testing dry heat sterilizers, ethylene oxide sterilizers
- Spores of non-toxicogenic strains of Clostridium tetani are used to test efficacy of dry heat (hot air oven, flaming, incineration)

IMMUNITY

- Prozone phenomenon is due to: Antibody excess
- Post-zone phenomenon is due to: Antigen excess
- Interaction absent in antigen-antibody complex formation: Covalent
- Anamnestic reaction: Seen in persons who have past typhoid/ who have had immunization against typhoid. Such patient develop antibodies when they contract fever/ malaria
- Proinflammatory cytokines that are present with dominance of cell mediated immunity: Interleukin-2, Interferon-gamma, Tumour necrosis factor-alpha, Interleukin-1
- Anti-inflammatory cytokines that are present with the dominance of humoral immunity: Interleukins - 4, 5, 6 & 10
- Most potent stimulator of Naïve T cells: Mature dendritic cells
- Enzyme responsible for respiratory burst of phagocytic cells: NADPH oxidase
- Thymectomy/removal of thymus, improves neuromuscular disorders like myasthenia gravis

Immunoglobulins

- Most prevalent: IgG
- First Ab (antibody) to be synthesized by fetus: IgM
- Fixes complement: IgM
- Produced after primary immunization: IgM
- Produced after re-immunization: IgG
- Related with secondary immune response: IgG
- Mediates reaginic hypersensitivity: IgE
- Major serum Ig: IgG
- Only Ig that crosses placenta: IgG
- Second most abundant Ig: IgA
- Ig that provides natural passive immunity to newborn: IgG
- Ig found in mucous secretions (saliva, tears, respiratory, genitourinary & gastro-intestinal tract and colostrum): IgA/Secretory antibody
- Prime mediator of the memory response: IgG
- Commercial gamma-globulin is almost: IgG

- Millionaire molecule: IgM, It is not transported across placenta, So presence in fetus/ newborn indicates congenital infection (syphilis, rubella etc.)
- Shortest t1/2: IgE
- Indicator of recent infection: IgM, As they are short lived
- Associated with atopy/ allergic conditions: IgE
- Ig seen in children with intestinal parasites: IgE
- Anaphylactic or skin sensitizing Ab: IgE
- IgE is found in: Respiratory & GI mucous secretions (like IgA)
- Enhance phagocytosis by opsonization: IgG, IgM
- IgG & IgM fix complement via classical pathway while IgA fixes complement via alternate pathway
- IgM is the most potent antibody in fixing complement

Hypersensitivity (HS) reactions

- Normally protective immune mechanism can sometimes cause detrimental reactions in the host

Type I

- Immediate HS
- IgE mediated release of histamine (mast cells & basophils)
- Prior sensitization to specific antigen (allergen) is there
- Anaphylaxis, atopy, eczema, urticaria, hay fever, asthma, theobald smith phenomenon, prausnitz kustner (PK) reaction, casoni's test
- Mast cells are important cells
- Histamine is an important mediator
- Eosinophils are important in late phase reaction of type I HS
- Most potent eosinophilic activating cytokine is IL-5
- IL-4 is important

Type II HS

- Antibody mediated
- Involves IgG or IgM, followed by complement fixation
- Transfusion reaction, erythroblastosis foetalis, glomerulonephritis, vascular rejection in organ grafts, myasthenia gravis, graves disease, autoimmune hemolytic anemia, Goodpasture's syndrome, rheumatic fever

Type III

- Antigen-antibody immune complex mediated, that deposits in post capillary venules of various tissues, followed by complement fixation
- Serum sickness, arthus reaction, schick test, polyarteritis nodosa, rheumatoid arthritis, SLE, hyperacute graft rejection, type II lepra reaction (ENL)

Type IV

- Initiated by activated T-lymphocytes
- T helper cells produces IL-2
- Delayed type HS (mediated by CD4-T cells)
- T-cell mediated cytotoxicity (mediated by CD8-T cells)
- Tuberculin test, lepromin test, sarcoidosis, TB, contact dermatitis, granulomatous inflammation, type I lepra reaction, graft rejection

Immunodeficiencies

- Humoral immunodeficiencies
  - o Common variable immunodeficiency: Late onset hypogammaglobulinemia, Infection with Giardia
- Cellular immunodeficiencies
  - o DiGeorge's syndrome: Thymus hypoplasia, Fallot's tetralogy
- Combined immunodeficiencies
  - o Ataxia telangiectasia
  - o Wiskott-Aldrich syndrome: X-linked Thrombocytopenia, Decreased cell mediated immunity
- Subacute chronic immunodeficiency: Adenosine deaminase deficiency
- Phagocytosis defects
  - o Chediak-Higashi syndrome: Decreased pigments, Photophobia, Nystagmus
  - o Lazy leucocyte syndrome: Peripheral neutropenia, Decreased phagocytosis

BACTERIOLOGY

- Peptidoglycan is thick in: Gram positive cells (thin in gram negative)
- Teichoic acid is present in: Gram positive cells (absent in gram negative)
- All cocci are gram positive except Neisseria & Moraxella
- Gram positive bacteria with spore formation are: Anthrax & Clostridia
- Capsulated organisms: Pneumococcus, Anthrax bacilli, Meningococci, V. parahemolyticus
- Flagella are detected by: Dark ground microscopy
- Capsules are detected by: Quellung reaction/ Indian ink

Bacterial genetics

- Multiple drug resistance is by the process of: Conjugation (horizontal gene transfer)
- Process of introduction of foreign gene into a host cell's genome is possible by:
- Transduction (it is a process by which DNA is transferred from one bacterium to another bacterium by a virus)
- Transposons: Jumping genes; Mobile genetic elements that can move themselves from one DNA to other

Exotoxin & Endotoxin

- Exotoxins are produced mostly by gram positive and some gram negative bacteria (Shiga's dysentery bacillus, vibrio ETEC, pseudomonas)
- Endotoxin is produced only by gram negative bacteria
- Mostly secreted by gram positive bacteria: Exotoxin; Endotoxin is secreted by gram negative bacteria
- Consist of lipopolysaccharides: Endotoxin; Exotoxin consist of polypeptides
- Highly toxic: Exotoxin; Endotoxin have low toxicity
- Heat stable: Endotoxin; Exotoxin is heat sensitive
- Highly antigenic: Exotoxin; Endotoxin is poorly antigenic
- Toxoids are used as vaccines: Exotoxin; No toxoids, so no vaccines from endotoxin
- Secreted by cell: Exotoxin; Endotoxin is not secreted from cell

Culture media & bacteria

- Loeffler's serum slope: Corynebacterium diphtheria
- Tellurite media: Corynebacterium diphtheriae
- Korthof media: Leptospira
- Skirrows media: Campylobacter jejuni
- Thayer martin media: N. gonorrhea
- Lowenstein jenson media: Mycobacterium TB
- Dorset egg medium: Mycobacterium
- BYCE medium: Legionella
- Bordet Gengou medium: B. pertussis

Colony appearances & bacteria

- Medusa head colonies: B. anthracis
- Frosted glass colonies: B. anthracis
- Swimming growth (fishy/ seminal smell): Proteus
- Fried egg colonies: Mycoplasma
- Draughtsman (concentric rings) colonies: Pneumococci
- Cigar bundle (globi) appearance: M. leprae
- Stalactite growth: Yersinia pestis

Important growth factors & bacteria:

- Tryptophan: Salmonella typhi
- Niacin: Mycobacterium TB, M. microti
- Factor V (NAD) & X (Hemin): H. Influenzae
- Factor X: H. ducreyi
- Factor V: H. parainfluenzae
- Cholesterol: Mycoplasma

AFB positive/ Positive Ziehl-neelsen staining:

- Mycobacteria
- Nocardia
- Bacterial spores

Urease positive bacteria

- Proteus
- H. pylori
- Klebsiella

Non-motile, non-sporing, non-capsulated bacteria

- Mycobacterium TB
- Actinomycetes
- C. diphtheriae

Virulence factors & bacteria

- Coagulase: Staph. aureus
- M-protein: Streptococci
- Capsular polysaccharide: Pneumococci
- Cord factor: Mycobacterium TB
- Lecithinase: Cl. welchii

Classification basis & bacteria

- Carbohydrate-C: Streptococci
- Mannitol fermentation: Shigella
- O & H antigens: Salmonella

Bacteria & their other names

- Pseudomonas pseudomallei: Whitmore bacillus
- Mycoplasma: Eaton agent
- Mycobacterium paratuberculosis: Johne's bacillus
- Mycobacterium intercellulare: Battey's bacillus
- Klebsiella pneumoniae: Friedlander's bacillus
- Haemophilus aegyptius: Koch weeks bacillus
- Corynebacterium pseudotuberculosis: Nocard bacillus

Bacteria & associated keywords

- Chinese letter arrangement: C. diphtheriae
- Hemophilus ducreyi: School of fish
- Mycoplasma: Fried egg colony
- Pneumococcus: Draughtsman colony
- Proteus: Swarming motility
- Satellitism: H. influenza
- Meta-chromatic staining: Corynebacterium
- Lancet shaped diplococci: Pneumococci
- Bean shaped diplococci: Neisseria
- Bipolar staining: Yersinia

Bacteria & associated test/reactions

- Anthrax/plague: Ascoli's thermoprecipitation test
- Rickettasiae: Xeno-diagnosis
- Clostridia: Naegler's reaction (due to lecithinase)
- V. cholerae: Cholera red reaction, Indole formation, Nitrates to nitrites conversion, String test
- Pseudomonas mallei: Strauss reaction
- Rickettsia mooseri: Neil Mooser reaction (Tunica reaction)
- Elek's test: C. diphtheriae
- Schick's test: C. diphtheriae
- Streptococci/ pneumococci: Dick test
- B. anthrax: Mc-fadyean's reaction
- Brucellosis: Milk ring test; Rose bengal card test
- Tuberculosis: Von- pirquet test; Koch's phenomenon

Bacteria & motility

- V. cholerae: Darting motility
- Proteus (gram negative): Swarming motility; clostridia tetani (gram positive) also shows swarming motility
- Fusobacterium: Spinning motility
- Listeria: Tumbling motility
- Spirocheates: Cork screw

Condition & causative bacteria

- Malignant pustule (cutaneous anthrax): Bacillus anthrax
- Undulant/ Malta/ Mediterranean fever: Brucella melitensis
- Weil's disease: Leptospira icterohemorrhagica
- Lyme's disease: Borrelia burgdorferi
- Epidemic relapsing fever: Borrelia recurrentis
- Trench fever: Bartonella henselae
- Pontiac fever: Legionella pneumophilia

Genetics

- **Conjugation:** Transfer of genetic elements after actual physical contact between a male donor bacterium and female recipient

- **Transposons:** Jumping genes consisting of inverted repeat sequences, responsible for transferable drug resistance
- **Transformation:** Transfer of genetic information through the agency of free DNA
- **Transduction:** Transfer of a portion of DNA from one bacterium to another through the agency of a bacteriophage

Some important terms

- **Quellung reaction:** When a suspension of a capsulated bacterium is mixed with its specific anticapsular serum, and examined under microscope, capsule becomes very prominent and appears swollen
- Chemical present in gram-positive bacterial wall but absent in gram-negative bacteria is: **Teichoic acid**

Mechanism of action of toxins

- ADP ribosylation of G-protein: Pertussis toxin
- Activation of cyclic amp: LT (ETEC), cholera toxin
- Activation of cGMP: Heat stable E. coli toxin
- Irreversible protein synthesis inhibition: Shiga toxin (shigella dysenteriae-1), EHEC, diphtheria toxin, exotoxin A (pseudomonas aeruginosa)

Arrangement of bacteria

Features	*Bacteria*
Chains	Streptococci
Chains (bamboo stick appearance)	Anthrax
Bunches	Staphylococci
Pairs	Pneumococci, enterococci
Pairs, mainly intracellular	Neisseria
Cuneiform or Chinese letter pattern	Diphtheria
Pairs at angle (oval cells) or short chains	Enterococci
Single or chains or bundles	Clostridium welchii
Diplococcus (pairs)	Morax-axenfeld bacillus
In globi, cigar bundle appearance	Leprosy bacilli

STAPHYLOCCCUS AURUES

- Factor responsible for Staph. aureus pathogenicity: Coagulase
- Food poisoning results due to: Preformed endotoxin
- IP of Staphy. aureus food poisoning: Less than 6 hours
- Staphy. aureus food poisoning is seen after ingestion of: Dairy products
- Conditions caused by Staph. aureus: Furuncle, Carbuncle, Sycosis barbae, Tropical polymyositis etc.

Staphylococcus

- Spherical cocci**,** Grape like clusters, Gram-positive
- Non-motile, non-sporing, Aerobes and facultative anaerobes
- Produce golden yellow pigment on nutrient agar slope-oil paint appearance
- Ferment sugar, producing acid but no gas
- On blood agar- beta hemolysis
- Mac Conkey's agar- pink colonies
- Mannitol is fermented anaerobically by S. aureus but NOT by other species
- Catalase positive S. aureus gives prompt phosphatase
- S. epidermidis is the most common cause of infection of central nervous system shunts

STREPTOCOCCI

- Factor responsible for pathogenicity of streptococci: M protein
- Lancefield classification is based on: C-carbohydrate
- Special feature of **streptococcus agalactiae**: Group B streptococci, Gram positive, Bacitracin resistant, CAMP
  test positive
- MC cause of acute meningitis in neonates: Group B streptococci (also E. coli); (H. influenza in childrens)

Streptococcus pyogenes

- Nonmotile, Nonsporing, Gram-positive

- Aerobes and facultative anaerobes
- Spherical, arranged in chains
- Catalase negative
- Do not ferment inulin
- Ferment sugar producing acid but no gas
- Does not grow on simple media, requires blood or serum, sugars
- Virulent forms give matt/granular colonies, while avirulent give glossy colonies
- Blood agar - Circular, small colonies with area of hemolysis around them

PNEUMOCOCCUS

- Most virulent type of pneumococcus: Type C
- Appearance of pneumococcal colonies: Draughtsman colonies
- Vaccine against pneumococcus is made from: Capsule
- Virulence of streptococcus is due to: Capsule
- Gross appearance of pneumococcus: Lanceolate, Flame shaped diplococcus
- Special feature: Gram positive, Quellung reaction seen

Pneumococcus

- Aerobes and facultative anaerobes
- Small, Lanceolate, Diplococci
- Capsulated, Gram-positive
- Blood agar - Under aerobic conditions, small, dome shaped, shiny colonies with greenish discoloration (alpha hemolysis), with central umbonation, giving carom coin or draughtsman appearance
- Under anaerobic conditions – they show beta hemolysis
- Catalase and oxidase negative, Sensitive to optochin
- Ferment inulin, bile soluble

NEISSERIA GONOCOCCUS

- Reactions shown by gonococcus: Ferments glucose, Don't ferment maltose
- Condition caused: Urethritis, Meningitis, Arthritis, Endocarditis
- Special feature of gonococcus: Intracytoplasmic, Gram negative

Other Neisseria

- Source of infection of N. meningitis: Carriers

Gonococcus

- Kidney shaped, Aerobic and facultatively anaerobic
- N. gonorrhea ferments glucose, but not maltose
- N. meningitides ferments both

Neisseria meningitides

- Gram-negative, aerobic, nonsporing, non-motile
- Strict aerobes
- Oxidase positive
- Weak hemolysis on based agar
- Exacting growth requirements
- Solid media - round, bluish grey smooth, glistening, butyrous

CORYNEBACTERIUM DIPHTHERIAE

- Toxin of C. diphtheriae is: Phage mediated
- Culture media for C. diphtheriae: Loeffler's serum slope, Tellurite media
- Special features of C. diphtheriae: Babes Ernest granules/ Volutin granules/ Metachromatic granules
- Daisy head colony is associated with: C. diptheriae gravis

Other corynebacterium

- Erythrasma is caused by: C. minutissimum
- Nocardia bacillus is also known as: C. pseudo tuberculosis
- C. parvum is used as an: Immunomodulator

Corynebacterium diphtheriae/ Klebs Loeffler bacillus

- Slender rod, clubbing at end, pleomorphic, nonsporing, non-motile, non-capsulated, gram-positive

- Bacilli are arranged in Chinese letter or cuneiform pattern
- Tellurite blood agar is the selective medium (Grey/ black)

B. ANTHRAX

- Colony characteristic for B. anthracis: Medusa head, Frosted glass appearance, String of pearl appearance
- Pulmonary anthrax is also known as: Wool sorters disease
- Special feature: Zoonosis, McFadyen's reaction positive, Painless malignant pustule (charbon)

Bacillus anthracis

- Aerobic and facultatively anaerobic
- Sporing
- Large capsulated bacilli (Polypeptide capsule)
- Arranged in long chains, giving bamboo stick appearance
- Gelatin swab culture - Inverted fir tree appearance
- String of pearls reaction - When grown solid media containing penicillin, cells become large spherical and in chains
- Grows on ordinary media
- Agar - Round, grayish colonies with frosted glass appearance which under low power resembles locks of matted hair, called medusa head appearance
- McFadyen's reaction- when blood films containing anthrax bacilli are stained with polychrome - Methylene blue, and examined under microscope, capsule is detected as amorphous purplish material around the bacilli

Bacteria & tests

Bacteria/ conditions	*Tests/ reactions*
Anthrax, plague	Ascoli's thermoprecipitation test
Rickettsiae	Xenodiagnosis
Clostridia	Naegler's reaction
Clostridium tetani	Green fluorescence on media with neutral red
Vibrio cholerae	Cholera red reaction, indole formation and nitrates to nitrite conversion
Pseudomonas mallei	Strauss reaction
Rickettsia mooseri	Neil Mooser reaction
H. influenza	Satellitism
Corynebacterium diptheriae	Elek's test, schick's test
Streptococcus	Dick test, schultz-charlton reaction
Bacillus anthracis	McFadyean reaction
Clostridium welchii	Stormy reaction in culture
Brucellosis	Milk ring test
Mycobacterium tuberculosis	Von-pirquet test, koch's phenomenon
Pneumococci	Francis test
Vibrio cholera	String test
Corynebacterium diphtheria	Metachromatic staining

CLOSTRIDIA

- Clostridium difficile (normal gut commensal) causes: Pseudomembranous colitis (particularly after antibiotic therapy)
- Clostridium perfringens causes: Gas gangrene/ myonecrosis, Gastroenteritis
- Clostridium tetani causes: Tetanus
- Arrangement of spores of C. tetani: Drumstick appearance; Spherical & terminal spores
- Motility of C. tetani: Motile with swarming tendency
- Effect of toxin of Clostridium botulinum: Blocks release of acetylcholine at neuro-muscular junction; CNS is NOT affected
- Feature of botulinsm: Symmetric descending paralysis

E. COLI

- MC cause for traveler's diarrhea: ETEC/ Enterogenic E. coli
- Most of the cases of hemolytic uremic syndrome (HUS) are caused by: EHEC/ Enterohemorrhagic E. coli

- Important cause of infant diarrhea: EPEC/ Enteropathogenic E. coli
- Only EPEC affects paediatric population, rest all strains can affect any age group
- Sereny test is positive in: EIEC/ Enteroinvasive E. coli
- Special feature of EIEC: Non-motile, Non-lactose fermenting

E. coli

- Gram-negative, straight rod, motile by peritrichous flagella
- Aerobe and facultatively anaerobe
- Hemolytic on blood agar
- MacConkey's medium - Bright pink colonies, due to lactose fermentation

PROTEUS

- Odour associated with proteus: Seminal/ fishy
- Special feature of proteus: Dienes phenomenon; Urease positive
- Effect of urease, produced by proteus: Urease hydrolyzes urea to ammonia, which results in alkalinization of urine;
- Hence high prevalence of UTI in long-term catheterized individuals

Proteus mirabilis

- Gram-negative, non-capsulated, pleomorphic, motile rod
- Cultures give a fishy or seminal odour
- Swarming growth
- Lactose fermenters
- Produces urease, rapidly hydrolyses urea to ammonia and carbon dioxide
- MacConkey's medium - Colorless colonies
- Weil –Felix reaction - Heterophilic agglutination due to the sharing of carbohydrates hapten by proteus and rickettsiae

SHIGELLA

- Division of shigella is done on the basis of: Mannitol fermentation
- Most virulent type is: S. dysenteriae
- Best test for S. dysenteriae: Stool culture
- Special feature: Non-motile; Lactose non-fermenters

Shigella

- Gram-negative, rods, non-motile, nonsporing, non-capsulated
- Aerobes and facultative anaerobes
- Grow on ordinary media
- Deoxycholate citrate agar/ DCA - Selective medium
- MacConkey's - Colorless colonies, EXCEPT Shigella sonnei which is late lactose fermenter

SALMONELLA

- Factor needed for growth: Tryptophan
- Virulence factor: O antigen; Used for classification
- Most immunogenic antigen: H. antigen
- Carriers are detected by: Vi agglutination; Vi antigen is not seen in normal population
- Special feature: Diazo reaction

Salmonella

- Gram-negative, motile with peritrichous flagella
- Aerobic and facultatively anaerobic
- Ferment sugars producing acid and gas, EXCEPT Salmonella typhi which is anerogenic
- MacConkey's agar and Deoxycholate citrate - colonies are colorless due to absence of lactose fermentation
- Wilson and Blair medium – jet black colonies, due to H_2S production
- Selenite F broth and tetrathionate broth are enrichment media

VIBRIO CHOLERAE

- Most cases of cholera are: Subclinical
- Isolation of V. cholerae was done by: Koch
- Motility of V. cholerae: Darting motility
- Action of toxin of V. cholerae is mediated by: cAMP
- Reservoir of V. cholerae: Humans
- V. cholerae survives: Boiling for 30 seconds, Cold temperature (ice for 4-6 weeks)
- Special features: Non-halophilic, Ferments glucose, Transported in alkaline medium

Vibrio cholera

- Comma shaped, actively motile by polar flagella, characteristic vibratory/ darting motility, like a swarm of gnats
- Venkatraman – Ramakrishnan medium and Cary Blair medium - Holding of transport medium
- Alkaline peptone water and Monsur's taurocholate tellurite peptone water are transport and enrichment medium
- TCBS is the preferred plating medium (yellowish green)

PSEUDOMONAS

- Effect of exotoxin A produced: Inhibition of protein synthesis
- Pyoverdin is: One of the pigment produced by P. aeruginosa
- Anti-pseudomonal drug: Piperacillin
- Diseases caused by P. aeruginosa: Shock with bullous lesions, Serious infections in burn patients etc.
- Multi-drug resistance is due to: Biofilm production (in cornea)

Other pseudomonas

- Melioidosis is caused by: P. pseudomallei

Pseudomonas aeruginosa

- Aerobic, nonsporing, gram-negative, motile by polar flagella
- Grows on simple media-colonies give musty or earthy smell
- Produces pigments: Pyocyanin - bluish green; Fluorescein/ pyoverdin - greenish yellow; Pyorubin - red, Pyomelanin –brown
- MacConkey's and DCA - Colorless colonies

YERSINIA PESTIS

- Special feature: Gram negative, Coccobacillus
- Pattern of growth: Stalactite growth
- Condition associated with Y. pestis: Plague
- MC form of plague: Bubonic plague
- DOC for prophylaxis: Tetracycline
- DOC for plague: Streptomycin

Yersinia pestis

- Reservoir of plague
- Gives safety pin appearance (Bipolar staining) [Similar safety pin appearance in Burkholderia pseudomallei]
- Ghee broth culture - Stalactite growth

HEMOPHILUS

- Factors required for growth: Factor V & X
- Appearance on culture: School of fish
- Special feature: Satellitism

Haemophilus influenzae/Pfeiffer bacillus

- Gram-negative, capsulated
- Fastidious growth requirements, require accessory growth factors, named X and V

Haemophilus ducreyi

- Shows bipolar staining
- Bacilli are arranged in whorls or parallel chains, giving school of fish or rail road track appearance

BORDETELLA

- Media used: Bordet gengou medium
- Incubation period of whooping cough: 1-2 weeks
- Culture characteristic: Thumb printing appearance

Bordetella pertussis/ Bordet Gengou bacillus

- Gram-negative, strict aerobes, produce toxins
- Capsulated
- Bordet Gengou glycerin-potato-blood agar: Selective medium
- Dome shaped, smooth, opaque, grayish- white colonies, bisected pearls or mercury drops appearance
- In culture films, thumb print appearance
- Colonies are surrounded by a hazy zone of hemolysis; confluent growth gives aluminum paint appearance

BRUCELLA

- Brucella causes: Malta fever/Undulant fever/ Mediterranean fever
- Special feature: NO person to person transmission, Zoonosis
- Tests for brucella: Rose bengal card test, Milk ring test

Brucella

- Gram-negative, strict aerobic
- Catalase, oxidase and urease positive
- Antigenic cross reactions between Brucella and Vibrio cholera
- Brucellosis is also known as Mediterranean fever, Malta fever, undulant fever
- Transmitted through unpasteurised milk

MYCOBACTERIUM TB

- M. bacilli was discovered by: Robert Koch
- Factor responsible for acid fastness Mycolic acid & cell wall
- Stain used for rapid diagnosis of M. bacilli: Auramine Rhodamine stain
- Factor which promotes virulence: Cord factor
- Special feature: Production of niacin

Mycobacterium tuberculosis

- Acid fast (Due to presence of mycolic acid)
- Generation time is 14-15 hours
- Lowenstein Jensen medium is the most widely used solid medium

Mantoux test

- 0.5 ml of PPD is injected intradermally, on the flexor aspect of forearm
- Result is read after 72 hours
- Positive tuberculin test indicates hypersensitivity to tuberculin protein due to infection with tubercle bacillus or BCG immunization
- Induration > 10 mm is Positive
- 5 mm or less is Negative

MYCOBACTERIUM LEPRAE

- Generation time of M. leprae: 12 days
- M. leprae can be grown in: Foot pad of mice
- M. leprae spreads by: Skin to skin contact
- Lepra cells are: Histiocytes

Other mycobacterium

- Buruli ulcer is caused by: M. ulcerans
- Swimming pool granuloma/ fish tank granuloma is caused by: M. marinum/ M. balanei

Mycobacterium leprae

- Gram-positive and acid fast
- **Bacteriological index:** Number of bacilli in tissues
- **Morphological index:** Live bacilli appear solid and uniformly stained, whereas dead bacilli appear fragmented (The percentage of uniformly stained bacilli is called morphological index)
- They agglomerate, as globi (giving a cigar bundle appearance)
- They are not cultivable (Can be grown in footpads of mice kept at 200 and in nine banded armadillo

TREPONEMA PALLIDUM

- Minimum organism needed for detection in dark ground microscopy: 10^4 organisms

- Specific test for T. pallidum: FTA-ABS
- VDRL is a type of: Slide flocculation test
- VDRL is positive in: Secondary syphilis
- Special feature: Levaditi stain

Treponema pallidum

- Thin, spiral
- It can be stained with silver impregnation method
- It can be seen in low microscope by negative staining with India ink.
- Morphology and motility can be seen under dark ground or phase contrast microscope

BORELLIA

- Lyme's disease/ erythema migrans is caused by: B. burgdorferi
- Relapsing fever is caused by: B. recurrentis

LEPTOSPIRA

- Leptospirosis is transmitted by: Rat urine
- Leptospirosis is associated with: Rat, Ricefields, Rain
- Weil's disease is caused by: L. icterio-hemorrhagica

Leptospira

- Generation time is 12-16 hours
- Actively motile
- Coiled appearance seen under dark ground microscopy
- Their ends are hooked, resembling umbrella handles

MYCOPLASMA

- Also known as Eaton agent
- Smallest free living organisms
- Prokaryotes, that are bounded by cell membrane
- As they lack cell wall, they show cellular pleomorphism & resistance to cell wall active antimicrobial agents (penicillins & cephalosporins)
- Appearance of colonies: Fried eggs colonies
- MC forms of mycoplasma: L forms

Mycoplasma

- Gram-negative
- Aerobic and facultatively anaerobic
- Require cholesterol for growth
- Devoid of cell wall, pleomorphic
- Show true branching
- Biphasic colonies, with a fried egg appearance
- Hemolytic

ACTINOMYCETES

- Gram positive
- Growth usually results in formation of clumps (grains/ sulfur granules)

LISTERIA MONOCYTOGENES

- Gram positive coccobacillus (in short chains)
- Survives & multiplies in phagocytes
- Test used: Anton's test

H. PYLORI

- Motility of H. pylori is due to: Spiral shape, Flagellae
- Route of transmission of H. pylori: Man to man, Faeco-orally, Oro-gastric route
- Gram negative
- Spiral, flagellate bacillus
- Produces Urease
- Urease protects it from acid by catalyzing conversion of urea to ammonia (buffer)

ANAEROBIC INFECTION

- Non-sporing anaerobic bacteria: Bacteroides fragilis, Fusobacterium, Peptostreptococcus, Actinomyces israelii

RICKETTSIAL DISEASE

- Rickettsial pox is caused by: R. akari

- Q fever is caused by: Coxiella burnetti
- Weil-Felix reaction: Tube agglutination test in which sera are tested for agglutinins to the O antigen of proteus vulgaris strains OX-19 & OX-2 and proteus mirabilis (OX-K)

Rickettsiae

- They are obligate intracellular parasites
- Transmitted by arthropod vectors

CHLAMYDIAE

- Detected by: Nucleic acid amplification test (NAAT)
- Obligate intracellular bacteria
- Gram negative
- Elementary body is metabolically inert (extracellular)
- Inclusion bodies in psittacosis: Levinthal Cole-Lillie bodies
- Inclusion bodies in conjunctivitis: Halber-staedter Prowazekii/ HP bodies

Chlamydiae

- Called energy parasites
- They are obligate intracellular parasites.
- Occur in two forms:
  - o Reticulate body/initial body: Intracellular, growing and replicative form
  - o Elementary body: Extracellular, infective form

VIROLOGY

- Virions: Extracellular infectious particles
- Capsid: Protein coat, surrounding nucleic acids
- Prions: Protein molecules, that can spread from cell to cell & effect changes in the structure of their normal counterparts (cellular proteins)
- E.g. Creutzfeldt-Jakob disease, Kuru, Gerstmann-Straussler disease, Mad cow disease, Fatal familial insomnia
- Structures absent in virus: Ribosomes, Mitochondria, Nucleus (but DNA/ RNA is present), Motility
- Usually DNA viruses are double stranded (exception is parvovirus which is single stranded DNA) & RNA viruses are single stranded (exception is rovers which is double stranded RNA)
- Smallest virus/ Virus with smallest genome: Parvo virus
- Virus with segmented RNA: Influenza virus
- Largest virus: Pox virus
- Largest RNA virus: Rhabdovirus
- Smallest RNA virus: Picorna virus

Inclusion bodies

- Molluscum bodies: Molluscum contagiosum
- Torres bodies/Councilman bodies: Yellow fever
- Warthin- Finkeldey cells: Measles
- Negri bodies: Rabies
- Guarneri bodies: Vaccinia
- Bollinger bodies: Fowl pox
- Cowdry A inclusion bodies (Lipschultz): Herpes, yellow fever
- Cowdry B inclusion bodies: Adenovirus, polio virus

Infectious mononucleosis

- Kissing disease is another name for infectious mononucleosis, as kissing is the predominant mode of transport.
- Paul - Bunnell test is used for diagnosing infectious mononucleosis

HERPES VIRUS

- Latent infection is characteristic of herpes group
- Viruses belonging to herpes group: HSV, Varicella zoster, EBV, CMV etc.
- HSV (herpes simplex virus) virus is a: Double stranded DNA virus
- MC cause of sporadic viral encephalitis: HSV
- Varicella zoster virus remains dormant in: Trigeminal (sensory) ganglion
- Infectivity of herpes zoster lasts: 6 days after the onset of rash

- Diseases caused by EBV: Oral hairy leukoplakia, Burkitt's lymphoma, Anaplastic nasopharyngeal carcinoma, T-cell lymphoma, Thymoma
- HHV-8 causes: Kaposi sarcoma
- HHV-6 causes: Roseola infantum & multiple sclerosis
- HHV-2 causes: Genital lesions
- More than 50% of renal transplants with fever, 1-4 months after transplantation have: CMV infection

Conditions & inclusion bodies

Condition	*'Bodies' seen*
Trachoma	Halberstaedter-prowazekii bodies
Buboes from LGV	Miyagawa's granulo-corpuscles
LGV	Lygranum antigen
Corynebacterium diphtheria	Babes-ernest granule
Trypanosomiasis	Morula cells with IgM deposits
Yellow fever	Councilman bodies and Torres bodies
Granuloma inguinale	Donovan bodies
Kala-azar	Leishmania Donovan bodies
Psittacosis	Levinthal-cole-lillie bodies
Measles	Warthin Finkeldey giant cells
Parkinsonism	Lewis bodies
Multiple bodies	Russel's bodies
Cytomegalovirus, herpes	Owl-eye inclusion bodies

ADENOVIRUS

- Adenovirus causes: Haemorrhagic cystitis, Epidemic keratoconjunctivitis

PICORNAVIRUS

- Picornavirus includes: Enterovirus, Rhinovirus
- Enterovirus-70 causes: Acute hemorrhagic conjunctivitis, Acute epidemic keratoconjunctivitis

POLIOVIRUS

- MC manifestation of polio is: Subclinical infection (90%)
- Inapparent infections are MC transmitted by: Feco-oral route
- Polio virus spreads by: Hematogenous route, Neural route
- Death in polio is mostly due to: Respiratory paralysis
- Most outbreaks are due to: Type 1 (most common)
- Most effective antigen (immunogenic): type 2
- Vaccine associated paralytic poliomyelitis is caused by: Type 3

INFLUENZA VIRUS

- Influenza virus type B causes: Reyes syndrome
- Feature of haemagglutinin & neuraminidase: Strain specific
- Antigenic variation seen with influenza virus: Antigenic drift & shift
- Antigenic drift (minor change): Small mutations in H & N
- Antigenic shift (major change)
- Bird flu virus is also known as: Avian flu influenza virus/ H5N1
- Swine flu (2009 outbreak) was due to: H1N1
- In influenza, virus antigen variation occurs mainly in: Type A
- Antigenic variation does not occur in: Type C (antigenically stable)

MEASLES VIRUS

- Measles virus belongs to: Paramyxovirus
- Infectivity period of measles: 4 days before rash, 5 days after rash appearance
- Conditions associated with measles virus: Hecht's pneumonia/ Primary giant cell pneumonia
- A rare, late complication: SSPE (subacute sclerosing panencephalitis)

MUMPS VIRUS

- MC complication of mumps in post-pubertal males: Orchitis
- Parotitis can be preceded by: Meningoencephalitis

- Special feature of mumps: One attacks gives lifelong immunity

RABIES VIRUS

- Rabies virus is: Enveloped virus with, ssRNA
- Rabies virus is inactivated by: Phenol, UV radiation, Beta propio lactone
- Negri bodies are pathognomonic of: Rabies encephalitis, They are present inside nerve cells
- Stains used for ante-mortem diagnosis: Fluorescent diagnosis

HEPATITIS VIRUS

- Special feature of hepatitis A virus (previously known as enterovirus 72): No chronic course
- Hepatitis A virus is inactivated by: Boiling, Formalin, UV radiation
- Hepatitis B virus contains: DNA dependent DNA polymerase, RNA dependent reverse transcriptase
- Reverse transcriptase is coded by: P gene
- Dane particle is: HBV
- HBV strain in India: Ayw, Adr
- Maximum perinatal transmission risk: HBV
- Serological marker of acute hepatitis B infection: HBsAg, Core antibody
- Epidemiological marker of Hepatitis B infection: Core antibody
- REMEMBER: HBcAg is NOT demonstrable in blood but, core antibody, anti-HBe appear in serum a week or 2 after appearance of HBsAg
- Indicator of high infectivity of hepatitis B infection: HBeAg, (indicator of intrahepatic viral replication)
- Feature of hepatitis B vaccine: Cell fraction derived
- Feature of hepatitis C virus: Linear, Single-stranded, Positive sense, Enveloped, RNA virus
- HCV belongs to: Flaviviridae
- MC cause of post-transfusion hepatitis: HCV
- HCV also causes: Chronic hepatitis
- HEV is transmitted: Enterically
- Highest mortality in pregnancy with hepatitis is with: HEV
- REMEMBER: Fulminant hepatic failure in pregnancy can also occur with HCV
- In pregnancy, HEV is also associated with: Hepatic encephalopathy
- Hepatitis viruses spreading by feco-oral route are: HAV, HEV

HIV

- HIV is: Single stranded, Positive sense, RNA virus
- HIV is found in: Blood, Semen, Saliva
- HIV consists of: 2 copies of ssRNA, RNA dependent DNA polymerase (reverse transcriptase) [compare with HBV], Integrase, Protease
- Seroconversion takes: 4 weeks
- MC mode of transmission: Hetero-sexual
- In hetero-sexual transmission: Male to female is commoner (as compared to female to male)
- Chances of transmission with accidental needle prick: 0.3%
- Retroviral sequence in host cell: RNA-DNA-RNA
- p24 antigen (used for early diagnosis) disappears after: 6-8 weeks of HIV infection
- CD4: CD8 ratio is: Reversed in HIV infection
- Reservoir of HIV infection: Macrophages
- Window period: Time period between, infection to appearance of antibodies in serum
- During window period, ELISA & western blot are: Negative
- MC cause of diarrhea in AIDS: Cryptosporidiosis (NOT cryptococcus)
- MC cause of meningitis in AIDS: Cryptococcus
- MC cause of oral ulcer in AIDS: Candida
- MC cause of TB in AIDS in tropical countries: Mycobacterium TB
- MC opportunistic infection in AIDS in India is: TB

ROTAVIRUS

- Feature of Rotavirus: DsRNA virus, Non-cultivable (does not grow in cell cultures), Detected by antigen in stools
- MC cause of infantile diarrhea: Rotavirus

HUMAN PAPILLOMA VIRUS

- Human papilloma virus (HPV) causes: Warts & genital warts, Cervical Ca, Vulval Ca, Penile Ca, Anal Ca, Perianal Ca
- HPV with high oncogenic potential: HPV 16, HPV 18, HPV 31, HPV 33

PRION DISEASE

- MC infectious prion diseases in humans: CJD
- In CJD: Spongiform transformation of the cerebral cortex & deep grey matter structures (Caudate, putamen nucleus) is seen
- Corneal transplant may transmit CJD
- Subacute spongiform viral encephalopathy (SSVE) is also known as bovine spongiform encephalopathy (Mad Cow disease)

OTHER VIRUS

- Dengue virus is: Flavivirus subtype, of Arbovirus group
- Hanta virus causes: Hanta virus pulmonary syndrome
- Conditions associated with respiratory syncytial virus/ RSV: Bronchiolitis (infants), Pneumonia (infants)
- HTLV-1 (RNA virus) causes: Adult T-cell leukemia

PARASITOLOGY

Tests & parasites

- Sabin Feldman dye test: Toxoplasmosis
- Casoni test: Hydatid cyst
- Frenkel's skin test: Toxoplasmosis

Diseases & causative parasites

- Biliary obstruction: Clonorchis sinensis
- Cirrhosis of liver, Katayama disease: S. japonicum
- Pipestem/periportal cirrhosis: S. mansoni
- Ground itch/Ancylostoma dermatitis: Necator
- Cutaneous larva migrans/ cutis & creeping eruptions: Ancylostoma braziliense & A. caninum
- Visceral larva migrans: Toxocara canis
- Ocular larva migrans: Toxocara canis
- Larva Curran's/ hyperinfection syndrome/ autoinfection: Strongyloides
- Malignant hydatid disease: Echinococcus multilocularis
- L. donovani causes: Visceral leishmaniasis
- Loa Loa causes: Calabar swelling

Other names of parasites

- Oriental liver fluke: C. sinensis
- Oriental lung fluke: P. westermani
- Oriental blood fluke: S. japonicum
- Smallest tapeworm: Echinococcus granulosus
- Dwarf tapeworm: H. nana
- Longest tapeworm: T. saginata
- Largest intestinal fluke/ trematode: F. buski

MALARIA

- In malaria, size of RBC is increased in: Vivax
- Infective agent of malaria is: Sporozoite

Falciparum malaria

- Gametocytes are seen in peripheral blood smear
- Parasitemia is highest
- Most virulent plasmodium species
- Exo-erythrocytic stage is absent
- Multiple infections of RBC's
- Splenic rupture is common

Plasmodium falciparum

- Resistance: Drug resistance widespread
- CNS involvement: Present
- Anaemia: Present
- Hypnozoites: Absent

- Incubation period: 12 days
- Stages: Only rings and gametocytes
- Special forms: Accole, wing, marginal
- RBC size: Not enlarged
- Dots: Maurer's dots
- Infection: Multiple infections per RBC

KALA AZAR

- NNN (Novy, Neal & Nicolle) medium is used
- Aldehyde test is positive in 12 weeks
- Hyper-gamma-globulinemia is seen

WUCHERIA BANCROFTI

- Wuchereria bancrofti causes: Lymphatic filariasis
- Habitat of Wuchereria bancrofti: Lymph vessels & lymph nodes

Occult filariasis

- Occult filariasis/ Mayers – Kouwenaar syndrome
- Cause: Microfilariae
- Organs involved: Lymphatic system, lungs, Liver and spleen
- Therapeutic response: Responds to DEC
- Microfilaria: Present in affected tissues
- Loa Loa: Microfilariae are detected in blood in daytime.

Classical filariasis

- Cause: Developing worms and adults
- Organs involved: Lymphatic system
- Therapeutic response: No response
- Microfilaria: Present in blood

ECHINOCOCCUS GRANULOSIS

- Hydatid disease/ Echinococcosis is caused by: E. granulosus
- Definitive host for hydatid disease: Dog
- ARA C-5 is used in diagnosis
- Hydatid cyst (& trichuriasis) are caused by ingestion of infected egg via feco-oral route from contaminated soil

ENTAMOEBA HISTOLYTICA

- Features of cyst of Entamoeba histolytica: Cyst has glycogen mass, Chromatoidal bars, Eccentric nucleus
- Extra-intestinal infection by E. histolytica most often involves: Liver (amoebic liver abscess)

MYCOLOGY

Classes of fungi

- Fungi which are spherical in tissue, but grow like moulds, when cultured at room temperature are: Dimorphic fungi, e.g. Histoplasmosis, Blastomycosis, Sporotrichosis, Coccidio-idomycosis
- Fungi without sexual stage: Fungi imperfectii/ deutero-mycetes e.g. candida, coccidioides immitis

Culture & staining

- Fungal cell membrane is stained by: PAS
- Culture media for fungi: Sabouraud's medium
- Non-culturable fungus: Rhinosporidium

Characteristic of fungi

Characteristic	*Fungi*
Thick walled spherules filled with endospores	**Coccidio-ido-mycosis**
Arthrospores	**Trichophyton, microsporum in hair**
Ergotism	**Claviceps purpura**
Fungi in walls of blood vessels and causes thrombosis and infraction	**Mucor**
Otomycosis, aspergilloma	**Aspergillus**
Miliary calcification, diagnostic tubercular spores	**Histoplasmosis**
Endospores (Valley fever or desert rheumatism)	**Phialophora**
Brain abscess	**Cladosporium bartineon**
Pear shaped conidia arranged in rosettes	**Sporothrix**

Friable polyps of nose, mouth and eye	**Rhinosporidiosis**
Asteroid bodies, cigar shaped yeast cells (cigar shaped globi)	**Sporotrichosis**
Sclerotic bodies	**Chromoblastomycosis**
Chlamydospores	**Candida**
Micro and macro-conidia	**Dermatophytes**

CANDIDA

- Candidiasis is an: Endogenous infection
- MC fungal infection in neutropenic patients: Candidiasis
- Reynolds Braude phenomenon is shown by: Candida
- Thrush is caused by: Candida (thrush is also known as oral candidiasis)

Yeast like fungi

- Partly yeast, partly hyphae
- Candida

CRYPTOCOCCUS

- Capsule of cryptococcus: Polysaccharide capsule
- Cryptococcus has predilection for: Brain
- Rapid & sensitive test for capsular polysaccharide in CSF cryptococcal infection: Latex particle agglutination test
- India ink (microscopy) wet mount is used for diagnosis of: Cryptococcus
- MC cause of acute meningitis in AIDS: Cryptococcus

Yeast

- Unicellular fungi
- Cryptococcus

COCCIDIOIDES IMMITIS

- Growth of coccidioides immitis: On Culture media, it grows as a white fluffy mould, Non-budding spherical form (spherule) in host tissue/ special conditions
- Coccidioides immitis reproduces in host tissue by: Forming small endospores, within mature spherules
- Coccidioides immitis causes: Valley fever/ Desert rheumatism

ASPERGILLUS

- Hyphae in Aspergillus fumigates: Branching hyphae/ Septate
- Portal of entry of Aspergillus fumigates: Lungs (can colonize the damaged bronchial tree, pulmonary cysts, cavities of patients with underlying lung tissue)

CHROMOBLASTOMYCOSIS

- Chromoblastomycosis is caused by: Cladosporium
- Diagnostic histological feature of chromoblastomycosis: Sclerotic bodies/ Thick walled, dark colored, rounded forms (copper pennies)

Other fungal infections

- Features of Mucormycosis: Angio-invasive, Uncommon, Largely confined to patients with serious pre-existing diseases (diabetic ketoacidosis)
- Pneumocystis carnii are: Obligate, Extracellular fungi
- Dermatophytes infects: Skin, Nail, Hair
- Mycetoma present as: Ulcer on leg, Indurated margin, Discharging sinus
- Feature of Blastomyces dermatitidis: Dimorphic fungi, seen as Broad based, budding, round yeast like cells, with thick wall

Moulds/ filamentous fungi

- True mycelia
- Dermatophytes

Dimorphic

- Yeast at 37 degrees and Mould at 22 degrees: Paracoccidioides, Histoplasma
- Filaments and yeasts at different temperature: Coccidioides, Blastomyces

CLINICAL QUESTIONS

1. **A gardener has multiple vesicles on hand and multiple eruptions along the lymphatics. Fungus responsible for such a presentation:**

   A. Sporothrix schenckii B. Cladosporium

   C. Histoplasma D. Candida

   Clinical presentation is suggestive of sporotrichosis.

   Sporotrichosis/ Rose Gardner's disease is a chronic subcutaneous pyogranulomatous disease caused by a thermally dimorphic fungus, Sporothrix schenckii.

   Lympho-cutaneous type is the most common type of sporotrichosis (80%) and is characterized by nodulo-ulcerative lesions (painless) occurring along the lymphatics.

   Answer: A i.e., Sporothrix schenckii

2. **25 years old male presented with diarrhea for 6 months. On examination, the causative agent was found to be acid fast with 10 micro meter diameter. Most likely agent is:**

   A. Cryptosporidium B. Isospora

   C. Cyclospora D. Giardia

   Clinical presentation is suggestive of diarrhoea due to Cyclospora.

   Cyclospora Cayetanensis causes prolonged diarrhea with abdominal pain, low-grade fever, and fatigue.

   The oocyts can be stained by Zeihl-Neelsen stain. Oocysts of Cyclospora are acid fast and stain red in color.

   The oocyst is a non-refractile sphere, measuring 8-10 micrometer in diameter.

   Answer: C i.e., Cyclospora

3. **A resident doctor sustained a needle stick injury while sampling blood of a patient who is HIV positive. A decision was taken to offer him post-exposure prophylaxis. Which one is the best recommendation?**

   A. Zidovudine + Lamivudine for 4 weeks

   B. Zidovudine + Lamivudine + Nevirapine for 4 weeks

   C. Zidovudine + Lamivudine + Indinavir for 4 weeks

   D. Zidovudine + Stavudine + Nevirapine for 4 weeks

   3 drugs are given (2 NRTI's + 1PI) for post-exposure prophylaxis.

   Zidovudine (300 mg twice a day), Lamivudine (300 mg twice a day) and Indinavir (800 mg thrice a day)/ Nelfinavir (750 mg thrice a day)

   Expanded regimen (NACO guidelines for post-exposure prophylaxis) is given for 4 weeks.

   Answer: C i.e., Zidovudine + Lamivudine + Indinavir for 4 weeks

4. **A 30 years old patient with CSF leak is presenting with neck rigidity, fever and seizures. What could be the probable infective agent?**

   A. Streptococcus pneumoniae

   B. N. meningitidis

   C. Listeria monocytogenes

   D. E. coli

   Clinical presentation is suggestive of meningitis.

   Neck rigidity/ stiffness, fever and seizures suggest the diagnosis of meningitis.

   Streptococcus pneumoniae is the leading cause of meningitis in all ages (except in neonates).

   Answer: A i.e., Streptococcus pneumoniae

5. **A teacher presents with profuse bloody diarrhoea and fever of 104 degrees F. Many children studying in the same school had similar episodes. Possible organism is:**

   A. Shigella dysenteriae

   B. Staphylococcus aureus

   C. Yersinia

   D. Entamoeba histolytica

   Clinical presentation is suggestive of diarrhoea due to Shigella dysenteriae.

   Dysentery phase of shigellosis is characterized by frequent passage of bloody mucopurulent stools with increased tenesmus and abdominal cramps.

It is preceded by fever, malaise, anorexia and vomiting.

Risk factors for shigellosis include overcrowding, poor hygiene and children less than 5 years.

It tends to occur as epidemics in developing countries such as Indian subcontinent and sub-Saharan Africa.

Answer: A i.e., Shigella dysenteriae

6. **A 14 years old boy is admitted with history of fever, icterus, conjunctival suffusion and hematuria for 20 days. Which serological test can be of diagnostic utility?**

A. Widal test

B. Microscopic agglutination test

C. Paul Bunnell test

D. Weil Felix test

Clinical presentation is suggestive of leptospirosis.

High grade fever, jaundice and raised liver enzymes, hemorrhages (pulmonary hemorrhage, petechiae and purpura, conjunctival hemorrhage) and raised urea - creatinine suggest the diagnosis of Weil's disease/ Hepato-renal-hemorrhagic syndrome.

It is caused by Leptospira interrogans.

MAT (microscopic agglutination test) detects antibodies against specific serovars of L. interrogans.

It is the gold standard method and the reference test for the diagnosis of leptospirosis.

Answer: B i.e., Microscopic agglutination test

7. **A 30 years old patient presented with history of jaundice for 10 days. His liver function tests showed bilirubin of 10 mg/ dL. SGOT/ SGPT: 1100/ 1450 and serum alkaline phosphatase: 240 IU. He was positive for HBsAg. Confirmatory test to establish acute Hepatitis B virus infection:**

A. IgM anti-HBc antibody B. HBeAg

C. HBV DNA PCR D. HBcAg

Presence of acute HBV infection is made by detecting IgM anti-HBc antibody.

Anti-HBc IgM is the first antibody to be elevated following HBV infection.

It appears within 1-2 weeks after the appearance of HBsAg and lasts for 3-6 months.

Its presence indicates acute hepatitis B infection.

Answer: A i.e., IgM anti-HBc antibody

8. **A 36 years old IT professional had a business trip to China where he ate crab. Now after coming back to India, he is having dyspnea, high-grade fever, cough and rusty sputum. Sputum is negative for mycobacterium tuberculosis. Most likely causative organism is:**

A. Fasciola hepatica

B. Fasciola buski

C. Paragonimus westermani

D. Clonorchis sinensis

Clinical presentation is suggestive of infestation of Paragonimus westermani.

Paragonimus westermani is endemic in the Far East – Japan, Korea, Taiwan, China etc.

Man acquires infection by eating undercooked crab or cray fish containing metacercariae.

Patient presents with cough, chest pain, and hemoptysis.

The viscous sputum is speckled with the golden-brown eggs.

Chronic cases may resemble pulmonary tuberculosis.

Answer: C i.e., Paragonimus westermani

9. **A child is presenting with constipation, dilated pupil and ptosis after eating outside food. Most probable cause of food poisoning:**

A. Cl. tetani B. Cl. septicum

C. Cl. perfringens D. Cl. botulinum

Clinical presentation is suggestive of botulism.

The manifestations of botulism are due to decreased acetylcholine in cranial nerve and parasympathetic nerve terminals.

Common symptoms include diplopia, dysphasia, dysarthria, descending symmetric flaccid paralysis of voluntary muscles, decreased deep tendon reflexes, constipation etc.

Food borne botulism results from consumption of foods contaminated with preformed botulinum toxin (home-made canned food).

Answer: D i.e., Cl. botulinum

10. A diabetic presented with bloody nasal discharge, orbital swelling and pain. Culture of periorbital pus showed broad aseptate hyphae. Which is the most probable organism?

A. Mucor　B. Candida

C. Aspergillus　D. Rhizopus

Clinical presentation is suggestive of mucormycosis.

Diabetic ketoacidosis is the most important risk factor for development of mucormycosis.

Acidosis causes release of iron from the sequestered proteins in serum.

Most common form of mucormycosis is rhinocerebral mucormycosis; starts as eye and facial pain, may progress to cause orbital cellulitis, proptosis and vision loss.

Histopathological staining of tissue biopsies shows broad aseptate hyaline hyphae with wide angle branching.

Answer: A i.e., Mucor

11. 24 years old AIDS patient develops chronic abdominal pain, low-grade fever, diarrhoea and malabsorption. Oocysts were demonstrated in stool. Likely cause of his diarrhea:

A. E. histolytica　B. G. lamblia

C. Microsporidia　D. Isospora belli

Clinical presentation is suggestive of diarrhoea due to Isospora.

Infection with Isospora belli results in abdominal discomfort, mild fever, diarrhoea, and malabsorption. The diarrhoea is usually watery and does not contain blood or pus and is self-limiting. However, protracted diarrhoea, lasting for several years can be seen in immunocompromised persons, particularly in the human immunodeficiency virus (HIV) infected. The staining technique used are modified Ziehl-Neelsen stain or Kinyoun acid fast staining of stool smear. In these methods, pink colored acid-fast large oocyst (>25 micrometers) can be demonstrated.

Answer: D i.e., Isospora belli

12. A patient presented to the hospital with severe hydrophobia. Which is the best test for making a clinical diagnosis of rabies:

A. RT-PCR for rabies virus

B. Negri bodies

C. Antibodies to rabies virus

D. Indirect immunofluorescence

RT-PCR for rabies virus is done for diagnosing rabies.

Reverse transcription-polymerase chain reaction (RT-PCR) can be used to amplify genes of rabies virus RNA from the brain tissue.

It is the most sensitive and specific assay available at present for the diagnosis of rabies.

Answer: A i.e., RT-PCR for rabies virus

13. A 48 years old woman develops fever and focal neurological signs. MRI shows a left temporal lobe lesion. Most appropriate test that can be used to confirm the diagnosis of HSV encephalitis in this patient is:

A. Brain biopsy

B. Tzanck smear

C. PCR assay for viral DNA in CSF

D. Serum IgM antibody detection

Polymerase chain reaction (PCR) is the most sensitive test for detecting HSV infections and can be used to differentiate between HSV-1 AND HSV-2.

Answer: C i.e., PCR assay for viral DNA in CSF

14. Serological testing of patient shows HBsAg, IgM anti-HBc and HBeAg positive. The patient has:

A. Chronic hepatitis B with low infectivity

B. Acute hepatitis B infection with high infectivity

C. Chronic hepatitis with high infectivity

D. Acute on chronic hepatitis B infection

Clinical presentation is suggestive of acute hepatitis B infection with high infectivity.

Acute hepatitis B infection with high infectivity is indicated by HBsAg positive, IgM anti-HBc positive and HBeAg positive tests.

Answer: B i.e., Acute hepatitis B infection with high infectivity

15. **A 25 years old sexually active woman presented with purulent vaginal discharge and dysuria for 7 days after an unprotected sexual intercourse with a new partner. Most sensitive investigation to determine the etiological agent:**

    A. A polymerase chain reaction for nucleic acids

    B. An enzyme immunoassay

    C. Gram stain

    D. Culture on selective medium

Clinical presentation is suggestive of non-gonococcal urethritis.

Non-gonococcal urethritis/ NGU is characterized by mucopurulent discharge followed by dysuria and urethral irritation.

Chlamydia trachomatis is the most common cause of NGU, responsible for 30-50% of cases of NGU.

Nucleic acid amplification test (NAAT) has revolutionized the diagnosis of chlamydial infections.

Various methods available (for NAAT) are polymerase chain reaction (PCR), ligase chain reaction (LCR), transcription mediated amplification (TMA) and strand displacement assay (SDA).

Answer: A i.e., A polymerase chain reaction for nucleic acids

16. **A patient of acute lymphocytic leukemia with fever and neutropenia develops diarrhea after administration of amoxicillin therapy. Likely causative organism:**

    A. Salmonella typhii

    B. Clostridium difficile

    C. Clostridium perfringens

    D. Shigella flexneri

Clinical presentation is suggestive of pseudomembranous colitis.

Clostridium difficile is responsible for a unique colonic disease – pseudomembranous colitis.

Clostridium difficile infection is associated with prolonged antimicrobial use.

This can result in disruption of the normal colonic flora, which enhances the susceptibility to Clostridium difficile infection. Cephalosporins (e.g., ceftriaxone) are frequently responsible for this condition.

Other antibiotics, such as clindamycin, ampicillin and fluoroquinolones (ciprofloxacin) are also implicated in hospital outbreaks.

Answer: B i.e., Clostridium difficile

17. **A 22 years old male presented with history of fever, sore throat and enlarged neck lymph nodes. He was ordered a Paul-Bunnell test with a suspicion of infectious mononucleosis. What is the immunological basis behind the use of this test?**

    A. Heterophile antibody test

    B. Complement mediated agglutination reaction

    C. Homophile antibody test

    D. Latex agglutination test

Pail Bunnell test is a heterophile antibody test.

Paul-Bunnell test (for infectious mononucleosis) is a tube agglutination test that uses RBCs sheep to detect heterophile antibodies in patient's serum.

Answer: A i.e., Heterophile antibody test

18. **A person presents with pneumonia. His sputum was sent for culture. The bacterium obtained was gram positive cocci in chains and alpha hemolytic colonies on sheep agar. Antibiotic utilized for confirming diagnosis:**

    A. Novobiocin   B. Optochin

    C. Bacitracin   D. Oxacillin

Clinical presentation is suggestive of pneumococcus, which is Optochin sensitive.

Streptococcus pneumoniae (commonly referred to as pneumococcus; a gram-positive cocci) is the leading cause of lobar pneumonia, otitis media in children and meningitis in all ages.

They are alpha hemolytic and may present as commensals in human upper respiratory tract.

They differ from alpha hemolytic viridans streptococci in many ways such as their shape (lanceolate-shaped diplococci), bile solubility, optochin sensitivity and presence of polysaccharide capsule.

Answer: B i.e., Optochin

19. A 20 years old male presents to the STD clinic with a genital ulcer. The gram stain of the smear from ulcer shows gram negative coccobacilli. Most appropriate media for culture would be:

A. Thayer-Martin media

B. Blood agar with X & V factors

C. Chocolate agar with isovitalex

D. Tellurite blood agar

Clinical presentation is suggestive of chancroid.

Hemophilus ducreyi is a pleomorphic gram-negative coccobacillus; occurs in groups or in parallel chains.

It is an etiologic agent of chancroid (or soft chancre), a sexually transmitted disease characterized by painful genital ulceration that bleeds easily.

H. ducreyi requires factor X (hemin), but not factor V for its growth.

Primary isolation is difficult. It can be grown on rabbit blood agar or chocolate agar enriched with 1% isovitalex and made selective by adding vancomycin.

Answer: C i.e., Chocolate agar with isovitalex

20. A farmer presenting with fever off and on for the past 4 years was diagnosed to be suffering from chronic brucellosis. Which of the following serological test would NOT help in making a diagnosis?

A. Standard agglutination test

B. 2-Mercapto-ethanol test

C. Complement fixation test

D. Coomb's test

As isolation of Brucella is difficult, serological tests are of paramount importance in diagnosis of brucellosis. Several tests have been developed, such as standard agglutination test, 2-mercaptoethanol (2ME) agglutination test, complement fixation test and ELISA.

Answer: D i.e., Coomb's test

21. A patient is having pneumonia. Sputum examination is showing gram positive branched organism which is strict aerobe and partial acid fast. Most likely organism:

A. Nocardia

B. Actinomycetes

C. Mycobacterium tuberculosis

D. Pneumococcus

Clinical presentation is suggestive of pneumonia due to Nocardia.

Nocardia species (named after Edmond Nocard, 1898) are gram-positive branching filamentous bacilli similar to Actinomyces; however, they differ from the later by being aerobic and acid fast.

Lobar pneumonia is the most common form of pulmonary nocardiosis, characterized by subacute onset of cough with thick, purulent sputum.

Answer: A i.e., Nocardia

22. A 15 years old girl was admitted to the infectious disease hospital with a provisional diagnosis of rabies. The most suitable clinical sample that can confirm the antemortem diagnosis is:

A. Serum for anti-rabies IgG antibody

B. Corneal impression smear for immunofluorescence

C. CSF sample for viral culture

D. Giemsa stain on smear prepared from salivary secretions

Direct immunofluorescence test (direct-IF) can be performed to detect rabies nucleoprotein antigens in specimens by using specific monoclonal antibodies tagged with fluorescein dye.

The best specimen is hair follicle of nape of neck (most sensitive).

Corneal impression smear can also be used.

It is usually positive in late stage with a sensitivity of 30%.

Answer: B i.e., Corneal impression smear for immuno-fluorescence

23. A 30 years old male presented with subcutaneous itchy nodules over the left iliac crest. On examination, they are firm, non-tender and mobile. Skin scrapings contains microfilariae and adult worms of:

A. Loa loa

B. Onchocerca volvulus

C. Brugia malayi

D. Mansonella perstans

Clinical presentation is suggestive of onchocercoma.

The subcutaneous nodule or onchocercoma is a circumscribed, firm, non-tender tumor, formed as a result of fibroblastic reaction around the worms.

They tend to occur over anatomical sites where the bones are superficial, such as scalp, scapulae, ribs, elbows, iliac crest, sacrum, and knees.

The nodules are painless and cause no trouble except for their unsightly appearance.

Answer: B i.e., Onchocerca volvulus

24. Gram-stained peri-orbital exudates in a severe pan-ophthalmitis with cellulitis in an elderly diabetic shows irregular branching, aseptate and broad hyphae. Most likely diagnosis:

A. Candida

B. Aspergillus

C. Penicillium

D. Apophysomyces species

Clinical presentation is suggestive of mucormycosis.

Apophysomyces elegans and Apophysomyces trapeziformis are able to cause mucormycosis, in humans, which is often fatal but very rare.

Most common form of mucormycosis is rhinocerebral mucormycosis; starts as eye and facial pain, may progress to cause orbital cellulitis, proptosis and vision loss.

Histopathological staining of tissue biopsies shows broad aseptate hyaline hyphae with wide angle branching.

Answer: D i.e., Apophysomyces species

25. A Veterinary doctor had pyrexia of unknown origin. His blood culture in special laboratory media was positive for gram-negative short bacilli which was oxidase positive. Most likely organism grown in culture is:

A. Pasteurella species
B. Francisella species
C. Bartonella species
D. Brucella species

Clinical presentation is suggestive of brucellosis.

Brucella is an obligate aerobic, fastidious, non-sporing, non-motile, non-capsulated small gram-negative cocco-bacillus, responsible for highly contagious febrile illness called brucellosis.

Classic triad of brucellosis include fever with profuse sweats, arthralgia/ arthritis and hepatosplenomegaly.

Brucella do no ferment carbohydrates, is catalase positive and oxidase positive (except some strains of Bacillus abortus, Bacillus neotomae and Brucella ovis).

Answer: D i.e., Brucella species

26. A person returns to Delhi from Bangladesh. After 2 days he had diarrhea. Stool examination shows RBC's in stools. Likely causative organism:

A. Enteropathogenic E. coli

B. Enterotoxigenic E. coli

C. Salmonella typhi

D. Shigella dysenteriae

Clinical presentation is suggestive of dysentery due to Shigella.

Dysentery phase of shigellosis is characterized by frequent passage of bloody mucopurulent stools with increased tenesmus and abdominal cramps.

It is preceded by fever, malaise, anorexia and vomiting.

Risk factors for shigellosis include overcrowding, poor hygiene and children less than 5 years.

It tends to occur as epidemics in developing countries such as Indian subcontinent and sub-Saharan Africa.

Wet mount preparation of feces shows large number of pus cells, erythrocytes and macrophages.

Answer: D i.e., Shigella dysenteriae

27. A 50 years old male has fever for the past 1 week with abdominal distension and loss of appetite. It is not responding to antibiotics and antimalarials. Widal test is negative but RK39 dipstick test is positive. Which drug can be used in such a patient?

A. Bedaquiline

B. Linezolid

C. Fluconazole

D. Liposomal Amphotericin-B

Clinical presentation is suggestive of Kala-azar.

The onset of Kala-azar is insidious.

The clinical illness begins with fever, splenomegaly and hepatomegaly.

A specific rapid immune-chromatographic dipstick (ICT) method for antibody has been developed using a recombinant leishmania antigen rk39 consisting of 39 amino acids conserved in kinesin region of Leishmania infantum.

The sensitivity of the test is 98% and specificity of 90%.

Liposomal amphotericin-B has been developed and used extensively to treat visceral leishmaniasis in all parts of the world.

Answer: D i.e., Liposomal Amphotericin-B

28. A patient comes to your clinic with complaints of multiple episodes of loose watery stool for 3 days. On probing, you discover that these episodes starting after ingestion of shellfish in a restaurant, 3 days back. Other people who had food from that restaurant had similar symptoms. Most common cause of such viral diarrhea:

A. Adenovirus

B. Calicivirus

C. Rotavirus

D. Norovirus

Clinical presentation is suggestive of Norovirus infection.

Ingestion of shellfish that have not been sufficiently heated – under 75 °C (167 °F) – poses a high risk for norovirus infection.

Norovirus infection is characterized by nausea, vomiting, watery diarrhoea, abdominal pain, and in some cases, loss of taste.

A person usually develops symptoms of gastroenteritis 12 to 48 hours after being exposed to norovirus.

Answer: D i.e., Norovirus

CHAPTER 6

PHARMACOLOGY

RAPID REVISION NOTES

Drugs & their groups

Drugs	*Group*
Phentolamine, phenoxybenzamine	**Alpha blockers**
Nifedipine, verapamil, diltiazem	**Calcium channel blockers**
Acetyl-cysteine, bromhexine	**Mucolytic agents**
Captopril, e3nalapril	**ACE (angiotensin converting enzyme) inhibitor**
Spironolactone	**Aldosterone antagonist**
Morphine, pethidine, methadone, fentanyl	**Opioid receptor agonist**
Neostigmine, physostigmine, pyridostigmine, edrophonium	**Acetyl-cholinesterase inhibitor**
Cimetidine, ranitidine, famotidine	**H_2 receptor blockers**
Terbutaline, metaproterenol, ritodrine	**Selective beta-2 agonist**
Epinephrine	**Non-selective alpha and beta agonist**
Iso-proterenol	**Non-selective beta agonist**
Phenyl-ephrine	**Selective alpha-1 agonist**
Clonidine	**Selective alpha-2 agonist**
Bromocriptine	**Selective dopamine-2 receptor agonist**
Pirenzepine	**Selective M1 receptor agonist**
Bethanechol	**Selective M2 receptor agonist**
Atropine	**Acetylcholine receptor blocker (muscarinic)**
Metoclopramide, domperidone, cisapride	**Dopamine antagonist**
Labetalol, timolol	**Alpha & beta blockers**
Propranolol, alprenolol, nadolol, pindolol, sotalol	**Non-selective beta blockers**
Atenolol, acebutolol, metoprolol	**Cardio-selective beta blockers**

GENERAL PHARMACOLOGY

Some important definitions

- Pharmacokinetics: Study of drug movement in the body/ effect of body on the drug
- Side-effects: Unwanted effect at therapeutic doses
- Agonist: Have affinity & maximal efficacy

- Antagonist: Have affinity & NO maximal efficacy
- Clearance: Measure of body's ability to excrete a drug
- Therapeutic window phenomenon: Optimal effect is exerted only over a narrow range of plasma drug concentration e.g. TCA, clonidine, glipizide
- Therapeutic index: Toxic dose/ Therapeutic dose (LD50/ ED50)
- Drug efficacy: Maximal effect that a drug may elicit; More important (than efficacy) in determining drug of choice
- Drug potency: Amount of drug required to produce a certain response
- Bioavailability: Fraction of drug that reaches in the blood

Transport of drugs

- Active transport of the drug is: Carrier mediated, requires ATP, saturation occurs
- Factors affecting drug absorption: Route of administration, vascularity, solubility
- Absorption of drug from gut is decreased by: Presence of food, first pass metabolism, increased expression of p-glycoprotein

Effects of pH

- pKa is: Numerically equal to the pH at which the drug is 50% ionized (but for every unit by which pH is changed, the ratio of unionized to ionized molecules changes 10 fold)
- If an acidic drug has pKa value of 4.5, then % of ionized drug at pH of 3.5 will be 10%
- Acidic drugs are more ionized at alkaline pH
- Acidic drugs are largely unionized at acidic pH & are absorbed from stomach
- A highly ionized drug is excreted mainly by the kidneys

Bioavailability (BA)

- BA can be determined from plasma concentration or urinary excretion data
- BA is determined by the area under the plasma concentration-time curve
- BA depends upon extent of absorption & extent of 1st pass metabolism in intestinal wall, portal blood or liver
- Bioavailability by intravenous route is: 100%

Microsomal enzyme inducers

- Phenytoin
- Phenobarbitone
- Rifampicin

Acetylation is the mode of metabolism for

- Isoniazid
- Hydralazine

First pass effect/ first pass elimination

- First pass metabolism (Metabolism of drug in liver, intestinal wall or portal blood) + excretion of drug into bile is known as first pass elimination
- First pass metabolism is seen with: Oral route, Rectal route
- Drugs showing high first pass metabolism are: Lignocaine, propranolol, salbutamol

Volume of distribution (VOD)

- Calculated as dose administered/ plasma concentration
- Factors influencing VOD: Drug plasma protein binding, lipid solubility, degree of blood flow, age, tissue affinity, pKa
- Apparent VOD may exceed total body fluid volume if a drug is: Sequestrated in body tissues

Blood brain barrier

- Drugs crossing blood brain barrier: Propranolol, physostigmine

Placental barrier

- Maximum transfer of drug across placenta occurs in 1st trimester
- Ion trapping of basic drugs occurs in the placenta
- Drugs crossing placental barrier: Warfarin, lithium, morphine
- Heparin & Insulin DO NOT cross placental barrier & hence are agents of choice in pregnancy

Half life (t1/2)

- Time taken for amount of drug in the body to decline by 50%
- Amount of drug excreted in 4th t1/2: 93.7%
- t1/2 can determine: Elimination time, Steady state plasma concentration, Dosing rate, Maintenance dose

Prodrugs

- Enalapril
- Sulindac
- Ticlopidine
- Clopidogrel

Zero order reaction

- Constant AMOUNT is excreted
- Rate of elimination INDEPENDENT of plasma concentration
- Variable t1/2
- Phenytoin
- Ethanol
- Salicylates

First order reaction

- Constant FRACTION of drug is eliminated
- Rate of elimination is directly DEPENDENT on plasma concentration
- t1/2 is constant

Teratogenic drugs

- Carbamazepine: Cleft lip, cleft palate
- Valproic acid: Neural tube defects
- Thalidomide: Phocomelia
- Chloramphenicol: Grey baby syndrome

Miscellaneous

- Drugs metabolized in liver are: Phenytoin, erythromycin, cimetidine, diazepam
- Drug metabolized in kidney: Penicillin G
- Duration of action of a drug administered intravenously depends upon: Protein binding, Clearance, distribution volume, lipid solubility, drug concentration
- Effect of displacement of protein bound drug: Raises plasma level of that drug
- Drugs bindings sites on protein are: Non-specific (one drug can displace other)
- Drugs bound to albumin: Phenytoin Warfarin
- Ionized drugs are mainly excreted by: Kidney
- Basic drugs are absorbed from: Proximal intestine
- Phase II of drug metabolism involves: Conjugation with glucuronide, sulfate, glutathione

Competitive antagonist

- Chemically resembles the agonist
- Reduces potency of the agonist
- Binds to the same receptor
- Maximal response can be obtained
- V_{max} is same, Km increases

Drugs & the enzyme they inhibit

- 5 Fluorouracil: Thymidine synthetase
- Omeprazole: Gastric H ATPase
- Phenelzine: MAO
- Pargyline: MAO
- Acetazolamide: Carbonic anhydrase
- Captopril: Angiotensin convertase
- Penicillin: Transpeptidase
- Aspirin: Cyclo-oxygenase
- Allopurinol: Xanthine oxidase
- Beta aminopropionitrile: Lysyl oxidase
- Sarin: Cholinesterase
- Statins: HMG-CoA reductase

CLINICAL TRIALS

- Phase I: Human pharmacology & safety
- Phase II: Therapeutic exploration & dose ranging, Determines efficacy
- Phase III: Therapeutic confirming
- Phase IV: Post marketing surveillance, No ethical clearance required

- Good clinical practice is not required for pre-clinical trials but is needed for phase I -IV

Drugs and ocular toxicity

Drugs	*Ocular effects*
Busulfan, chlorambucil, phenothiazines, glucocorticoids	**Cataracts**
Oral contraceptives	**Corneal oedema**
Vitamin D, indomethacin, chloroquine, mepacrine	**Corneal opacities**
Mydriatics, sympathomimetics	**Glaucoma**

DRUGS & SIDE EFFECTS

- Drug deposited in retina: Chloroquine
- Drug deposited in muscle: Digoxin
- Drugs causing hepatitis: Halothane Rifampin, INH, pyrazinamide
- Drugs causing intrahepatic cholestasis: Phenothiazines, TCA
- Hepatotoxins: CCl_4, Paracetamol
- Bleomycin & pulmonary changes: Pulmonary fibrosis (stimulation of alveolar macrophages)
- Drugs causing pulmonary fibrosis: Bleomycin, Busulfan
- Cardiotoxic drugs: Doxorubicin, Daunorubicin
- Drugs causing osteoporosis: Glucocorticoids, Heparin
- Drugs with low safety margin: Lithium, Aminoglycosides, Digoxin
- Drugs causing hyperuricemia: Pyrazinamide, Ethambutol
- Drugs causing hirsutism: Minoxidil, Phenytoin
- Drugs causing extra-pyramidal side effects: Haloperidol, Levodopa

CHOLINERGIC SYSTEM

General facts

- Acetylcholine release is inhibited by: Botulinum
- Acetylcholine use is not possible because: It is rapidly degraded

Acetyl-cholinesterase inhibitors

- Edrophonium (diagnosis of Myasthenia gravis)
- Neostigmine/ Pyridostigmine (treatment of urinary retention, ileus, reversal of neuromuscular blockade)

Organophosphate poisoning

- Pupils in Organophosphate poisoning: Pin point pupils
- Treatment of organophosphate poisoning: Atropine & Pralidoxime (reactivates cholinesterase)

ANTICHOLERGIC DRUGS

Uses of atropine

- Organophosphate poisoning
- Mushroom/ Inocybe poisoning
- Treating brady-arrhythmias

Atropine

- Mydriasis
- Cycloplegia
- Decreases: Respiratory secretions, acid secretion in stomach, motility of gut
- Can cause acute angle closure glaucoma in eyes with narrow angles
- Can cause urinary retention in elderly with BPH
- Can cause hyperthermia in infants

ADRENERGIC SYSTEM

Alpha1 agonist

- Phenylephrine
- Methoxamine

Alpha2 agonist

- Clonidine
- Methyldopa

Beta1 agonist

- Isoproterenol (beta1 = beta2)
- Dobutamine (beta1 > beta2)

Beta2 agonist

- Salmeterol
- Terbutaline
- Ritodrine

Alpha1 blockers

- Prazosin
- Tamsulosin

Alpha2 blockers

- Yohimbine
- Mirtazapine (antidepressant)

Beta1 blocker

- Acebutolol
- Atenolol
- Betaxolol
- Bisoprolol
- Esmolol
- Metoprolol

Beta1 & Beta2 blocker

- Dilevalol
- Labetalol
- Carvedilol (alpha1, beta1, beta2 blocker)

Timolol

- Mainly used for glaucoma
- No miosis
- It can precipitate asthma
- Contraindicated in: Asthma, Heart block

Esmolol

- Cardioselective
- No intrinsic activity
- Shortest acting beta blocker (10 minutes)

Adrenergic Receptor Location

- Alpha 1: Post-junctional
- Alpha 2: Pre and Post-junctional
- Beta 1: Heart
- Beta 2: Bronchi

SEROTONIN RECEPTORS

5HT 1A agonist

- Buspirone (antianxiety)

5HT 1B agonist

- Sumatriptan (migraine)
- DOC for acute severe migraine: Sumatriptan

5HT 4 agonist

- Cisapride (increases gastric motility)

5HT 2A antagonist

- Cyproheptadine
- Ketanserin

5HT 2A/2C antagonist

- Clozapine

5HT 3 antagonist

- Ondansetron

PROSTAGLANDIN

- Role of prostaglandins: Cytoprotective for stomach, Contract uterus
- PGE1 (Misoprostol): Treatment of NSAID induced ulcer, Maintains ductus arteriosus
- PGF 2alpha (Latanoprost): Treatment of glaucoma

Thromboxanes

- Platelet aggregator

Actions of Prostaglandins

- PGE_1/PGI_2: Vasodilation, inhibition of platelet aggregation
- PGE_2: Vasodilation, bronchodilation, uterine contraction

- PGF_2 alpha: Uterine contraction, bronchoconstriction, vasoconstriction
- TXA_2: Vasoconstriction, bronchoconstriction, platelet aggregation

Uses of prostaglandin drugs

- PGE_1 (Alprostadil): Causes vasodilation, Useful in erectile dysfunction
- PGE_1 analogue (Misoprostol): Gastric cytoprotection, Useful in preventing peptic ulcers caused due to NSAIDS
- PGE_2 (Dinoprostone): Causes contraction of uterus, Useful as abortifacient, cervical ripening

NSAIDS

- Aspirin inhibits: Cox inhibitor (irreversible)
- Selective Cox2 inhibitor (they lack anti-platelet actions): Coxibs i.e. Lumiracoxib, valdecoxib
- Preferential Cox2 inhibitors: Nimesulide, Nabumetone
- NSAID with good tissue penetration: Diclofenac
- NSAID with good concentration in synovial fluid: Ketorolac
- Drug used in acetaminophen toxicity: N-acetyl cysteine

KETOROLAC

- Non-narcotic
- Non-steroidal
- Acts on opioid receptors

THIAZIDES

- Mechanism of action of thiazides: Inhibit Na+/Cl- transporter n DCT
- Side effects of thiazides (chlorothiazide, indapamide): Hyperglycemia, Hypercalcemia
- Thiazides are used in the treatment of hypercalciuria but they themselves cause hypercalcemia & renal calculi

LOOP DIURETCIS

- MOA of loop/ high ceiling diuretics (frusemide, ethacrynic acid): Inhibit Na+/ K+/ 2Cl- transporter on thick ascending limb of loop of Henle
- Frusemide is a: Sulfamoyl derivative
- Uses of frusemide:
  - o DOC for acute hypercalcemia
  - o Acute pulmonary edema (2nd DOC after morphine)
- Side effects of frusemide:
  - o Hyperuricemia
  - o Hypocalcemia
  - o Hyperlipidemia
- Main side effect of ethacrynic acid: Ototoxicity

POTASSIUM SPARING DIURETIC

- They (spironolactone, triamterene) act on: Distal tubule & collecting duct
- Spironolactone antagonizes the (sodium retaining) effect of: Aldosterone
- Active metabolite of spironolactone is: Canrenone
- Side effects of spironolactone:
  - o Fatal hyperkalemia (particularly when administered with other potassium sparing diuretics)
  - o Gynaecomastia

MANNITOL

- MOA of Mannitol: Increases blood viscosity, Increases perfusion
- C/I of mannitol:
  - o Acute tubular necrosis
  - o Anuria
  - o Pulmonary edema

Drugs for raised intracranial tension

- Intravenous mannitol
- Frusemide

DOC for diabetes insipidus

- Desmopressin (intranasally)

DOC for SIADH

- Demeclocycline

BIGUANIDE

- Effects of metformin (biguanide) on glucose metabolism:
    - o Increased glycolysis
    - o Decreased gluconeogenesis
- Feared complication of metformin: Lactic acidosis
- Metformin is C/I in: Renal failure
- Special features of metformin:
    - o It does not cause weight gain (so particularly used in obesity
    - o Obesity is NOT a C/I)

ALPHA GLUCOSIDASE INHIBITOR

- MOA of Acarbose & Miglitol (alpha glucosidase/ starch inhibitor):
    - o Decreases progression of impaired glucose tolerance to overt disease
    - o Reduces fibrinogen level also
- Special features of Acarbose & Miglitol:
    - o They are euglycemics
    - o They do not cause hypoglycemia

SULFONYLUREA

- Features of hypoglycemia seen with sulfonylureas (tolbutamide):
    - o Severe
    - o Prolonged for days
    - o Fatal (elderly & in heart failure)

PIOGLITAZONE

- Effects of Pioglitazone (thiazo-lidine-diones) are:
    - o Acts by binding to PPARs (peroxisome proliferator activator receptors)
    - o Increases insulin sensitivity

REMEMBER

- Oral hypoglycemic agent causing cholestatic jaundice: Chlorpropamide

INSULIN

- t1/2 of Insulin: 5 minutes
- Effect of Insulin on potassium: Promotes entry of potassium into the cell
- Difference between human & pork insulin: Human insulin differs from pork insulin by 1 amino acid
- Humulin is: Human insulin

Rapid acting insulin

- Insulin aspartate
- Lispro insulin
- Insulin glulisine

Long acting insulin

- Insulin glargine

Intermediate acting insulin

- Lente/Insulin – zinc suspension (7 Ultra Lente + 3 Semilente): 20- 24 hours
- NPH- Neutral Protamine Hagedorn/ Isophane: 20-24 hours

CORTICOIDS

- Maximum mineralo-corticoid activity is shown by: Aldosterone
- Maximum gluco-corticoid activity is shown by: Dexamethasone
- Androgen receptor blocker is: Cyproterone
- Anti-estrogen drug is: Clomiphene
- MOA of tamoxifen:
    - o Oral selective estrogen receptor modulator
    - o Decreases FSH
- Agents used for Ca breast:
    - o Tamoxifen

- o Exemestane
- o Letrozole (aromatase inhibitor)
- S/E of danazol are:
  - o Acne
  - o Weight gain
  - o Occasionally hot flushes

FLUTAMIDE

- Flutamide & nilutamide are: Anti-androgens
- Use of flutamide:
  - o Metastatic prostate cancer

FINASTERIDE

- MOA of finasteride is: Selective 5 alpha reductase type-1 inhibitor
- Use of finasteride:
  - o BHP

THEOPHYLLINE

- MOA of theophylline & doxophylline:
  - o Inhibits phospho-di-esterase 4 (PDE4)
  - o Increases cAMP concentration
  - o Blocks adenosine receptors
  - o Beta2 agonist
  - o Stimulator of mucociliary movement
- Factors decreasing theophylline levels:
  - o Smoking
  - o Microsomal enzyme inducers
- Factors which increase plasma levels of theophylline:
  - o Erythromycin
  - o Ciprofloxacin
  - o Cimetidine

MONTELEUKAST

- MOA of Montelukast (leukotriene receptor antagonist/ LTRA):
  - o CysLT1 antagonist
  - o Blocks action of leukotriene D4 on the cysteinyl leukotriene receptor (CysLT1) in the lungs
- Uses of montelukast:
  - o Used in maintenance therapy of asthma
  - o Relief of seasonal allergies
  - o NOT useful in acute attacks

STEROIDS

- Steroids in asthma (NO role in acute attacks/ status asthmaticus) act by:
  - o Anti-inflammatory/ reduce airway inflammation
  - o Increase lipocortin levels
  - o Blocks phospholipid breakdown
- Commonly used steroids in asthma:
  - o Budesonide
  - o Fluticasone
  - o Triamcinolone
- S/E of inhaled steroids: Oropharyngeal candidiasis
- S/E of topical steroids: Glaucoma
- S/E of parenteral steroids: Posterior subcapsular cataract

Remember

- MOA of sodium cromoglycate (used for prophylaxis): Inhibitor of mast cell degranulation
- Zafirlukast (LTRA) is taken: Once daily
- Zileuton inhibits: 5 Lipo-oxygenase
- Anticholinergic bronchodilators:
  - o Ipratropium
  - o Tiotropium

Antidotes of some drug poisonings

Antidotes	*For poisoning of*
N-acetyl cysteine	Phenacetin/ paracetamol
Diphenhydramine	Promethazine
Promethazine	Phenothiazines
Heparin	Ergotamine & EACA

Glucagon	Beta-blockers
Ethyl alcohol	Methyl alcohol, ethylene glycol
EDTA	Lead (acute & chronic)
Dimercaprol	Arsenic, gold, copper, mercury
Cobalt edetate	Cyanide
Calcium gluconate	Fluoride poisoning
Benztropine	Extra-pyramidal symptoms
Arginine or ammonium chloride forced diuresis	Phencyclidine

ANTIMICROBIAL DRUGS

Mechanism of action

- Drugs which inhibit cross-linking (transpeptidases) & impair cell wall synthesis:
  - o Penicillins
  - o Cephalosporins
  - o Vancomycin
  - o Imipenem
  - o Aztreonam
- Drugs binding to 30s ribosomal unit & inhibiting protein synthesis:
  - o Aminoglycosides
  - o Tetracyclines
- MOA of sulfonamides & trimethoprim: Inhibits nucleotide synthesis of tetra-hydro-folate
- MOA of Amphotericin B: Disrupts fungal cell membrane by binding to ergosterol
- MOA of quinolones: Blocks DNA topo-isomerases

PENICILLIN

- Penicillinase-resistant (resist degradation by staphylococcal penicillinase) drugs:
  - o Methicillin (acid labile)
  - o Cloxacillin
- Quinupristin & Dalfopristin are used in (bacteriostatic): Vancomycin resistant enterococcus faecium (VREF)
- Imipenem is inhibited by: Dehydropeptidase (hence given along with cilastatin)
- Special features of aztreonam: Can be safely used in patients allergic to penicillin & related group of drugs (because of lack of cross reactivity)
- Linezolid is used in:
  - o Methicillin-resistant Staphylococcus aureus (MRSA)
  - o No effect on gram negative bacteria

Procaine penicillin

- Plasma concentration is more
- Painless injection
- Small dose 0.5-1 MU
- Short duration of action
- Allergic phenomenon common
- Can be fortified with aqueous penicillin G

Benzathine penicillin

- Plasma concentration is less, so only prophylactic use
- Painful injection
- Allergic phenomenon not common
- Large dose 0.6-2.4 MU
- Very long duration of action
- Not fortified with aqueous penicillin G

VANCOMYCIN

- Glycopeptides antibiotics include:
  - o Vancomycin
  - o Teicoplanin
- S/E of vancomycin: Red man syndrome
- DOC for MRSA infection: Vancomycin
- Drug used for pseudomembranous colitis: Vancomycin

CLINDAMYCIN

- MOA of clindamycin: Binds to 50s ribosomal subunit & inhibits protein subunit
- Drug implicated in pseudomembranous colitis: Clindamycin

CEPHALOSPORIN

- Cephalosporin effective against gram negative entero-bacteriaceae (3rd generation):
  - o Cefoperazone (anti-pseudomonal activity)
  - o Cefixime
- 4th generation cephalosporin:
  - o Cefepime
  - o Cefpirome

1st Generation Cephalosporins

- Parenteral: Cefazolin
- Oral: Cephalexin, Cephradine, Cefadroxil

2nd Generation Cephalosporins

- Parenteral: Cefuroxime
- Oral: Cefaclor, Cefuroxime axetil

3rd Generation Cephalosporins

- Parenteral: Cefotaxime, Ceftizoxime, Ceftriaxone, Ceftazidime, Cefoperazone
- Oral: Cefixime, Cefpodoxime proxetil, Cefdinir, Ceftibuten

4th Generation Cephalosporins

- Parenteral: Cefepime

MACROLIDES

- Azithromycin is effective against:
  - o Chylamydia
  - o Mycoplasma
  - o Ureaplasma
  - o Legionella
- Macrolides cause GIT distress as they stimulate: Motilin receptors
- Drug used in penicillin allergies: Erythromycin

TETRACYCLINE

- MOA of tetracycline: They bind to 30s ribosomal subunit
- Complication arising due to use of outdated tetracycline: Fanconi's syndrome
- S/E of doxycycline: Photo-dermatitis
- Tetracycline group drug causing pigmentation: Minocycline
- S/E of tetracycline:
  - o Teratogenic
  - o Super-infections
  - o Tooth discoloration

CHLORAMPHENICOL

- MOA of chloramphenicol: Binds to 50s subunit & blocks elongation of peptide chain

AMINOGLYCOSIDE

- MOA of aminoglycosides:
  - o Inhibits translation
  - o Bactericidal
  - o Distributed only extracellularly
- Framycetin, sisomicin belong to: Aminoglycosides
- Streptomycin is used in: Plague/ tularemia
- S/E of aminoglycosides:
  - o Teratogenic
  - o Ototoxic
  - o Vestibulotoxic
  - o Nephrotoxic
  - o Causes neuromuscular blockade (should not be used in myasthenia gravis)
- One of the most resistant aminoglycoside to bacterial inactivating enzyme: Amikacin

FLUOROQUINOLONE

- Longest acting quinolone: Sparfloxacin
- Most phototoxic quinolone: Sparfloxacin
- Quinolone is avoided in: Children (causes arthropathy)

DRUG OF CHOICE

- DOC in cholera: Doxycycline

- DOC in toxoplasmosis: Cotrimoxazole
- DOC in MRSA: Vancomycin
- DOC in syphilis: Penicillin G
- DOC in legionella: Azithromycin/ Levofloxacin
- DOC in LGV: Azithromycin
- DOC in gonorrhea: Ceftriaxone
- DOC in P. carinii: Cotrimoxazole
- DOC in actinomycosis: Penicillin-G
- DOC in plague: Streptomycin
- DOC in kala-azar: Pentamidine
- Oral drug for kala-azar: Miltefosine

CHEMOPROPHYLACTIC AGENT OF CHOICE

- Chemoprophylactic agent for cholera: Tetracycline
- Chemoprophylactic agent for Rheumatic fever: Benzathine penicillin

Pathogenic agents & Chemoprophylaxis

- Streptococci: Penicillin
- Neisseria meningitides: Rifampicin /Ciprofloxacin
- Clostridium perfringens: Metronidazole
- Clostridium tetani: Penicillin
- Yersinia pestis (Plague): Tetracycline/ Cotrimoxazole
- Bordetella pertussis (whooping cough): Erythromycin
- Mycobacterium tuberculosis: Isoniazid and Rifampicin
- Leptospira: Doxycycline

ANTI-MALARIAL

- Drug used for chloroquine resistant malaria: Mefloquine
- Halofantrine is effective against: Chloroquine resistant plasmodium falciparum & plasmodium vivax
- Lumefantrine & pyronaridine act as: Antimalarial
- S/E of chloroquine:
  - o Retinal toxicity
  - o Corneal deposits
  - o Blurred vision
  - o Pigmentary bulls eye retinopathy
  - o Myopathy

Chemoprophylaxis of vivax and Chloroquine *sensitive* falciparum malaria

- Chloroquine 300 mg of base once Weekly, started one week before exposure and continued for 4 weeks after returning

Chemoprophylaxis of chloroquine *resistant* falciparum malaria

- Mefloquine 250 mg base once weekly.

PRIMAQUINE

- Primaquine is effective for: Radical cure of plasmodium vivax
- Primaquine is ineffective against: Plasmodium falciparum
- S/E of primaquine: Hemolysis in G6PD deficiency

QUININE

- DOC for cerebral malaria: Quinine
- S/E of quinine: Hypoglycemia
- Special feature of quinine: Can be given safely in pregnancy (chloroquine can also be given in pregnancy)

KETOCONAZOLE

- MOA of ketoconazole:
  - o Inhibits fungal lanosterol 14-demethylase
  - o Impairing ergosterol synthesis

AMPHOTERICIN B

- MOA of amphotericin B: Forms micropores in fungal cell membrane (it has affinity for ergosterol)
- Amphotericin B intravenously, is given along with: Glucose solution
- S/E of amphotericin B: Hypokalemia
- Parenteral amphotericin B is indicated in the treatment of:

- o Cryptococcosis (caused by cryptococcus neoformans C)
- o Fungal septicemia
- o Cryptococcal meningitis (cryptococcus neoformans)

ANTI-VIRAL

- Antiviral more active against CMV: Ganciclovir
- Structurally idoxuridine is:
  - o Thymidine analogue
  - o Cannot be given orally

Viral Condition & Drug of choice

- H. simplex encephalitis: Acyclovir
- Neonatal herpes simplex: Acyclovir
- Herpes simplex keratitis: Trifluridine/ Vidarabine
- Herpes simplex oro-labialis: Penciclovir

ANTI-HIV

- Abacavir belongs to: Nucleoside reverse transcriptase inhibitors
- Nevirapine & Efavirenz belong to: Non-nucleoside reverse transcriptase inhibitor
- Saquinavir & Nelfinavir belong to: Protease inhibitor
- Peripheral neuropathy is commoner with:
  - o Stavudine
  - o Didanosine
  - o Zalcitabine
- S/E of zidovudine:
  - o Myelosuppression
  - o Megaloblastic anemia
- S/E of didanosine: Pancreatitis

ART

- Nucleotide RTI**:** AZT, Lamivudine, Abacavir
- Non NRTI: Nevirapine
- Nucleotide analogue: Tenofovir
- Protease inhibitor: Indinavir
- Fusion inhibitor: Enfuvirtide

ANTI-TUBERCULAR

- Tuberculocidal anti-TB drugs:
  - o INH
  - o Rifampicin
  - o Pyrazinamide
  - o Streptomycin

Most effective drug for specific populations of M. tuberculosis

- Spurters: Rifampicin
- Dormant: No drug is effective
- Rapid growers: Isoniazid
- Slow growing: Pyrazinamide

INH

- MOA of Isoniazid/ INH: Inhibits mycolic acid synthesis
- S/E of INH:
  - o Peripheral neuritis (common in slow acetylator)
  - o Hepatotoxicity (common in elderly & alcoholics; rare in children)
- Anti-TB drug showing maximum resistance in India: INH
- Special features about activity of INH:
  - o Bacteriostatic against resting bacilli
  - o Bactericidal against rapidly multiplying organism (both intracellularly & extracellularly)
- INH associated hepatitis is more with:
  - o Daily alcohol consumption
  - o Concomitant rifampin administration
  - o Slow INH acetylators
- Treatment of INH related peripheral neuritis:
  - o Peripheral neuritis with INH administration is due to interference with pyridoxine (vitamin B6) metabolism.

- So 10-50 mg of pyridoxine is to be administered daily

RIFAMPICIN

- S/E of rifampicin:
  - Respiratory syndrome
  - Abdominal syndrome
  - Flu like syndrome
  - Cutaneous syndrome

Adverse reactions of Rifampicin

- Cutaneous syndrome – chills, fever, headache
- Abdominal syndrome – nausea, vomiting, abdominal cramps
- Hepatitis
- Respiratory syndrome – breathlessness

Remember

- S/E of ethambutol: Retrobulbar optic neuritis

PYRAZINAMIDE

- S/E of pyrazinamide:
  - Hepatotoxicity
  - Hyperuricemia
  - Hyperglycemia
- Pyrazinamide is used for: Short course therapy for TB
- Special feature of pyrazinamide: Levels in CSF are high
- MOA of pyrazinamide: Similar to INH (inhibition of mycolic acid cell wall synthesis), but intracellular action

ANTI-LEPROTIC

- Most rapidly acting drug against leprosy bacillus: Rifampicin
- Most potent drug against leprosy bacillus: Rifampicin
- S/E of clofazimine:
  - Reddish black discoloration of skin
  - Acneiform eruptions

Treatment of Paucibacillary leprosy

- Rifampicin 600 mg monthly and Dapsone 100 mg daily
- Treatment for 6 months
- Follow up for 2 years

Treatment of Multibacillary leprosy

- Rifampicin 600 mg and Clofazimine 300 mg monthly
- Dapsone 100 mg and Clofazimine 50 mg daily
- Treatment for 2 years
- Follow up for 5 years

DAPSONE

- DOC for leprosy: Dapsone
- S/E of dapsone: Hemolysis in G6PD deficient

ANTI-PARASITIC DRUGS

Drug of choice

- DOC for cysticercosis/ Taenia solium: Praziquantel
- DOC for dracunculiasis: Metronidazole

ANTIHYPERTENSIVES

- Beta blockers are used in:
  - Angina
  - Migraine prophylaxis
  - Hypertension
- Angiotensin receptor blockers (losartan) have utility & tolerability similar to ACE inhibitors EXCEPT: They do not cause cough/ angioedema

Arteriolar dilators

- Hydralazine
- Minoxidil
- Calcium channel openers

Venodilators

- Nitrates

- Glyceryl trinitrate
- Isosorbide dinitrate

Mixed dilators

- ACE inhibitors
- Losartan
- Prazosin
- Phentolamine
- Nitroprusside

ACE INHIBITORS

- ACE inhibitors cause cough because of: Bradykinin
- C/I of ACE inhibitors:
  - Patients with single kidney
  - Bilateral renal artery stenosis
  - Pregnancy
  - Pheochromocytoma

NITROPRUSSIDE

- DOC for malignant hypertension: Nitroprusside (as it dilates both arterioles & veins)
- Special features of nitroprusside:
  - Increase guanylate cyclase
  - No central effects
  - Raised nitric oxide level with nitrates & hydralazine co-administration

REMEMBER

- Special feature of Diazoxide: Inhibits labour
- Special feature of hydralazine: Causes drug induced lupus
- MOA of minoxidil: Potassium channel opener
- DOC for hypertension in pregnancy: Methyldopa
- DOC for hypertensive crisis in pregnancy: Hydralazine
- Anti-hypertensive's absolutely C/I in pregnancy: ACE inhibitors
- Drugs associated with prolonged QT syndrome/ Torsades de pointes:
  - Quinidine
  - Cisapride
  - Procainamide etc.

ANTI-ARRYTHMIC DRUGS

- Lignocaine is classified as: Class Ib antiarrhythmic
- Potassium channel blockers are classified as: Class III antiarrhythmic agents

Drug of choice

- DOC for ventricular arrhythmias: Lidocaine
- DOC for PSVT: Adenosine
- DOC for WPW syndrome: Procainamide

DRUGS USED IN HEART FAILURE

- DOC in acute heart failure: Frusemide
- Special features of nesiritide
  - Recombinant brain natriuretic peptide (BNP)
  - Has shorter half life

DIGOXIN

- Therapeutic level of digoxin: 0.5 to 1.5 ng/ml
- Toxic level of digoxin: More than 2.4 ng/ml
- MOA of digoxin:
  - Inhibits Na+/K+ ATPase
  - Increases ventricular contractile force
- Route of excretion of digoxin: Kidneys
- C/I of digoxin: HOCM
- Digoxin toxicity consists of:
  - Hypokalemia (classical finding)
  - Hypomagnesemia

NITRATES

- Effects of nitrates on CVS physiology:

- Decrease preload & afterload
- Decrease myocardial oxygen consumption

- S/E of nitrates:
  - Reflex tachycardia
  - Hypotension
- Long acting nitrates are NOT used chronically as: Tolerance develops (due to –SH group)

HYPOLIPIDEMIC DRUGS

- MOA of Statins: HMG CoA reductase inhibition
- MOA of Niacin:
  - Raises HDL level
  - Lowers triglycerides & LDL level

Hypolipidemic drug & Mechanism of action

- Statins: Decrease cholesterol synthesis by inhibition of rate Limiting HMG-CoA reductase
- Bile acid Sequestrants: Decrease bile acid absorption, increased hepatic conversion of cholesterol to bile acids
- Fibric acid derivatives, Gemfibrozil: Increased activity of lipoprotein lipase, Decreased release of fatty acids from adipose tissue
- Nicotinic acid: Decreases production of VLDL, Decrease lipolysis in adipocytes

DRUGS ACTING ON GIT

- Proton pump inhibitor with an additional enzyme inhibiting activity: Omeprazole
- Ulcer protective drug is: Sucralfate

CANCER CHEMOTHERAPY

- Uses of cetuximab: Acts against epidermal growth factor receptor (EGFR) positive colorectal cancer (as a single agent)
- Trastu-zumab/ Herceptin is used for: Breast Ca
- Drug used in CML & GIST (gastro-intestinal stromal tumours): Imatinib (tyrosine kinase inhibitor)

HEPARIN

- Structurally, heparin is a: Polysaccharide
- S/E of heparin:
  - Osteoporosis
  - Hyperkalemia
- Drug used in heparin overdose: Protamine sulphate
- Anticoagulant of choice in HIT (heparin induced thrombocytopenia) is: Argatroban
- Anticoagulant of choice in pregnancy is: Heparin

WARFARIN

- Warfarin inhibits: Vitamin K dependent clotting factors (2,7,9,10)
- Warfarin induced skin necrosis is due to: Protein C deficiency
- Monitoring of warfarin is done by: INR

GOUT

- Drugs used in acute gout:
  - NSAIDs
  - Colchicine
  - Steroids
- Uricosuric drugs are:
  - Probenecid
  - Sulfinpyrazone

ALLOPURINOL

- Allopurinol inhibits: Xanthine oxidase
- DOC in chronic gout: Allopurinol

COLCHICINE

- MOA of colchicine: Inhibits microtubule polymerization & stabilizes tubulins in microtubules
- Special feature of colchicine: Neither analgesic nor anti-inflammatory
- MC S/E of colchicine: Bloody diarrhea

Drugs & neurotoxicity

Drugs	*Toxicity*
Hypervitaminosis A, oral contraceptives, tetracyclines, glucocorticoids, amiodarone	**Pseudo-tumour cerebri**
Polymyxins, aminoglycosides	**Exacerbate myasthenia gravis**

DRUGS ACTING ON CNS

- TCA:
  - Amitriptyline
  - Clomipramine
- Tetracyclic antidepressants (second generation): Maprotiline
- SSRI's: Fluoxetine
- Extra-pyramidal side effects are:
  - Parkinsonism (responds to levo-dopa)
  - Akathisia (severe restlessness)
  - Tardive dyskinesia
  - Acute dystonia

TCA

- Early features of overdose of TCA manifests as: Anticholinergic activity (dry mouth, dilated pupils, sinus tachycardia, blurred vision)
- Akathisia (restlessness) is commonly caused by:
  - Haloperidol
  - May respond to beta blockers (propranolol)

CLOZAPINE

- Most serious adverse effect of clozapine: Agranulocytosis
- Extrapyramidal side-effects are rare with: Clozapine

CARBAMAZEPINE

- Apart from epilepsy, carbamazepine is also indicated in:
  - Maniac depressive psychosis
  - Trigeminal neuralgia
  - Atypical pain syndromes
- S/E of carbamazepine: Increased ADH secretion (hyponatremia)

Mechanism of action of antiepileptics

- Phenytoin, Carbamazepine, Lamotrigine, valproate: Prolongation of Na+ channel inactivation
- Barbiturates, benzodiazepines, Vigabatrin, gabapentin, valproate: Facilitation of GABA mediated Chloride channel opening
- Ethosuximide, Trimethadione, Valproate: Inhibition of T type of Calcium current

REMEMBER

- Bromocriptine is a: Dopamine agonists
- Tolcapone is a: Catechol-O-Methyl Transferase/ COMT inhibitor
- S/E of phenytoin:
  - Gum hypertrophy
  - Hydantoin syndrome
  - Cerebellar atrophy
  - Megaloblastic anemia
  - Lymphoma
  - CNS depression

Drug of choice

- DOC for myoclonic epilepsy: Valproate
- DOC for partial seizures: Carbamazepine

AMIODARONE

- S/E of amiodarone:
  - Pulmonary fibrosis
  - Hyperuricemia
  - Hypothyroidism/ hyperthyroidism

CYCLOSPORIN

- MOA of cyclosporin (immunosuppressant): Decreases clonal proliferation of T-cells by reducing IL-2 release
- Cyclosporin acts on: CD4 + T-cells
- S/E of cyclosporin:
  - Nephrotoxicity

- o Hypertension
- o Hyperkalemia
- o Hypertrichosis
- o Tremors

TACROLIMUS

- MOA of Tacrolimus:
  - o Inhibits IL-2 (same as cyclosporin)
  - o Acts mainly on T-cells
- Tacrolimus belongs to: Macrolide antibiotic
- Use of tacrolimus: Organ transplantation
- S/E of tacrolimus:
  - o Glucose intolerance
  - o Nephrotoxicity

BROMOCRIPTINE

- Bromocriptine inhibits: Prolactin secretion
- Bromocriptine is indicated in:
  - o Galactorrhea (due to hyperprolactinemia)
  - o Infertility (due to hyperprolactinemia)
  - o In acromegaly
  - o Idiopathic/ post-encephalitic parkinsonism (along with levo-dopa/ carbi-dopa)

OCTREOTIDE

- Octreotide is used in:
  - o Varices/ esophageal bleeding
  - o May be used in AIDS patients with secretory diarrhea (who have failed to respond to antimicrobial or antimotility agents)

PROPYL-THIOURACIL

- Less potent
- Safe in pregnancy
- t½ 1-2 hr.
- No active metabolites
- Peripheral conversion of t4→t3 prevented
- Useful in thyroid storm

Drugs & inhibitors of their metabolism

Drugs	*Metabolism inhibited by*
Warfarin, quinidine, nifedipine, lidocaine, theophylline, phenytoin	**Cimetidine**
Cyclosporin, warfarin, carbamazepine, triazolam, theophylline	**Erythromycin**
Phenytoin, tolbutamide	**Clofibrate**
Warfarin	**Excess alcohol**
Phenytoin	**Isoniazid**
Cyclosporine	**Ketoconazole**
Warfarin	**Metronidazole**
Warfarin, phenytoin, tolbutamide	**Phenylbutazone**
Prednisolone	**Cyclosporine**
Azathioprine, 6-mercaptopurine	**Allopurinol**

CLINICAL QUESTIONS

1. **A young male with urinary tract infection was given some antimicrobial agent. This agent has the tendency of causing arthropathy in children and causing tendon rupture. What is the mechanism of this antimicrobial drug given to the patient?**

   A. DNA gyrase inhibitor

   B. DHFRase inhibitor

   C. Inhibition of synthesis of mycolic acid in bacterial cell wall

   D. Inhibition of protein synthesis

   The drug discussed in the question is ciprofloxacin (prototype of fluoroquinolones/ FQ).

   Tendinitis and tendon rupture is one important adverse effect of ciprofloxacin.

   Risk of tendon damage is higher in patients above 60 years of age and in those receiving corticosteroids.

   The FQ should be stopped at the first sign of tendinitis.

   On the basis of the finding that administered to immature pups, ciprofloxacin (and other FQ) caused cartilage damage in weight bearing joints, the FQs were contraindicated in children.

   The FQs inhibit the enzyme bacterial DNA gyrase (primarily active in gram negative bacteria), which nicks double stranded DNA, introduces negative supercoils and the reseals the nicked end.

   This is necessary to prevent excessive positive supercoiling of the strands when they separate to permit replication or transcription.

   Answer: A i.e., DNA gyrase inhibitor

2. **A young patient consumed 8 tablets of 0.25 mg of Digoxin and developed features of digoxin toxicity. His heart rate was 55 beats/ minute and ECG showed third degree AV block. Such a patient is best managed by:**

   A. Phenytoin

   B. DC shock

   C. Digoxin Fab fragment

   D. Lidocaine

   For AV block and bradycardia caused due to digoxin toxicity, atropine 0.6-1.2 mg i.m. may help; otherwise, cardiac pacing is recommended. But these options are not there in the question.

   Digoxin antibody was developed for measuring plasma concentration of digoxin by radioimmunoassay, it has been found effective in treating toxicity as well.

   Digoxin specific antibody cross-reacts with digitoxin also.

   The Fab fragment has been marketed in Europe as DIGIBIND.

   Cardioversion by DC shock is contraindicated in digitalis toxicity because severe conduction defects may be unmasked in the digitalis intoxicated heart.

   Answer: C i.e., Digoxin Fab fragment

3. **A known case of depressive illness consumed large number of TCA tablets and presented to the Emergency department with altered sensorium, dryness of mouth, sweating, postural hypotension and urinary retention. ECG was done which showed wide QRS complex. Important step in management of such a patient:**

   A. DC cardioversion
   B. Sodium bicarbonate
   C. Lidocaine
   D. Adenosine

   Treatment of TCA side effects is primarily supportive with gastric lavage, respiratory assistance, fluid infusion, maintenance of BP and body temperature.

   Acidosis must be corrected by bicarbonate infusion.

   Diazepam may be injected to control convulsions and delirium.

   Most important is the treatment of cardiac arrhythmias, for which propranolol/ lidocaine may be used.

   This seems a controversial question as both sodium bicarbonate and lidocaine are used in TCA overdose, but since arrhythmias may be responsible for sudden death in these patients, so administration of antiarrhythmic is an important step in management.

   Also, correction of acidosis will automatically correct arrhythmias.

   Answer: B i.e., Sodium bicarbonate

4. **A female suffering from carcinoma of ovary was started on Cisplatin. Later on, she presented to the Emergency department with the complaints of several episodes of vomiting. She was given some anti-emetic drug, which resulted in the development of muscle dystonia. Which anti-emetic drug was probably given?**

A. Ondansetron B. Metoclopramide

C. Scopolamine D. Domperidone

Clinical presentation is suggestive of intake of metoclopramide.

Metoclopramide is generally well tolerated.

Sedation, dizziness, loose stools, muscle dystonias (especially in children) are the main side effects.

Long-term use can cause parkinsonism, galactorrhoea and gynecomastia, but it should not be used to augment lactation.

Answer: B i.e., Metoclopramide

5. **A 50 years old male who was recently diagnosed as pulmonary TB, was started on ATT. Later on, he presented with the complaints of tingling and numbness over fingers. He is also a chronic alcoholic. This patient should be managed by starting:**

A. Vitamin B_1 B. Vitamin B_3

C. Vitamin B_6 D. Vitamin B_{12}

Clinical presentation is indicative of INH associated neurotoxicity.

INH is well tolerated by most of the patients.

Peripheral neuritis and a variety of neurological manifestations (paresthesias, numbness, mental disturbances, rarely convulsions) are the most important dose-dependent toxic effects.

These are due to interference with production of the active coenzyme pyridoxal phosphate from pyridoxine, and its increased excretion in urine.

Pyridoxine given prophylactically (10 mg/ day) prevents the neurotoxicity even with higher doses.

Prophylactic pyridoxine must be given to diabetics, chronic alcoholics, malnourished, pregnant, lactating and HIV infected persons, but routine used is not mandatory.

INH neurotoxicity is treated by pyridoxine 100 mg/ day (in the given question).

Answer: C i.e., Vitamin B_6

6. **A known case of COPD was started on I/V theophylline after which he developed diuresis. Such an action of theophylline is mediated through which receptors:**

A. Phosphodiesterase receptor

B. Adenosine receptor

C. Beta-1 adrenergic receptor

D. Beta-2 adrenergic receptor

Theophylline increased urine output in diuretic-dependent critically ill children and the diuretic effect may have been potentiated by concurrent use of dopamine.

Adenosine receptor antagonism may be a more likely mechanism for the diuretic effect of theophylline than phosphodiesterase inhibition.

Answer: B i.e., Adenosine receptor

7. **A patient on anti-tubercular drug therapy developed tingling sensation on lower limb. Which of the following drug should be used for management?**

A. Thiamine B. Folic acid

C. Pyridoxine D. Vitamin B_{12}

Isoniazid/ INH interferes with the utilization of pyridoxine and increases its urinary excretion, causing pyridoxine deficiency, which manifests as peripheral neuritis and variety of neurological manifestations (paraesthesias, numbness, mental disturbances), accounting for most important dose dependent toxic effects of INH.

Answer: C i.e., Pyridoxine

8. **An obese diabetic patient was on Metformin monotherapy, but his sugar levels were not well controlled. He is allergic to sulpha drugs and does not comply to injectables. He has history of pancreatitis and family history of bladder carcinoma. In view of the raised glucose levels, which others anti-diabetic drug should be added?**

A. Liraglutide B. Sitagliptin
C. Canagliflozin D. Pioglitazone

Practically all the glucose filtered at the glomerulus is reabsorbed in the proximal tubules.

The major transporter, which accomplishes this, is SGLT2, whose inhibition induces glucosuria and lowers blood glucose in type 2 DM, as well causes weight loss.

Members of this group are dapagliflozin and canagliflozin.

Answer: C i.e., Canagliflozin

9. **A medical student presented with protracted vomiting. For this, he was given an anti-emetic following which he developed abnormal posturing. Which drug is responsible?**

A. Metoclopramide B. Ondansetron
C. Domperidone D. Pantoprazole

Extrapyramidal side effects of metoclopramide include dystonia.

This is because of blockade of central D2 receptors.

Answer: A i.e., Metoclopramide

10. **A patient with infertility was prescribed bromocriptine by the gynecologist. What could be the cause?**

A. Hypogonadotropic hypogonadism
B. Premature ovarian failure
C. Hyperprolactinemia
D. Polycystic ovarian syndrome

Bromocriptine and Cabergoline are the first line of drug for most cases of hyperprolactinemia (due to microprolactinoma) presenting as galactorrhoea, amenorrhoea and infertility in women; gynecomastia, impotence and sterility in men.

Answer: C i.e., Hyperprolactinemia

11. **A patient is on indinavir, lamivudine and ketoconazole. He developed breast hypertrophy, nephrolithiasis, hyperlipidemia and central obesity. Identify the drug responsible drug:**

A. Lamivudine B. Indinavir
C. Ketoconazole D. Nevirapine

Adverse effects of indinavir include nephrolithiasis and cholelithiasis.

Answer: B i.e., Indinavir

12. **Manufacturer of a drug company labels that the drug contains 500 mg of paracetamol. On analysis, it was found to contain only 200 mg of drug. Such a drug is known as:**

A. Orphan drug B. Counterfeit drug
C. Spurious drug D. Unethical drug

A counterfeit medicine is one, which is deliberately and fraudulently mislabeled with respect to identity and/ or source. Counterfeiting can apply to both branded and generic products and counterfeit products and may include products with the correct ingredients, wrong ingredients, without active ingredients, with insufficient quantity of active ingredients or with fake packaging.

Answer: B i.e., Counterfeit drug

13. **A patient developed acute biliary colic for which an analgesic was given. However, this drug increased the severity of the pain. Which analgesic drug was administered?**

A. Nefopam B. Morphine
C. Diclofenac D. Paracetamol

Morphine can worsen the biliary colic as it causes spasm of sphincter of Oddi (biliary sphincter) and can cause acute rise in intra-biliary pressure. So, morphine should be used cautiously in patients with gall bladder and biliary tract dysfunction.

Answer: B i.e., Morphine

14. **A boy was planning to travel by a bus, but he is a known case of motion sickness. Which drug can be given to prevent an episode of motion sickness?**

A. Fexofenadine
B. Promethazine
C. Levocetirizine
D. Sumatriptan

Anticholinergic and H_1 antihistaminic drugs are more effective in motion sickness as vestibular apparatus send impulses to brain via cholinergic muscarinic and H_1 histaminic receptors. Among antihistaminics, first generation/ old antihistaminics (promethazine) are preferred over second-generation antihistaminics (Levocetirizine, fexofenadine etc.).

Answer: B i.e., Promethazine

15. A patient on lithium therapy developed hypertension. He was started on thiazides to control hypertension. After few days, he developed coarse tremors and other features indicating lithium toxicity. Most likely mechanism of such a toxicity:

A. Thiazides increase tubular reabsorption of lithium

B. Thiazides potentiated action of lithium

C. Thiazides inhibited metabolism of lithium

D. Thiazides and lithium acts on same receptors

Thiazides (diuretics) promote proximal tubular reabsorption of lithium, as they cause loss of sodium ions.

By promoting lithium reabsorption, thiazide may precipitate lithium toxicity.

Answer: A i.e., Thiazides increase tubular reabsorption of lithium

16. A known case of schizophrenia is responding well to haloperidol, but later on, he developed symptoms of parkinsonism. Drug of choice to treat this complication:

A. Anticholinergic B. Bromocriptine

C. Levodopa D. Tolcapone

Haloperidol has high tendency to cause extra-pyramidal effects (drug induced parkinsonism).

Central anti-cholinergics are the only effective drugs for this complication.

They act by reducing unbalanced cholinergic activity.

Answer: A i.e., Anticholinergic

17. Deficiency of which enzyme results in 5-fluoro-uracil induced mucositis, myelo-suppression and neuro-psychiatric manifestations:

A. CYP2D7

B. Dihydro-folate reductase

C. Tetra-hydro-folate reductase

D. Dihydro-pyrimidine dehydrogenase

Patients with dihydro-pyrimidine-dehydrogenase deficiency are at increased risk of developing 5-fluoro-uracil related toxicity as this enzyme is the rate limiting step (and initial step) in the breakdown of 5-fluoro-uracil.

Answer: D i.e., Dihydro-pyrimidine dehydrogenase

18. A known case of COPD and type II diabetes underwent a surgery. Post-operatively, he developed urinary retention. Drug used for short-term relief in such a patient:

A. Tamsulosin B. Bethanechol

C. Methacholine D. Atropine

Because of the presence of Chronic obstructive pulmonary disease, case of post-operative urinary retention should be managed with tamsulosin.

Post-operative urinary retention is better managed by bethanechol (M_3 muscarinic agonist) but it can result in bronchoconstriction as well because of stimulation of M_3 muscarinic receptors in respiratory system, so it is avoided in a patient with COPD.

Answer: A i.e., Tamsulosin

19. During surgery, a patient was administered a nicotinic receptor acting competitive neuromuscular blocker drug. Which drug is indicated to reverse the effect of this drug at the end of operation?

A. Carbachol B. Physostigmine

C. Neostigmine D. Suxamethonium

Neostigmine is the commonly used drug for reversal of non-depolarizing/ competitive neuromuscular drug (physostigmine can also be used) because it increases the concentration of acetylcholine by inhibiting its breakdown by the enzyme cholinesterase.

So, it antagonizes competitive blockers action.

Answer: C i.e., Neostigmine

20. A known case of rheumatoid arthritis was started on some drug, but he developed blurring of vision and corneal opacity after 2 years of use. Which drug was the patient taking?

A. Methotrexate B. Amiodarone

C. Chloroquine D. Sulfasalazine

Corneal deposits and visual loss are few commoner side effects of chloroquine/ CQ.

Prolonged use of CQ causes retinal damage (Bull's eye retinopathy) and may cause visual loss.

Answer: C i.e., Chloroquine

21. A known case of bipolar disorder was taking lithium since, 6 months. After keeping fast for few days, she developed seizures, coarse tremors, weakness of limbs and confusion. What investigation should be done?

A. MRI of brain

B. EEG

C. Estimation of serum lithium levels

D. Serum electrolytes estimation

Any factor which causes reduction in glomerular filtration rate/ GFR with cause lithium toxicity, which manifests as seizures, confusion, coarse tremors and weakness of limbs. Reduction in GFR may result from dehydration as seen in fasting conditions.

Answer: C i.e., Estimation of serum lithium levels

22. A patient developed tremors, rigidity, bradykinesia and sialorrhea on taking fluphenazine for few weeks. Such a patient is best managed by:

A. Haloperidol B. Trihexyphenidyl

C. Clozapine D. Atropine

Clinical presentation is suggestive of drug induced parkinsonism.

Fluphenazine use can cause drug induced parkinsonism which manifests as tremors, bradykinesia, excessive salivation (sialorrhoea) and rigidity.

Drug induced parkinsonism is best managed by central anticholinergics like benzhexol (trihexiphenidyl), benztropine etc.

Answer: B i.e., Trihexyphenidyl

23. A 50 years old male with renal failure under renal transplant surgery and was prescribed a nucleotide derivative. Which is the drug of therapeutic importance in this case?

A. Cytarabine B. Azathioprine

C. Methotrexate D. 5-fluorouracil

Azathioprine primarily suppresses cell mediated immunity (CMI) and is used mainly in auto-immune disease (rheumatoid arthritis, ulcerative colitis) as well as in organ transplantation.

Answer: B i.e., Azathioprine

24. A 54 years old chronic smoker, who use to smoke around 50 packs per year, presented with lesions suggestive of oral leukoplakia. Which drug can regress the lesions?

A. Alpha-tocopherol B. Isotretinoin

C. Beta-carotene D. Selenium

Isotretinoin causes dramatic improvement in acne.

It is also effective in the prevention and treatment of skin cancers.

Oral leukoplakia, actinic keratosis and other premalignant lesions can be treated, but benefit-risk ratio is not clear.

Answer: B i.e., Isotretinoin

25. A newborn is having cleft lip, cleft palate and inter-atrial septal defect. Mother took some drug during pregnancy. Which drug could it be?

A. Erythromycin B. Paracetamon

C. Chloroquine D. Isotretinoin

Isotretinoin is highly teratogenic; up to 25% exposed fetuses had birth defects – craniofacial, heart and CNS abnormalities (Accutane embryopathy).

Answer: D i.e., Isotretinoin

26. A patient who was given primaquine, developed dark coloured urine. Likely cause is:

A. Glcose-6-phosphatase deficiency

B. Glucose-6-phosphate-dehydrogenase deficiency

C. Galactose-6-phosphatase deficiency

D. Galactose-6-phosphate dehydrogenase deficiency

The most important toxic potential is dose related haemolysis, methemoglobinemia, tachypnea and cyanosis.

These are due to the oxidant property of primaquine.

Its metabolites are more potent in this regard.

However, in normal individual doses <60 mg (base) produces little haemolysis.

Those with G-6-PD deficiency are highly sensitive and haemolytic anemia can occur with 15-30 mg/ day.

Answer: B i.e., Glucose-6-phosphate-dehydrogenase deficiency

27. A girl on sulphonamides developed abdominal pain and presented to the emergency with seizures. Most likely diagnosis:

A. Acute intermittent porphyria

B. Congenital erythropoietic porphyria

C. Infectious mononucleosis

D. Anaphylaxis

Clinical presentation is suggestive of acute intermittent porphyria.

Drugs that lead to increased activity of the hepatic P450 system, such as phenobarbital, sulfonamides, estrogens, and alcohol, are associated with acute intermittent porphyria.

Answer: A i.e., Acute intermittent porphyria

CHAPTER 7

FORENSIC MEDICINE

RAPID REVISION NOTES

X-rays for age determination

Age	*Region to be X-rayed*
15-16 years	Elbow
16-17 years	Ankle
17-18 years	Upper end of femur
18-19 years	Knee
17-19 years	Shoulder & wrist
20-50 years	Pubis
14-25 years	Sternum fusion takes place below upwards

INQUEST

- Investigation into cause of death (conducted in cases of murder, suicide, accidents & suspicious deaths):Inques
- Coroner's inquest was done in: Mumbai
- Commonest type on inquest done in India: Police inquest
- In case of death in lock-up, inquest is carried out by: Magistrate
- Written document issued by the court (served on the witness under a penalty in all cases by the police officer to attend the court for giving evidence on a particular day & time): Subpoena
- Fee paid to a witness at the time of serving summons (to cover the expenses for attending the court): Conduct money
- Telling lies by a witness under oath OR Failure to tell what he knows/ believes to be true: Perjury
- Mental ability to make a valid will: Testamentary capacity
- McNaughton's rule is for: Criminal responsibility
- Dying declaration: Written/ oral statement of a person, who is dying, due to some unlawful act, relating to his death
- Dying deposition: A magistrate records the statement, Has more legal value
- Punishment by a judicial magistrate of 1st class: 3 years imprisonment, Fine upto 5,000
- Punishment by a session court: Any sentence authorized by law, but death sentence must be confirmed by higher court
- In India, a death sentence can be commuted (exchange a penalty for a less severe one) by: President
- Amnesty (the formal act of liberating someone) for capital punishment vest (have power & authority) with: President

Types of inquest

- Police inquest
- Magistrate's Coroner's inquest
- Medical examiners inquest (Best system of inquest)

Magistrate's inquest is done in

- Prison death
- Police custody death
- Police firing death
- Dowry death
- Exhumation
- Police interrogation death

Dying deposition

- Recorded by magistrate
- Recorded under oath
- Presence of accused and it's lawyer necessary
- Superior

Dying declaration

- Recorded by magistrate or doctor
- No oath necessary
- Presence of accused and it's lawyer is not necessary
- Inferior

Type of consent

- Implied consent: When he conduct of the person indicated that he has given permission for the act to be done, without expression it verbally or in writing
- Expressed consent: When the person is asked for the consent for an act, then he expresses his consent
- Informed consent: Consent has been given after knowing all the pros and cons of the act for which the consent is being taken.

EXHUMATION

- Exhumation is done after a written order from: 1st class judicial magistrate
- It is conducted in: Day-light
- Maximum time limit for exhumation: NO time limit

IMPORTANT TERMS

- Expert witness: Person who is qualified/ experienced in a scientific/ technical subject (Doctor, Firearm expert, Finger print expert)
- Privileged communication: Statement communicated by a doctor to concerned authorities to protect the interests of community e.g. A person with some infectious disease working as a cook, A driver found to be colour blind, Syphilitic taking bath in a pool
- Novus actus interveniens: A doctor is responsible for his actions & also for its consequences e.g. A doctor leaving a scissor in the abdomen
- Professional negligence/ Malpraxis: It is the absence of reasonable care & skill or willful negligence on part of a doctor
- Therapeutic misadventure: Case in which a patient dies due to some unintentional act done by a doctor or hospital
- Corpus delicti: Elements of any criminal offence; body of offence, essence of crime
- Cephalic index: Determination of race, 70-75 in dolico-cephalic skull (aryans)
- Res ipsa loquitur: Evidence speaks for itself
- Respondent superior: An employer is responsible for the negligent acts of his employee, provided it is done under the direct supervision of the employer
- Res judicata: When a judgment delivered by a court of law in a particular Cases used as a precedent in another case of similar nature
- Compos mentis: Sound state of mind.
- Cheiloscopy / Figura linearum labiorum: Study of lip prints
- Poroscopy (Locard's method): Identification by examination of pores on the ridges of fingers and hands
- Dactylography (Henry- Galton system)/Dermatoglyphics: Study of finger prints
- Gustafson's method: Age estimation of adults over 21 years of age by studying the physiological changes in each of the dental tissues

- Portrait parle/ Bertillon's method: Scientific indexing and filing of the physical description of a person for the purpose of his future identification

Tests used for bloodstains

- Benzidine
- Phenolphthalein (Kastle-Meyer)
- Takayama's hemochromogen
- Teichmann
- Hemin
- Spectroscopic
- Leucomalachite green
- Luminal

Tests used to detect seminal stains

- Barberio's test
- Florence test
- Acid phosphatase test
- Creatinine phosphokinase
- Semen specific glycoprotein
- ELISA (SEMA assay for seminal vesicle specific antigen)

Importance of age

Age	*Medico-legal importance*
<7 years	No offence
7 years	A person is declared dead if not seen for 7 years
<12 years	Cannot give consent to inflict harm
<18 years	Cannot give consent to inflict harm which may lead to grievous injury
<14 years	No employment in factories (Factory act)
<15 years	Rape; coitus even with wife
<16 years	Rape; coitus with others; even with consent
<16 years	Juvenile

DENTITION

- It is a best method to study age upto: 14 years
- Factor delaying dentition: Hypothyroidism
- Eruption of primary teeth is completed by: 2-2.5 years
- Mixed dentition is seen in: 6-11 years
- First permanent molar appears at: 6 years
- Gustafson's method: Age estimation of adult over 21 years depending upon physiological age changes in dental tissue

Deciduous teeth eruption (in months)

- Lower central incisor: 6
- Upper central incisor: 7
- Upper lateral incisor: 8
- Lower lateral incisor: 9
- First molar: 12
- Canines: 18
- Second molar: 24

Permanent teeth eruption (in years)

- First molar: 6
- Central incisor: 7
- Lateral incisor: 8
- First premolar: 9
- Second premolar: 10
- Canines: 11
- Second molar: 12
- Third molar: 17-30

Skeleton

Type	*Cephalic index*	*Race*
Dolicho-cephalic	70-75	Aryans, Negroes
Mesati-cephalic	75-80	Europeans, Chinese, Indians
Brachy-cephalic	80-85	Mongolian

DACTYLOGRAPHY

- Study of fingerprints is known as: Dalton system of dactylography
- First used in India by: Sir William Herschel

- REMEMBER: Even 2 identical twins don't have identical finger prints
- MC type of fingerprints: Loops
- Permanent loss of fingerprints occur in: Leprosy, Electrical injury

Accuracy in sexing adult skeletal

- Entire skeleton: 100 percent
- Pelvis: 95 percent
- Skull alone: 90 percent
- Pelvis plus skull: 98 percent
- Long bones alone: 80 percent

POSTMORTEM HYPOSTASIS

- Post-mortem hypostasis starts as: Blotchy discoloration
- After death, post-mortem hypostasis gets fixed after: 5-6 hours

Postmortem lividity (colour & cause)

- Cherry red: Carbon monoxide
- Pinkish: HCN
- Bright red: Cold
- Dark brown: Phosphorus
- Brown: Potassium cyanide, sodium cyanide
- Brown: Aniline, carbon dioxide
- Greenish blue: Hydrogen sulphide
- Red: Drowning

RIGOR MORTIS

- Muscles affected in rigor mortis: All muscles (voluntary/ involuntary)
- Rigor mortis first appears in: Involuntary muscle (heart)

Postmortem caloricity is seen in

- Sunstroke
- Cholera
- Septicemia
- Tetanus
- Alcohol poisoning
- Strychnine poisoning
- Rabies

Cadavers spasm/ Instantaneous rigor

- Stiffening of muscles immediately after death without being preceded by primary relaxation
- Seen when the muscles of the body were in a state of strong contraction immediately before death

PUTREFACTION

- Late sign of death: Putrefaction, Adipocere formation, Mummification
- First sign of putrefaction:
    - o Externally: Greenish discoloration of flank over caecum
    - o Internally: Greenish discoloration of undersurface of liver
- Last organ to putrefy in males: Prostate, Testis
- Last organ to putrefy in females: Non-gravid uterus, Ovaries
- Putrefactive changes in liver: Honey coombing, Foamy liver
- Putrefaction is delayed by: Arsenic, Carbolic acid

ADIPOCERE FORMATION

- Adipocere formation is also known as: Saponification
- Climate for adipocere formation: Warm, Humid
- Adipocere formation is: Hydrolysis & hydrogenation of fat

MUMMIFICATION

- Mummification is: Desiccation, Dehydration, Shrinkage of cadaver (preserving body features)
- Mummification is seen in: Dry air condition, Wind, High temperature

ABRASION

- MC type of abrasions: Graze
- Brush burn/ Friction burn: Dragging over ground; A type of graze
- Patterned abrasion: Pressure injury

BRUISE

- Blue colour of bruise is due to: Deoxyhemoglobin, Seen after few hours to 3 days
- Green colour of bruise is due to: Hematoidin, Seen at 5-6 days

Colour changes in bruise (time, colour & cause)

- 0: Red (Blood)
- Few hours - 3 days: Blue
- 4 days: Bluish-black to brown (Hemosiderin)
- 5-6 days: Green (Hematoidin)
- 7-12 days: Yellow (Bilirubin)
- 14 days: Normal

Abrasion

Graze/ friction burns/ brush burns	Scrapping injury over a large surface
Scratch	Due to sharp objects
Pressure/ Imprint abrasion/ Patterned abrasion	Due to direct pressure/ impact

WOUNDS

- Tentative cuts/ Hesitation marks: Suicidal attempts
- Gaping of wound is determined by: Langerhan's lines
- Healing of clean, incised wound is by: Primary intention
- Incised looking wounds: Lacerated wounds over scalp
- Depth is maximum in: Stab wound

SKULL INJURIES

- Coup injuries: Skull Injury is located beneath the area of impact
- Contre coup: Skull Lesion is present in an area opposite the side of impact
- Pond fracture: Indented fracture of skull, in children
- Gutter fracture: Oblique bullet wound
- Fracture a la signature/ Depressed fracture: Outer table of skull driven into diploe, Due to heavy object, with small surface area

Grievous hurt

- Emasculation
- Permanent privation/ loss of sight of either eye
- Permanent privation/ loss of heating of either ear
- Privation of any member of any joint
- Destruction or permanent impairing of power of any member of joint
- Permanent disfiguration of head or face
- Fracture or dislocation of bone or tooth
- Any hurt which endangers the life or which causes the sufferer to severe bodily pain makes him unable to follow his ordinary pursuits for a period of 20 days.

FIREARM

- Choking (firearm): Constricting device at the muzzle end of a shotgun
- Contents of black gun powder: Potassium nitrate, Sulfur, Charcoal
- Smokeless powder: Nitrocellulose
- Tandem bullets: 2 bullets in succession
- Abraded collar/ Grease collar/ Dirt collar: Entrance wound of gun shot
- Dermal nitrate test detects: Gun powder/ gunshot residues

Bullets

- Tandem bullets/ Piggyback bullet: Bullets ejected one after another, as the previous one was stuck in the barrel
- Dumdum bullet: Nose cut off
- Ricochet: Before striking the aim, strikes some other object, to get rebound and hit the target
- Frangible bullets: Designed to fragment upon impact, often to the point of disintegration

Entry wound

- Smaller than the diameter of bullet
- Inverted edge
- Abrasion present
- Grease collar present
- Burning, stinging, tattooing, blackening present in close shot wounds
- Bleeding and tissue extrusion are less

Exit wound

- Larger than diameter of bullet
- Everted edge
- Abrasion absent
- Grease collar absent
- Burning, stinging, tattooing, blackening absent
- Bleeding and tissue extrusion are more

CAFÉ CORONARY

- Café coronary is common in: Mostly overdrunk, Deeply intoxicated, with depressed gag reflex
- Cause of death in café coronary: Asphyxia/ Reflex cardiac arrest from stimulation of vagus (laryngeal nerve)

Asphyxial deaths

Description	*Term*
Homicide by hanging by large group of people	**Lynching**
Strangulation with forearm	**Mugging**
Strangulation with sticks	**Bansdola**
Strangulation by twisting lever like a tourniquet	**Garroting**
Manual strangulation	**Throttling**
Mechanical obstruction to airways (other than by hanging, strangulation or throttling)	**Suffocation**
Closing the external respiratory orifice by hand or other means	**Smothering**
Closing the mouth and nose with cloth etc., and tying it around head or stuffing it into mouth	**Gagging**
Obstruction within the airways	**Choking**
Death due to entry of water into lungs	**Wet drowning**
Death due to laryngeal spasm (no entry of water into lungs)	**Dry drowning**
Death in half an hour to two days after resuscitation due to secondary changes in lungs	**Secondary drowning**
Death by vagal inhibition and cardiac arrest	**Immersion syndrome**

HANGING

- Constricting force in hanging: Weight of the body
- In typical hanging, the knot usually comes to lie under the: Chin
- Partial hanging: Bodies are partially suspended
- Le facies sympathique is associated with: Hanging
- Ligature marks are a type of: Printed abrasion
- Special feature of hanging: Saliva may be found dribbling from the angle of mouth
- Cause of death in judicial hanging: Fracture dislocation at C2-C3 or C3-C4

DROWNING

- Signs of drowning: Fine copious frothy discharge from mouth & nose, Diatoms in bone marrow, Goose skin/ cutis anserina, Paltauf's haemorrhage
- MC type of drowning: Accidental
- Gettler's test is done for: Drowning, It estimates the chloride content of the blood in both sides of heart
- Emphysema aquosum signifies: Wet drowning
- Edema aquosum is seen in drowning of unconscious
- Diatoms: Unicellular algae, suspended in water, Their presence in bone marrow & brain signifies drowning

BURNS

- Arborescent burns: Filigree/ Lichtenberg burns
- Joule burns: Electricity burns
- Crocodile skin appearance of skin: Suggestive of high voltage electric burns

- Pugilistic attitude is due to: Protein coagulation
- Pugilistic attitude is seen in: Burns
- Heat hematoma: Occurs between skull & duramater
- Features of antemortem burns:
  - o Line of redness present (line of redness is absent in postmortem burns)
  - o Vesicles contain chloride, albumin (Postmortem vesicles contains air)
  - o Soot in upper respiratory passage (Soot is absent in upper airways in postmortem burns)
  - o Carboxyhemoglobin in blood (Carboxyhemoglobin in blood is absent in postmortem burns)
  - o Enzymes are increased (enzymes are not increased in post mortem burns)

HEAT INJURIES

- Heat cramps/ miners cramps/ Stokers cramps/ Fireman's cramps:
  - o Caused by rapid dehydration of body
  - o Through the loss of water and salt in the sweat
  - o Seen in workers in high temperature
  - o There is profuse sweating
- Heat prostration/ Heat exhaustion/ Heat syncope/ Heat collapse:
  - o Condition of collapse without increase in body temperature
  - o Follows exposure to excessive heat
  - o Precipitated by muscular work & unsuitable clothing
- Heat hyperpyrexia/ Heat stroke:
  - o Hyperpyrexia is fever above 41.5 degree C
  - o Heat stroke is rectal temperature greater than 41 degree C and neurological disturbances

Abnormal sexual perversions

Description	***Term***
Sexual gratification by teasing partner	**Sadism**
Murder acts as a stimulus for sexual act	**Lust murder**
Eating dead body	**Necrophagia**
Sexual gratification by getting teased	**Masochism**
Sexual intercourse with dead body	**Necrophilia**
Sexual satisfaction by contact with articles of opposite sex	**Fetichism**
Peeping tom	**Voyeurism**
Contact with other person to obtain sexual gratification	**Frotteurism**
Sexual pleasure by witnessing the act of urination	**Undinism**
Wearing clothes of opposite sex	**Transvestism**

TOXICOLOGY

- Spinal poison are:
  - o Nux vomica
  - o Gelsemium
- Universal antidotes:
  - o Animal charcoal: 2 parts
  - o Magnesium oxide: 1 part
  - o Tannic acid: 1 part
- Hemodialysis is done for: Barbiturates, Aspirin, Methanol (alcohol)
- Widmark formula is related with: Alcohol
- Diwali poisons: Mercury, Phosphorous

Hemodialysis is not useful in Poisoning by following

- Digoxin
- Kerosene
- Benzodiazepines
- OPC

Contraindication for emesis

- Corrosive
- Irritant
- Convulsive
- Volatile
- Comatose
- Heart disease
- Pregnant women

Contraindication for gastric lavage

- Very old
- Corrosive
- Convulsants
- Unconsciousness
- Heart disease
- Peptic ulcer

Antidotes of some poisons

- Acids: Weak noncarbonated alkalies
- Alkalies: Weak vegetable acids- citric acid, acetic acid
- Silver nitrate: Sodium chloride
- Mercuric chloride: Egg albumin
- Arsenic poisoning: Freshly prepared ferric oxide
- Opium: Potassium permanganate, naloxone
- Dhatura: Neostigmine
- Strychnine: Barbiturate
- Oxalic acid: Calcium gluconate
- Phenol/carbolic acid: 20 percent alcohol for gastric lavage
- Aspirin: Stomach wash with magnesium oxide
- Yellow phosphorus: Stomach was with 0.1 percent solution of copper sulphate
- Lead: Stomach wash with magnesium or sodium sulphate, calcium disodium EDTA I/V
- Mercury: Egg albumin, BAL or penicillamine I/V
- OPC: Atropine, oximes

MERCURY POISONING

- Chronic mercury poisoning:
  - Erethism
  - Shaking palsy
  - Acrodynia (pinkish rash starting from tips of fingers)
- Acute mercury poisoning mainly involves: Kidney (PCT)

Poisons & Active principle

- Abrus precatorius / Rati: Abrin (Used by jewelers in olden days To measure gold and silver; Local effect similar to viper snake bite)
- Ricinus communis/ Castor: Ricin [Castor oil (Erandel oil)]
- Croton tiglium / purging croton / jamalgota: Carotene and Carotenoids (purgative)
- Semecarpus anacardium / Marking nut: Semicarpol and Bhilawanol (Used in laundries for making on clothes)
- Calotropis / madar: Calotropin, Calotoxin, Gigantin, uscharin
- Capsicum annum: Capsicin, Capsaicin
- Aconite/ Mitha vish: Aconitine [Pupils show hippus reaction (alternate constriction and dilatation]

ARSENIC POISONING

- Arsenic poisoning:
  - Aldrich Mees lines (nail)
  - Mimicks cholera poisoning
  - Rain drop pigmentation
  - Golden hair
  - Earliest sign: Gradual emaciation
  - Red velvety stomach mucosa
- Arsenophagist's: People who can tolerate high doses of arsenic
- Special features of arsenic poisoning:
  - Retardation of putrefaction
  - Detected in completely decomposed bones, ash & charred bodies and
  - Delayed rigor
- Tests for arsenic poisoning:
  - Marsh's test
  - Reinsch's test
  - Gutzeit test
  - Urinary excretion (> 100 mg/ day)
  - Atomic absorption spectroscopy

- Management:
  - o BAL
  - o Penicillamine
  - o Freshly prepared hydrated ferric oxide

LEAD POISONING

- Features of lead poisoning (ABCDE):
  - o Anemia
  - o Basophilia (punctate)
  - o Burtonian line
  - o Constipation
  - o Death
  - o Encephalopathy
- Burtonian line is: Appears at the gingiva-tooth border after prolonged high level exposure
- MC feature: Colic & constipation
- Early manifestation of chronic lead poisoning: Facial pallor
- Diagnostic measures:
  - o Urinary Coproporphyrin (> 150 mcg/ l)
  - o Urinary Amino-Levulinic acid (> 5 mg/ l)
  - o Lead in blood (> 70 mcg/ 100 ml)
  - o Urinary lead (> 0.8 mg/ l)
  - o Basophilic stippling of RBCs
- Management:
  - o Penicillamine (industrial/ poisoning in children)
  - o DMSA/ succimer (DOC)

Colloquial/ street names of some substances of abuse

- Mitha vish (sweet poison): Aconite
- Siddhi/Bhang: Leaves and stems of cannabis sativa (2% cannabinol)
- Majun: Sweetmeat preparation of Bhang
- Ganja: Flowering tops of female plants of C. sativa (5-10% cannabinol)
- Reefer: Cigarette preparation of Ganja
- Charas: Resinous extract form leaves and flowers of C. sativa (20-50% cannabinol)
- Speed ball/ Brown sugar/ Smack: Heroin

Poisons

Poison	*Tissue affected*
Phenol, oxalic acid & mercury	**Nephro-toxic**
Arsenic, alcohol, phosphorous, chlorpromazine	**Hepato-toxic**
Mercury, phosphorus	**Diwali poison**
Abrus, aconite, snake venom, strychnine	**Arrow poison**
Opium	**Somniferous poison**
Alcohol, chloroform, ether	**Inebriant poison**
Belladonna, cannabis, datura, hyoscyamus	**Deliriant poison**
Arsenic, cannabis, cocaine, opium	**Aphrodisiac**
Abrus, snake and scorpion venom, creatine, ricin	**Toxalbumin**
Nux vomica, gelsemium	**Spinal poison**
Aconite, oleander, digitalis, quinidine, tobacco, HCN	**Cardiac poison**
Curare, conium	**Peripheral poison**
CO, CO_2, HCN, H_2S	**Asphyxiant**
Cobra, krait, scorpion venom	**Neurotoxic**
Viper, scorpion venom	**Haemotoxic**
Sea snake venom	**Myotoxic**

SALICYLIC ACID POISONING

- Increased anion gap metabolic acidosis with respiratory alkalosis & ketosis suggests salicylates poisoning
- Platelet dysfunction (inhibition of aggregation)
- Prolonged clotting time
- Reye's syndrome can occur in children below 15 years of age on consumption of aspirin
- Treatment:
  - o Stomach wash with sodium bicarbonate
  - o Forced alkaline diuresis
  - o Peritoneal/ hemodialysis

SULPHURIC ACID POISONING

- Effects of sulphuric acid poisoning:
  - o Stomach mucosa is stained black
  - o Perforation of stomach is common
- Fatal period for sulphuric acid: 12-16 hours
- Special feature of sulphuric acid: Vitriolage (Throwing of H_2SO_4 on other individual)

Viscera preservation

- Saturated solution of salt: All poisonings, including carbolic acid, except acids
- Rectified spirit: Acid poisoning (except carbolic acid)
- 10 percent formalin: Preservation for histopathological examination
- Potassium oxalate + sodium fluoride: Blood preservation in alcohol poisoning case
- Sodium citrate + sodium fluoride: Blood preservation in oxalic acid, ethylene glycol
- Potassium oxalate + sodium nitrite: Blood preservation in fluoride poisoning case

CARBOLIC ACID POISONING

- Carboluria is seen with: Carbolic acid poisoning (urine turns green or black on exposure to air)
- Appearance of stomach in carbolic acid poisoning: Stomach looks leathery
- Special feature of carbolic acid poisoning: Retards putrefaction

SNAKE VENOM

- Russel's viper venom is: Hemolytic
- Cobra krait venom is: Neurotoxic
- Sea snake venom is: Myotoxic

Signs and symptoms of acute dhatura poisoning

- Flushed skin (red as beet)
- Hyperthermia (hot as hare)
- Inhibition of secretions (dry as bone)
- Dilation of pupils with loss of accumulation (blind as bat)
- Restlessness, delirium (mad as wet hen)

EPIDEMIC DROPSY

- Adulteration of mustard oil with argemone oil (which contains sanguinarine & dihydrosanguinarine)
- Features:
  - o Diarrhoea
  - o Marked edema/ generalized anasarca
  - o Glaucoma's

RAPE

Criteria of rape in India

- Unlawful intercourse by a man
- With his wife under age of 15 years
- With any woman under 16 years
- With any other woman above 16 years, against her will
- In case of rape- semen sample should be collected within 2 days

SEXUAL OFFENCES

- Indecent assault:
  - o Offence committed on a female with the intention or knowledge to outrage her modesty
  - o Such assaults are punishable under Sec. 354 IPC
- Incest:
  - o Sexual intercourse by a man with a woman who is closely related to him by blood
  - o In India, incest as such, is not an offence

Derivatives of cannabis sativa

Hash oil	Resinous mix lipid soluble plant extract	THC content 70-90%
Charas/ Hashish	Resinous exudates from flowering tops	THC content 25-40%
Ganja	Small leaves and brackets of inflorescence	THC content 15-25 %
Bhang	Dries leaves, flowering shoots, cut tops	THC content of 1-15 %

CANNABIS SATIVA

- Active content: THC/ Tetra-Hydro-Cannabinol
- Distorted perceptions (during trip)
- Run amok: Depression followed by impulse to murder

HYDROGEN CYANIDE POISONING

- Characteristic bitter almonds smell
- Postmortem staining: Cherry red color
- Mechanism of action of HCN: Inhibition of cytochrome oxidase & carbonic anhydrase which leads to histotoxic/ cytotoxic hypoxia
- Management:
    - o Amyl nitrate
    - o Sodium nitrite (converts hemoglobin to methaemo-globin)
    - o Sodium thiosulphate
    - o Hydroxy-cobalamin

CLINICAL QUESTIONS

1. **A MBBS doctor referred a patient to a radiologist for chest X-ray. In turn, MBBS doctor received a cheque from radiologist. This is referred to as:**

A. Medical dichotomy B. Conduct money

C. Vicarious liability D. Criminal negligence

Dichotomy is an unethical act. It defines that a physician shall not give solicit, or receive nor shall he offer to give, solicit or receive any gift, gratuity, commission or bonus in consideration of, or return for the referring, recommending or procuring any patient for medical, surgical or other treatment.

Answer: A i.e., Medical dichotomy

2. **A young male farmer presented with the complain of excessive sweating following consumption of some unknown poison. On examination, there is bradycardia and hypotension. Treatment is by:**

A. Acetylcholine B. Atropine

C. Edrophonium D. Dexamethasone

Clinical findings suggest the diagnosis of organophosphate poisoning. Atropine sulfate is given, which arrests the muscarinic effects of post-ganglionic parasympathetic (peripheral) activity (muscarinic receptor antagonist) and arrests CNS effects. Edrophonium, physostigmine and succinylcholine are avoided.

Answer: B i.e., Atropine

3. **Headache, behavioural changes, schizophrenia like psychosis, visual hallucination and paranoid symptoms are seen in intoxication of:**

A. Cocaine B. Alcohol

C. Amphetamines D. Cannabis

Acute intoxication of amphetamine causes paranoid hallucinatory syndrome, which closely mimics paranoid schizophrenia. There may be auditory or visual hallucinations in a setting of clear consciousness.

Answer: C i.e., Amphetamines

4. **A verbal statement recorded by the magistrate without any oath, by an assaulted person narrating the sequence of events responsible for his/ her condition is known as:**

A. Dying declaration B. Dying deposition

C. Summon D. Inquest

Dying declaration can be recorded by anyone (doctor, police, magistrate etc.). Oath is not administered as it is believed that a dying person would not lie.

Answer: A i.e., Dying declaration

5. **A 45 years old lady attended the skin OPD with photosensitive lesion on malar area of the face. The type of consent given for examination of face, in such a case is:**

A. Informed consent B. Implied consent

C. Expressed content D. Written consent

Implied consent means consent is presumed be there. If a patient has come to the doctor for treatment, it is presumed that he has given consent for routine physical examination (inspection, palpation, percussion and auscultation).

Answer: B i.e., Implied consent

6. **A child complains of pain in the anal region after being sodomized. Anal swabs were taken and treated with a card to obtain yellow crystals. Such a test is known as:**

A. Hensley test B. Acid phosphatase test

C. Barberio's test D. Florence test

In Barberio's test, yellow needle shaped rhombic crystals of spermine picrate are formed, when a saturated aqueous or alcoholic solution of picric acid is added to spermatic fluid.

Answer: C i.e., Barberio's test

7. **A patient is dependent on cocaine. He is consistently scratching skin and have scratch marks on skin. This phenomenon is known as:**

A. Withdrawal phenomenon

B. Locard's principle

C. Uthoff phenomenon

D. Magnan's phenomenon

A patient with chronic overuse of cocaine presents with persecutory delusions and tactile hallucinations (formication). Tactile hallucinations are manifested as bugs crawling under the skin (cocaine bugs/ Magnan's symptoms).

Answer: D i.e., Magnan's phenomenon

8. A person was brought for autopsy. His relatives said that he has tattoo marks but no tattoo marks were visible. Which site should be explored to confirm the presence of tattoo?

A. Spleen
B. Lymph nodes
C. Brain
D. Liver

Lymph nodes near tattoo marks show pigment deposition as the pigment from tattoo goes to the draining lymph node of that area, where tattoo was made. So microscopic examination of lymph node would help in detection of tattoo pigment.

Answer: B i.e., Lymph nodes

9. Nothing is an offence, which is done by a person who, at the time of doing it, by reason of unsoundness of mind, is incapable of knowing the nature of the act, or that he is doing, what is either wrong or contrary to law. This is defined as:

A. Durham's law
B. McNaughten's law
C. Curren's law
D. Locard's principle

Rule states that an accused person is not legally responsible for that act, if it is clearly proved that at the time of committing the act, the person has such an abnormality of the mind, that he did not know the nature and quality of the act he was doing, or that whatever he is doing, is wrong.

Answer: B i.e., McNaughten's law

10. An adult came to casualty with complaints of rapid heart rate. On examination, everything else was normal except for episodic tachycardia and occasional extra-systole and amblyopia. What could be the reason?

A. Cannabis
B. Nicotine
C. Atropine
D. Cocaine

Features of chronic nicotine poisoning include amblyopia, blindness, irregularity of the heart rate with extra-systoles etc.

Answer: B i.e., Nicotine

11. A 70 years old male presents with amblyopia, external chest pain, episodic tachycardia and extra-systoles on ECG. What is the cause?

A. Cocaine poisoning

B. Arsenophagia

C. Cannabis ingestion

D. Chronic nicotine poisoning

In chronic nicotine poisoning, there may be occasional attacks of chest pain suggestive angina pectoris.

Answer: D i.e., Chronic nicotine poisoning

12. A 40 years old female presented to the emergency with extensive burns. Patient had grade III burns on face, neck, back, upper arms and forearms with singeing of hairs. Which is NOT a proof of inhalational burns?

A. Black colored soot deposition on posterior part of the tongue

B. Hoarseness and stridor of voice

C. Singeing of eyebrows and facial hairs

D. Yellow coloured sputum

In cases of burn injury, there is no yellow-coloured sputum production. Blackish coal particles are embedded in frothy mucus, which covers the congested mucosa.

Answer: D i.e., Yellow coloured sputum

13. A patient presented to the emergency with overdose of some drug. There was increased salivation and increased bronchial secretions. On examination, the blood pressure was 80/ 60 mm Hg. RBC cholinesterase level is <50% of normal. What should be used in management?

A. Physostigmine B. Neostigmine

C. Protamine sulphate D. Atropine

Muscarinic manifestations of organophosphate poisoning include salivation, lacrimation, urination, defecation, gastrointestinal distress and emesis (SLUDGE). There is also increased bronchial secretions. RBC cholinesterase level of less than 50% of normal suggest organophosphate poisoning. Atropine is the drug of choice in organophosphate poisoning and it should be continued until the tracheobronchial tree is cleared of secretions and most secretions are dried.

Answer: D i.e., Atropine

CHAPTER 8

PSM

RAPID REVISION NOTES

Incubation period/ IP

Disease	*IP*
Influenza	1-3 days
Anthrax	1-3 days
Cholera	1-5 days
Diphtheria	2-6 days
Plague	2-6 days
Yellow fever	3-6 days
Tetanus	6-10 days
Measles	10 days
Pertussis	7-14 days
Polio	7-14 days and above
Chicken-pox	2-3 weeks
Rubella	2-3 weeks
Mumps	2-3 weeks
Hepatitis A	15-45 days
Hepatitis B	45-180 days

CONCEPT OF HEALTH & DISEASE

Indicator of health

- Morbidity indicators: Incidence & prevalence, notification rates, attendance rates of hospital, admission & readmission rates, discharge rates, duration of hospital stay, spell of sickness etc.
- Disability indicators: Sullivan's index (expectation of life free of disability), disability adjusted life year/ DALY (measures burden of disease in a defined population & effectiveness of interventions), health adjusted life year/ HALE

Physical quality of life index (PQLI)

- Includes literacy rate, infant mortality rate & life expectancy at the age of 1 year

Human development index (HDI)

- Includes life expectancy at birth (longevity), adult literacy rate & mean years of schooling (knowledge) & real GDP per capita in purchasing power parity in US dollars (income real)
- Value ranges between 0 to 1
- HDI value in India is 0.619
- Measures average achievements in basic dimensions of human development

Concept of disease causation

- Components of epidemiological triad: agent, host & environment
- Determinants of disease behaviour in a community: Infectiousness, density of aggregation of population, standard of hygiene & size of reservoir of infection

Iceberg diseases

- Waterline in iceberg diseases represents the demarcation between apparent & inapparent cases
- Submerged portion of the iceberg: Constitutes latent, inapparent, presymptomatic, carriers & undiagnosed cases
- Diseases showing iceberg phenomenon: Rubella, polio, Japanese encephalitis, influenza, mumps, hepatitis A & B, diphtheria etc.
- Iceberg phenomenon is NOT seen in: Rabies, tetanus, measles

Levels of prevention

- Primary prevention: Has 2 main components – health promotion & specific protection
- Health promotion includes: Health education, environmental modifications, nutritional interventions, life style & behavioral changes (Process of advising a patient to change his lifestyles in order to prevent any risk factor for a disease)
- Specific protection example include: Vitamin A prophylaxis; Iron & folic acid supplementation
- Primary prevention in coronary artery disease includes: Changing harmful lifestyles by education to prevent coronary artery disease; exercise in high risk area, BP monitoring, Salt restriction
- Immunization, chemoprophylaxis, marriage counseling are primary level of prevention
- Primordial prevention in myocardial infarction include: Maintenance of normal body weight, change in life style, change in nutritional habits
- Primordial prevention is done in population which has not developed risk factor
- Secondary level of prevention example includes: Sputum for AFB, amniocentesis in early pregnancy & Pap smear (screening test) [early diagnosis & treatment], benzathine penicillin prophylaxis for rheumatic fever
- Example of disability limitation (tertiary prevention): Resting affected limb in neutral position

Surveillance

- Epidemiological surveillance: Set of questions are constructed in such a way that it takes into account all the important epidemiological factors of a given disease
- Sentinel surveillance: Detects missing/ hidden cases (to find the total amount of disease in a population)
- Active surveillance: Calculates true morbidity
- Diseases under WHO/ international surveillance: Rabies, polio, salmonellosis, louse borne typhus fever, malaria, relapsing fever, human influenza

International classification of disease/ ICD

- Denoted as ICD-10
- Done every 10 years
- ICD-10 is arranged in 21 major chapters
- Conducted by WHO
- Poisoning is included in chapter XIX
- Each chapter has 3 character categories
- First character code is a letter
- Accepted for national & international use
- Provides the basis for use in other health fields

Miscellaneous

- Socialized medicine results in: Elimination of competition among physicians in search of clients, Ensures social equity (universal coverage by health services), provision of free medical care supported by state
- Most important component of level of living is: Health
- First country to implement compulsory sickness insurance: Germany
- Germ theory of disease was propounded by: Louis Pasteur

EPIDEMIOLOGY

Case fatality rate (CFR)

- Good index of the severity/ lethality of an acute disease

- Represents killing power of a disease
- Closely related to virulence
- Very useful for acute diseases (NOT chronic diseases)
- CFR is calculated as: Total number of deaths due to disease ×100/ Total number of cases of the disease
- It is a proportion

Incidence

- Increases in new cases in a community indicates: Increase in incidence rates
- Calculated as: Number of new cases in a given period × 1000/ Population at risk during that period
- Incidence is a rate

Prevalence

- In a stable situation: Prevalence = Incidence × duration
- Prevalence: Describes the balance between incidence, mortality & recovery
- If prevalence is very low as compared to the incidence for a disease, it indicates: Either the disease is very fatal or easily curable
- Factor increasing prevalence of a disease: Longer duration of illness
- If a disease has 4 times more incidence in females as compared to males, but the prevalence is same; it implies: Increase fatality in females OR less fatality in males
- Calculated as = Incidence X Duration
- It is a proportion
- Numerator is a part of the denominator

Epidemic

- First thing to be done in an epidemic is: Confirmation of the occurrence of epidemic
- Search for new cases in epidemic is done till: Twice the incubation period of the disease since occurrence of the last case

Point source/ Single exposure epidemic

- A type of common source epidemic
- All cases occur abruptly & simultaneously (explosive epidemic)
- All cases occur within a specified period (in one incubation period)
- Rapid rise & rapid fall
- One single peak only
- Explosive
- NO secondary waves & NO plateau phase
- Bhopal gas tragedy is an example

Propagated epidemic

- Spread depends upon herd immunity
- Person to person transmission occurs
- Secondary waves are SEEN
- Slow rise

Trend of disease

- Secular trend means: Changes in pattern of the disease over a long period of time
- Seasonal trend is shown by: Measles, varicella (chicken pox), rubella, gastroenteritis, cerebral meningitis
- Cyclical trend is related to: Herd immunity variations, antigenic variations, buildup of susceptible (NOT related to environmental conditions)
- Cyclic trend is shown by: Measles

Cross-sectional studies

- Observational study
- Not expensive
- All cases seen at one point of time (for example, many populations participating in the examination at the same time to calculate/ identify some particular feature)
- Follow up is not a necessary feature
- More useful for chronic diseases
- It tells about the distribution of a disease (NOT etiology, so cause & effect relationship can't be established)
- Prevalence can be calculated

Longitudinal studies

- Measure incidence

- Identifies risk factor
- Studies natural history of the disease

Case control studies/ Retrospective study

- A type of analytical study
- Rapid/ quick results are obtained
- Proceeds from effect to cause so one can study multiple causal associated factors at a time
- Useful in rare diseases
- Inexpensive, cost effective
- No risk to subjects
- Risk factor can be identified
- Problem of bias is common
- Odds ratio/cross product ratio can be estimated (NOT relative risk)
- Calculated as = ad/bc (where 'a' is number of cases with risk factor present, 'b' is control with risk factors, 'c' is cases with no risk factors & 'd' is control with absent risk factors)
- Odd's ratio (in case control study) measures association between disease & risk factor

Cohort study/ Prospective study

- Type of analytical study
- Measures incidence rate, relative risk (risk ratio), attributable risk (risk difference) & population attributable risk
- Best design (amongst epidemiological studies) to test the association between risk factors & disease is: Cohort study (though most reliable study is randomized controlled trial)
- In cohort study, non-smokers were found to have carcinoma lung. This indicates: Etiology of lung carcinoma is multifactorial
- Expensive
- Bias is unlikely to invalidate cohort studies used to assess risk of exposure because: Exposure is usually determined prior to disease occurrence

Relative risk (RR)

- Relative risk can be calculated as: Incidence of the disease among the exposed/ incidence of disease among non-exposed
- RR of more than 1: indicates positive association; O is no association & -1 hints towards no association between the factor & the disease
- RR is a direct measure of the strength of association between suspected cause & effect

Attributable risk (AR)

- Attributable risk can be calculated as: Incidence of disease in exposed – incidence of disease among the unexposed X 100/ incidence of disease in exposed
- AR measures the extent which is attributed by risk factor to disease
- AR means potential of prevention

Population attributable risk (PAR)

- Calculated as = Incidence in total population – incidence in non-exposed X 100/ Incidence in total population
- Community physician takes action based on: PAR

Randomized trial

- Essential purpose of randomization in randomized control trials is: To eliminate the selection bias & confounding factors
- In a controlled trial to compare 2 treatments, the main purpose of randomization is to ensure that: The two groups will be similar in prognostic factors
- Methods of randomization: Computer drawn randomization, lottery, random number table
- While analyzing a data, allocation into similar groups is done to ensure: Comparability
- Non-biased study is: Randomized controlled trials

Non randomized trials

- Degree of comparability is low (NOT high)
- Experiment can serve as its own control or can utilize a natural control
- Several trials may be needed before evaluation is considered conclusive
- Pre-post clinical trials: They use patients as his/ her own control

Bias

- Berksonian bias is: Selection bias
- Basic types of bias in epidemiological study: Investigation bias, subject bias, analyzer bias
- Interviewer bias can be reduced by: Allowing equal interview time
- Recall/ memory bias is more common with: Case control studies
- Hawthorne effect/ attention bias is seen in: Cohort study
- Bias can be eliminated by: Matching, blinding, randomization

Double blinding

- In double blind clinical drug trials: Study subjects & the investigators are not aware of the treatment study subjects are receiving
- Purpose of double blinding in clinical trials is to: Avoid observer & subject bias

Causation & association

- Goitre is prevalent at higher altitude is an example of: Indirect association
- Temporal association: Suspected cause preceding the observed effect
- Most difficult criterion to establish causal association in etiology of as disease: Specificity of association

Miscellaneous

- Denominator of crude birth rate is: Mid-year population
- Denominator in crude death rate is: Mid-year population
- Yardstick for assessment of standards of therapy is: Survival rate
- Direct Standardization is used to compare the mortality rates between 2 countries due to the difference in: Age distributions
- Best to compare vital statistics of the two populations is: Age standardized death rate
- In crude death rate, population is taken on: 1st July
- Parameter estimating the burden of a disease in the community is: Proportional mortality rate
- Disease rate is: Disease occurrence in a specified time period

INFECTIOUS DISEASE EPIDEMIOLOGY

Reservoir

- Soil is a reservoir for: Tetanus, anthrax, coccidiomycosis
- Animal reservoir is seen in: Rabies, yellow fever, influenza
- Human reservoir is seen in: Salmonella typhimurium, N. gonorrhoea, T. pallidum, hookworm

Carriers

- Incubatory carriers are seen in: Measles, polio, pertussis, mumps, influenza
- Healthy carriers are seen in: Cholera, diphtheria
- Chronic carriers are seen in: Malaria, diphtheria, gonorrhoea

Incubation period (IP)

- IP of less than 6 hours is seen in: Staphylococcal food poisoning, B. cereus (emetic form)
- Proxy measure of IP are: Latent period, serial interval, generation time (NOT period of communicability)
- IP helps in determining: Period of quarantine, identification of source of infection, immunization (NOT period of isolation)
- Disease highly transmitted during IP is: Pertussis, measles, chicken pox

Secondary attack rate (SAR)

- Denominator while calculating secondary attack rate is: All susceptible amongst close contact
- Calculated as: Number of exposed persons developing disease within the range of the IP X 100/ total number of exposed or susceptible contact
- SAR is a measure of: Communicability

Modes of transmission

- Vertical transmission is by: Placenta
- Biological transmission of filarial parasite in culex mosquito is: Cyclodevelopmental

- Transovarial transmission is a feature of: Scrub typhus
- Type of transmission in the case of plague in rate flea: Propagative
- Vector transmits agent by: Contamination of body fluids with vectors, scratching-in of infected faces, regurgitation

Host defence

- Active & passive immunity should be given together in: Tetanus, rabies, hepatitis-B
- Post exposure active immunization is done for: Rabies, measles, hepatitis-B, diphtheria, tetanus
- Congenital passive immunity/ maternal passive immunity is found in: Polio, measles, rubella, mumps

Vaccines

- Toxoid is prepared from: Exotoxin
- Killed vaccines are: DPT, IP (Salk-inactivated polio vaccine), hepatitis-B
- Vaccine administered by subcutaneous route: Measles
- Vaccine with highest efficacy: Measles (90% after a single dose)
- Vaccine not to be given in immunodeficient state: Rubella, trivalent oral polio vaccine
- Vaccine contraindicated in a patient on intensive chemotherapy: MMR, BCG
- Dose of OPV, given at birth, in case of institutional deliveries is: Zero dose of OPV

Vaccines & strains

- Mumps: Jeryll Lynn strain
- Measles: Edmonston Zagreb strain (commonest), Schwartz strain
- Chicken pox: OKA strain
- OPV & IPV: P1, P2, P3 strains (monovalent or trivalent)
- Rubella: RA 27/3
- BCG: Danish 1331

Vaccines & preservatives/ stabilizers

- Thiomersal is preservative in: DPT, influenza, pneumococcal
- Kanamycin is preservative in: Measles
- BCG has no preservative at all
- Stabilizer in oral polio vaccine: Magnesium chloride

Live vaccines

- Two live vaccines cannot be administered simultaneously
- Live vaccines are: BCG, oral polio vaccine, chicken pox vaccine, MMR, yellow fever (17-D)

Pregnancy & immunization

- Vaccine contraindicated in pregnancy: Live viral or bacterial vaccines (MMR, yellow fever, BCG, varicella)
- Vaccine which can be given: Inactivated viral vaccines (Influenza, hepatitis A & B)

Herd immunity (HI)

- HI provides protection to: Non-immunized persons
- Depends on clinical & subclinical cases
- Influenced by immunization
- Depends on the presence of alternative host
- HI is NOT constant
- % of HI necessary to prevent epidemic spread of diphtheria is: 70%
- HI is not useful in: Tetanus (HI is only relevant for contagious diseases)
- HI is affected by the presence & distribution of alternative animal hosts

Immunization programme

- Vaccines included in expanded programme of immunization (EPI): BCG, DPT, OPV, measles
- Measles vaccine is given at the age of: 9 months
- Vaccine in universal programme of immunization (UPI) which aims at preventing blindness: Measles
- Age group of children surveyed in WHO recommended EPI cluster sampling for primary immunization coverage is: 12-23 months
- Mass immunization is indicated in: Cholera, influenza, TB

- Ring immunization is: Given around 100 yards of detected case

Conditions & recommended immunization

- For 9 month old un-immunized child presenting for the first time: BCG, DPT-1(1st shot), OPV-1, measles
- For 3 years old un-immunized child presenting for the first time: DT-1, OPV-1, measles, vitamin-A
- 11 months old child with 2 doses of DPT & polio presents after 5 months of last dose: Repeat the whole course
- 37 weeks pregnant women presenting for the first time in antenatal clinic: Give a dose of tetanus toxoid (TT) & explain to her that it will not protect the newborn & she should take the second dose after 4 weeks even if she delivers in the meantime
- After administering live vaccine, immunoglobulins are given after: 2 weeks

Immunoglobulin

- When an antigen is administered for the 1st time to animal or a human being, who has never been exposed to it, the first antibody to develop is: IgM
- Secondary response is mediated by: IgG
- Binary exposure to an antigen results in sudden increase in: IgG

Cold chain

- Vaccine which requires most stringent conditions for storage/ most heat sensitive: OPV
- Vaccine which must be stored in the freezer compartment of the fridge: OPV, measles, BCG, yellow fever
- Vaccines not to be frozen are: DPT, TT
- Frozen DPT vaccine should be: Discarded
- Reverse cold chain is used for: Carrying stool samples of polio patients from a PHC to the laboratory
- Vaccine which can be stored at minus 10 degree Celsius temperature: Polio, measles

Isolation

- Isolation period should be: Period of communicability
- Isolation is strictly recommended for: Pneumonic plague, diphtheria, cholera
- Isolation is also done for (though less effective): Polio, typhoid, hepatitis A, mumps
- In salmonellosis, isolation is recommended till: 3 consecutive stool cultures are negative

Quarantine

- Quarantine is related to: Maximum incubation period
- It is NOT synonymous with isolation
- Absolute quarantine is restriction during the incubation period
- Exclusion of children form schools is an example of modified quarantine
- Quarantine should not be longer than the longest incubation period
- Internationally quarantinable diseases are: Plague, cholera, yellow fever

Chemoprophylaxis

- Drug of choice for chemoprophylaxis in contacts of a patient of pneumonic plague is: Tetracycline
- Tetracycline is also used for chemoprophylaxis of: Cholera
- Chemoprophylaxis is indicated for: Cholera, plague, meningococcemia (Sulfadiazine), malaria, bacterial conjunctivitis, diphtheria
- Mass chemoprophylaxis in endemic area is recommended for: Yaws, trachoma, filarial

Sterilization

- NOT a complete sterilization agent: Absolute alcohol
- Sharp instruments are sterilized by: Hot air oven

Disinfection

- Phenol coefficient indicates: Efficacy of a disinfectant
- Disinfectant used for blood spills: Sodium hypochlorite
- Best disinfectant for cholera stools: Cresol
- Amount of bleaching powder necessary to disinfect choleric stools: 50 gm/ litre
- Disinfection of sputum is done by: Boiling, autoclaving, burning

- Pasteurization is: Precurrent/ prophylactic disinfection
- Disinfection by autoclaving is NOT recommended for: Sharp instruments, glass syringes

Miscellaneous

- Subclinical cases are seen in: Rubella, influenza, polio, hepatitis, typhoid, mumps
- Latent infection occurs in: Herpes simplex, Brill-Zinsser disease, ancylostomiasis
- Human dead end diseases are: Bubonic plague, Japanese encephalitis, hydatid disease
- WHO surveillance is done for: Malaria, plague, relapsing fever
- International notification is a must for: Plague, cholera, yellow fever
- Bleaching powder: Unstable compound on storage
- Savlon contains: Chlorhexidine & cetrimide
- Epidemiological studies are carried for a period of: Twice the incubation period
- Bacteria is not shed in: Latent infection

Definitions (Cases)

- Primary case: First case of communicable disease introduced into the population
- Index case: First case to come to the attention of investigators
- Secondary case: Cases developing from contact with primary case

SCREENING FOR DISEASE

High risk screening

- It is the most economical & best screening
- It is the screening strategy for prevention of blindness from diabetic retinopathy (according to NPCB)

Criteria for screening

- Screening test is not useful when: Incidence is low in the community
- Least important for a screening test: High specificity (it's a quality for diagnostic test)
- Validity of a test is based upon: Accuracy, sensitivity, specificity (NOT precision)
- Levey-Jennings chart is used for monitoring: Accuracy (also precision)

Sensitivity & specificity

- Specificity of a test refers to ability of a test to detect: True negative
- Sensitivity means the ability to detect: True positive
- Sensitivity is inversely proportional to specificity
- Usefulness of a screening test in a community depends upon: Sensitivity
- When a diagnostic test is used in series mode then: Specificity increases but sensitivity decreases
- Sensitivity can be calculated as: True positives/ true positive + false negative
- Specificity can be calculated as: True negative/ true negative + false positive

Predictive value

- Reflects diagnostic power/ accuracy of the test
- Diagnostic power of a test to correctly exclude a disease is known as: Negative predictivity
- Denominator for calculating positive predictive value of a screening test: True positive + false positive
- Positive predictive value is most affected by: Prevalence
- If a test is done on 2 communities A & B, and more false positives are found in community A. This indicates: Prevalence is less in A community
- Too much false positives in a test is due to: Test have more sensitivity or prevalence & positive predictive value of test is low (high specificity gives large number of false negatives)
- Positive predictive value is calculated as: Sensitivity X prevalence/ (sensitivity X prevalence) + (100-specificity) (100-prevalence)
- Negative predictive value can be calculated as: Specificity X (100-prevalence)/ [specificity X (100-prevalnece)] + [(100-sensitivity) + prevalence]
- Predictive value of a positive test is calculated as: Total positives/ true positives + false positives

LEVELS OF PREVENTION

- Prevention of the emergence/ development of the risk factors, in the population, in which they have not appeared yet: Primordial prevention
- Disability limitation & Rehabilitation: Tertiary prevention
- Action halting the progress of disease at early stage & preventing its complication (includes early diagnosis & treatment): Secondary prevention
- Action taken prior to onset of disease, which lessens the possibility of occurrence of the disease (health promotion & specific protection-immunization, chemoprophylaxis): Primary prevention
- Spectacle usage in refractive error: Tertiary prevention
- Source reduction in malaria: Primordial prevention
- Defluoridation of water: Primary prevention
- Pap smear: Secondary prevention
- Salt restriction in non-communicable disease: Primordial prevention
- Cessation of smoking: Primordial prevention
- Marriage counselling: Primary prevention
- Immunization: Primary prevention
- IOL implantation in cataract surgery: Secondary prevention
- Physiotherapy in a case with poliomyelitis: Tertiary prevention

TERMS & PERSONS

- Theory of contagion: Fracastorius
- Social medicine: Jules Guerin
- Road to health chart: David Morley

MUST KNOW TERMS

- Provision of free medical services to people at GOVERNMENT expenses: State medicine
- Provision of medical services & professional education by STATE, but the programme is operated & regulated by PROFESSIONAL GROUPS rather than government: Socialized medicine
- Any loss/ abnormality of psychological, physiologic or anatomical structure or function (e.g. loss of foot, defective vision): Impairment
- Because of impairment, affected person may be unable to carry out certain activities, which may be considered normal for his age, sex (cannot walk): Disability
- Time interval between receipt of infection & maximal infectivity: Generation time
- Period between diagnosis by early detection/ screening & diagnosis by other means: Lead time
- Number of new cases during a specified time in a defined population: Incidence
- Gap between onset of primary case (1st case introduced) & secondary case (develops from primary case): Serial interval

INDICES

- Infant mortality rate, Life expectancy at ONE year, Literacy rate: Physical Quality of Life Index/ PQLI
- Average achievements in basic dimensions of human development: Human Poverty Index (HPI)
- Expectation of life free of disability: Sullivan's index
- Life expectancy at BIRTH, but includes an adjustment for time spent in poor health: Health Adjusted Life Expectancy/ HALE
- Burden of disease & effectiveness of interventions/ Years of life lost to premature death: Disability Adjusted Life Year/ DALY
- Education, Purchasing power, Life expectancy: Human Developmental Index/ HDI
- Education, Occupation, Income: Kuppuswamy's index

CASE CONTROL STUDY/ RETROSPECTIVE STUDY

- Suitable for rare diseases
- Rapid
- Inexpensive
- Yields Causal association, Odd's ratio

COHORT STUDY/ PROSPECTIVE STUDY

- Yields incidence
- Attributable & relative risk

DOUBLE BLIND STUDY

- Patient does not know which treatment they are receiving, Investigator does not know which treatment they are giving

Blinding

- Single blind: Participant is not aware whether he belongs to study group or the control group
- Double blind: Neither the doctor nor the participant is aware
- Triple blind: Participant, investigator and the person analyzing are unaware

Sterilization

Substances	*Mode*
Milk	**Holter method, flash method**
Destruction of viruses	**H_2O_2, $KMnO_4$, hypochlorite, beta-propiolactone**
Knives & scissors	**Chemical, hot air**
Rapid mass sterilization of syringes	**Infra-red rays**
Face mask, metal instruments, plastic tubes, polythene	**Glutaraldehyde**
Fabrics, cardiac catheters, heart lung machine, respirators, dental equipment	**Ethylene oxide**
Rooms, walls, furniture	**Formalin**
Faeces, urine, sputum	**Bleaching powder**
Bandages	**Gamma rays**
Glassware's, petridish, syringes, sharp instruments, swabs	**Hot air**

STERILIZATION & DISINFECTION

- Disinfectant kills all pathogenic micro-organisms
- Antisepsis: Inhibits growth of bacteria in wounds/ tissues
- Bacteriostatic agent: Agent, added to colony, inhibits growth & vice versa
- Pasteurization by flash method: 72° C, 15-20 sec
- Most resistant to sterilization: Prions
- Hot air oven is used for: Glassware, Liquid paraffin, Dusting powder, Forceps, scissors, scalpel
- Endoscopes are sterilized by: Glutaraldehyde
- Cidex is: 2% glutaraldehyde
- Disposable syringes are sterilized by: Gamma rays
- Vaccines are sterilized by: Heat inactivation
- Hospital dressings are best disinfected by: Incinerator (not done for sharp)
- Reidel walker coefficient: Determines germicidal efficiency of disinfectants (as compared to phenol)
- Tyndallization: Intermittent sterilization
- Bacterial spores are destroyed by: Autoclaving
- Cold sterilization is by: Gamma rays

BIOLOGICAL TRANSMISSION

- Propagative: Plague bacilli in rat flea
- Cyclopropagative: Malaria parasite in mosquito
- Cyclodevelopmental: Microfilaria in mosquito

Biological transmission

- Malaria: Cyclopropagative
- Filaria: Cyclodevelopmental
- Plague: Propagative
- Yellow fever: Propagative

MATERNAL & CHILD HEALTH

Cleans of safe delivery

- For elimination of NeoNatal Tetanus
- Clean delivery surface
- Clean hands (birth attendants)

- Clean cord cut (blade/ instrument)
- Clean cord tie
- Clean cord stump (no applicant)

Causes of maternal mortality (in descending order)

- Hemorrhage
- Anemia
- Sepsis
- Obstructed labour

Baby Friendly Hospital Initiative

- Have a written breastfeeding policy that is routinely communicated to all health care staff
- Train all health care staff in skills necessary to implement this policy
- Inform all pregnant women about the benefits and management of breastfeeding
- Help mothers initiate breastfeeding within one half-hour of birth
- Show mothers how to breastfeed and maintain lactation, even if they should be separated from their infants.
- Give newborn infants no food or drink other than breast milk, unless medically indicated.
- Practice rooming in- that is, allow mothers and infants to remain together 24 hours a day.
- Encourage breastfeeding on demand
- Give no artificial teats or artificial (also called dummies or soothers) to breastfeeding infants.
- Foster the establishment of breastfeeding support groups and refer mothers to them on discharge from the hospital or clinic

IMMUNIZATION

- Ring immunization: Given around 100 yards of a case detected
- BCG, DPT & Polio: Included in UIP
- Live vaccines:
  - o Long duration of immunity,
  - o Contain major & minor antigen
  - o Immunoglobulins can be given 2 weeks after live vaccine,
  - o BCG, Yellow fever (17D) etc.
- Killed vaccine: Salk polio, Pertussis etc.
- Fragment vaccine: Hepatitis B
- Freeze dried vaccine: Yellow fever, Measles, OPV etc.
- Strain used in BCG: Danish 1331
- Strain used in OPV: Sabin strain
- Strain used in Chicken pox: Oka strain
- Reconstituted vaccines: BCG, Measles, Yellow fever
- Vaccine C/I in pregnancy: MMR
- BCG (live attenuated vaccine) is given: Intradermally
- TY21 A (vaccine) is given for: Typhoid
- There is NO vaccine for Dengue fever yet
- Influenza vaccine is administered as: Nose drops
- HPV vaccine is: Both bivalent & quadrivalent

Live attenuated vaccines

- BCG
- Plague
- Typhoral
- OPV
- Yellow fever
- MMR
- Epidemic typhus
- Chicken pox
- Influenza

Killed vaccines

- Typhoid
- Cholera
- Pertussis
- Rabies
- IPV
- Influenza
- Hepatitis B
- Plague

EPI schedules as recommended by Govt. of India

- Birth- 15 days: BCG+ OPV (Zero dose)
- 6-8 weeks: OPV1 + DPT1
- 10- 12 weeks: OPV2 + DPT2
- 14- 16 weeks: OPV3 + DPT3
- 9 months (completed): Measles vaccine
- 15-18 months: 1st booster of OPV+DPT
- 4-6 years: OPV+DPT 2nd booster
- 16 years: Tetanus toxoid booster

BCG vaccine

- WHO recommends Danish 1331 strain
- It is reconstituted with normal saline
- Mantoux test becomes positive after 8 weeks

Secondary attack rate/ SAR

Disease	*SAR*
Small pox	**35-40%**
Measles	**80%**
Mumps	**86%**
Whooping cough	**90%**
Chicken pox	**90%**

MEASLES

- Caused by: RNA paramyxo virus (measles virus)
- Special feature: Kopliks spot
- Incubation period: 10-14 days
- Rash appears on: 4th day of fever
- Rare complication of measles: SSPE
- Measles vaccine is produced in India by: Serum institute, Pune
- Protective effect of measles vaccine is exerted within: 11-12 days of administration
- Measles vaccine has high efficiency
- Contamination of measles vaccine can cause: TSS (toxic shock syndrome)

RUBELLA

- Risk to fetus is maximum if mother gets infected during: 6-12 weeks of pregnancy
- Congenital rubella syndrome: Deafness, Cardiac malformations, Cataracts
- Rubella vaccine is given: To girls, between 11-14 years of age
- Recommended vaccination strategy for rubella vaccine: 15-49 years women

RABIES

- Symptoms appear in: About 10 days (4 days – 8 weeks)
- "Fixed strain" of virus: It has got short, fixed & reproducible IP, when injected intracerebrally
- Immunofluorescence is used for diagnosing Rabies
- Vaccine recommended by WHO: HDC vaccine
- Post exposure schedule (cell culture vaccine): 6 doses; 0, 3, 7, 14, 28 days; Booster on 90th day

Rabies categorization & preventive measures

- Category 1: Touching / licking intact skin
- Category 2: Minor scratches/ abrasion, lick on broken skin (Only vaccine)
- Category 3: Bites, scratches, contamination of mucus with licks (Immunoglobulin and vaccine)

YELLOW FEVER/ YF

- Caused by: Flavivirus
- Status in India: Absent (virus is absent)
- In YF, quarantine is done for: 6 days

POLIO

- IM injections & tonsillectomy should be avoided during polio epidemic because: Risk of paralytic polio increases
- Cause of death in polio: Respiratory paralysis
- Pulse polio was introduced in India in: 1995
- Pulse polio is given to children below: 5 years

- A country is said to be polio FREE if there is no case confirmed for last: 5 years
- In AFP/ acute flaccid paralysis, examination for residual paralysis should be done after: 60 day

Polio immunization

- Pulse polio immunization: 2 doses of OPV are given at an interval of 6-8 weeks, to children less than 5 years of age. On a fixed day, throughout the nation, irrespective of their immunization status
- Intensified pulse polio immunization: In the 3 days following PPI, unimmunized children are visited in their homes and vaccinated
- Mop-up round: 2 extra doses of OPV are given to children below 3 years of age irrespective of their immunization status, within a period of 7-14 days
- Ring immunization: Outbreak response immunization, carried out around 5 km radius of case of acute flaccid paralysis. A minimum of 5000 children under 5 years of are given 2 doses of OPV at an interval of 6 weeks. The first dose is to given within 48 hours of notification of case of AFP

Diseases subject to international health regulations

- Paralytic polio
- Malaria
- Louse borne typhus fever
- Relapsing fever
- Viral influenza

HIV

- Subtype most prevalent in India: C
- Seroconversion takes: 4 weeks
- MC mode of transmission of HIV: Heterosexual mode (male to female)
- Risk of transmission by accidental needle prick: 0.3%
- Retroviral sequence in host cell: RNA-DNA-RNA
- p24 antigen disappears after: 6-8 weeks of HIV infection
- Cells attacked in HIV: CD4 cells
- CD4: CD8 ratio is: Reversed
- Cells acting as reservoir of infection: Macrophages
- Window period: Time period between infection to appearance of antibodies in serum
- During window period, both ELISA & western blot are: Negative

Vaccines contraindicated in HIV/AIDS patient

- OPV
- Varicella
- Rotavirus
- MMR
- BCG

BORDETELLA PERTUSSIS

- Media used: Bordet Gengou
- IP: 1-2 weeks
- Culture characteristic: Thumb printing appearance

BRUCELLOSIS

- Zoonotic disease (NO person to person transmission)
- Test done: Rose Bengal Card test, Milk ring test

Zoonoses

- Anthropozoonoses: Infection transmitted from Vertebrate animal to man (Rabies, plague, anthrax)
- Zooanthroponosis: Infection transmitted from Man to vertebrate animals (Human TB in cattle)
- Amphixenosis: Infection maintained in both man and lower Vertebrate animals that may be transmitted in either directions (T. cruzi, S. japonicum)

Characteristic of zoonoses

- Direct: Direct transmission from animal to human with/ without mechanical vector /fomite
- Cyclozoonoses: More than one vertebrate host present
- Metazoonoses: Transmitted biologically via invertebrate vector
- Saprozoonoses: Transmitted via non- animal reservoir
- Anthropozoonoses: Transmitted via vertebrate vector

Disease transmitted by mosquito

Disease	*Vector*
Malaria	**Anopheles mosquito**
Filariasis (caused by wuchereria bancrofti), Japanese encephalitis	**Culex mosquito**
Yellow fever, dengue, hemorrhagic fever, filariasis (caused by wuchereria bancrofti)	**Aedes mosquito**
Filariasis (caused by brugia malayi)	**Mansonoides**

MALARIA

- Dengue is caused by: Aedes (prefers stagnant water)
- Size of RBC is increased in: Vivax malaria
- Infective agent of malaria is: Sporozoite
- Not seen in peripheral blood smear of falciparum: Schizont

P. falciparum

- Splenic rupture is common
- Parasitemia is highest
- Most virulent species of malaria
- Exoerythrocytic stage is absent
- Multiple infection of RBC's are seen

Mosquitos, Breeding place & Diseases transmitted

- Anopheles (Clean stagnant water): Malaria
- Culex (Polluted stagnant water): Bancroftian filariasis, Japanese encephalitis, West Nile fever, viral arthritis.
- Aedes (Artificial collections of water): Dengue, Yellow fever, Chikungunya
- Mansonites (Ponds with aquatic plants): Malayan filariasis, Chikungunya

National malaria eradication program (API > 2)

- Routine spraying: Done
- Entomological assessment: Done
- Active and passive surveillance: Done
- Presumptive and radical treatment: Given
- Follow-up smear after 1 year: Not done

National malaria eradication program (API <2)

- Routine spraying: Not done
- Entomological assessment: Not done
- Active and passive surveillance: Done
- Presumptive and radical treatment: Given
- Follow-up smear after 1 year: Done

Period of communicability/ POC

Disease	*POC*
Cholera	Infectious for a period of 9-10 days
Hepatitis A	Greatest 2 weeks before to 2 weeks after the onset of symptoms
Polio	1 week before and 1 week after the onset of symptoms
Whooping cough	1 week after exposure to about 3 weeks after the onset of paroxysmal stage
Diphtheria	Varies from 14-28 days after the onset of disease
Influenza	1 day before to 3-4 days after the onset of illness
Mumps	4-6 days before the onset of symptoms and 1 week or more thereafter
Rubella	1 week before and 1 week after the appearance of rash
Measles	4 days before and 5 days after rash
Chicken-pox	1-2 days before the appearance of rash ad for 4-5 days thereafter
Small-pox	Till scabs fall off

TB

- Mycobacterium TB was discovered by: Robert Koch
- Acid fastness is due to: Mycolic acid & cell wall
- Prevalence of TB in community is assessed by: Tuberculin test

- Ghon focus is related to: Primary pulmonary TB
- Primary TB may be associated with:
  - o Fibrocaseous lesion
  - o Phlyctenular conjunctivitis
- Category II of DOTS includes: Previously treated smear positive (relapse, failure, default)
- Defaulter is: Has not taken drugs for more than 2 months consecutively any time after starting treatment
- Case finding in RNTCP is based on: Sputum microscopy
- Standard dose of PPD for Mantoux test: 5 TU
- DOTS means:
  - o Short term treatment under supervision
  - o Alternate day treatment given

LEPROSY

- Generation time of lepra bacilli: 12 days
- Lepra bacilli can be grown in: Foot pad of mice
- Spreads by: Skin to skin contact
- Lepra cells are: Histiocytes
- Leprosy is a public health problem when prevalence is: 1:10,000
- Classification system/ index related to leprosy:
  - o Ridley Jopling's classification
  - o Dharmendra's index
- Lepromin test indicates: Prognosis

Leprosy survey (Prevalence, Rate & Survey type)
- Low (<1/1000): Contact
- Moderate (1/1000): Group
- High (> 10/ 1000): Mass

PLAGUE

- Causative agent of plague: Yersinia pestis
- Staining done in a case of plague: Wayson's staining
- Most contagious type of plague: Pneumonic plague
- Specific flea rate: Average number of fleas of each species/ rodent
- Best indicator of potential explosiveness of plague outbreak: Total flea index

Disease transmitting agents

Disease	*Vector*
Relapsing fever	**Soft tick**
Viral encephalitis, tularemia, tick paralysis	**Hard tick**
Guinea worm disease, diphyllobothrium latum	**Cyclops**
Scrub typhus	**Trombiculid mite**
Onchocerciasis	**Black fly**
Plague, endemic typhus, chiggerosis, hymenolepis	**Rat flea**
Epidemic typhus, relapsing fever, trench fever	**Louse**
Sleeping sickness	**Tse-tse fly**
Kala-azar, oriental sore, sand-fly fever	**Sand-fly**

RICKETTSIAL DISEASE

- Brill Zinser disease is: Delayed manifestation of epidemic typhus
- Vector for Epidemic typhus (R. prowazekii): Louse
- Vector for Endemic typhus (R. typhi): Rat flea
- Vector for Scrub typhus (R. tsutsugamushi): Mite

Disease & Vector

- R. prowazekii: Epidemic typhus, Brill-Zinser disease (Louse)
- R. typhi, R. felis: Endemic typhus (Rat flea/ Cat flea)
- R. rickettsii: Rocky mountain, Spotted fever (Tick)
- Orientia tsutsugamushi: Scrub typhus (Trombiculid mite)
- R. Quintana: Trench fever (Louse)
- R. akari: Rickettsial pox (Mite)
- Coxiella burnetii: Q-fever

OBESITY

- Indices for obesity:

- BMI (Quetelet's index)
- Corpulence index

- BMI is calculated as: Weight/ height^2
- Abdominal fat accumulation is assessed by: Waist/ hip ratio

IUCD

- IUCD acts by:
    - Causes aseptic endometritis
    - Prevents fertilization
    - Interferes implantation
- CuT 200 is inserted postnatally after: 8 weeks
- CuT380A should be replaced after every: 10 years
- If CuT 200 is implanted in myometrium, treatment is: Hysteroscopic removal
- Contraceptive 'TODAY' contains: 9 nonoxynol
- MINERA is: Progesterone IUCD

ORAL CONTRACEPTIVE PILLS

- OCP of choice in lactating females: Minipill
- After discontinuing OCP, fertility returns after: 6 months
- Levonorgestrel/ NORPLANT mechanism of action: Makes endometrium unreceptive
- OCP are protective against:
    - Endometriosis
    - Uterine Ca
    - RA
    - Ovarian Ca
    - PID
    - Ectopics (indirectly)
- Natural family planning methods:
    - Symptothermic method (most effective)
    - Cervical mucus method/ Billing method

STERILIZATION

- Criteria for sterilization:
    - Age of female between 22-60
    - Couple should have at least 2 children
- MC site for female sterilization is: Isthmus
- Pomeroy's method of female sterilization: Isthmus ampulla portion is ligated

Chemical qualities of water

Chemical	*Upper level*	*High level indicate*
Oxygen absorbed in 3 hours	1 mg/ L at 37 degrees	Organic matter
Nitrate	1 mg/ L	Old contamination
Nitrites	Zero	Pollution of recent origin
Albuminoid ammonia	0.1 mg/ L	Measure of decomposable organic matter
Free & saline ammonia	0.05 mg/L	Sewage contamination of recent origin
Total hardness	2 mEq/L	
Chlorides	600 mg/L	
Streptococcus faecalis		Recent faecal pollution

WATER

- Recommended level of fluoride in drinking water is- 0.5-0.8 mg/ litre
- Recommended fluorine concentration in water: 1.5 ppm
- Hardness level of water: 50
- Ortho-toluidine test: Determines both free & combined chlorine
- Horrock's apparatus: Measures chlorine demand of water

Characteristics of Waste

- Sullage: Waste water from domestic sources not containing human excreta

- Sewage: Waste containing human excreta
- Market refuse: Solid waste matter from markets containing putrid vegetable and animal matters

ENDEMIC FLUOROSIS

- Features:
  - o Mottling of dental enamel
  - o Chalky white appearance (Caries)
- Intervention: Nalgonda technique (NEERI, Nagpur)

ESSENTIAL FATTY ACID

- Examples of EFA:
  - o Linoleic acid
  - o Linolenic acid
  - o Arachidonic acid
- Rich sources of linoleic acid:
  - o Safflower oil
  - o Sunflower oil
- Sources of omega-3 Poly Unsaturated FA:
  - o Mustard oil
  - o Ground nut oil
  - o Fish oil

Important terms

- Net protein utilization= Digestibility coefficient × Biological value/ 100 = Nitrogen retained X 100/ Nitrogen intake
- Protein energy ratio: Energy from protein/ Total energy in diet
- Protein efficiency ratio: Weight gain per unit protein consumed
- Amino acid score: mg of amino acid per gram of protein (mg. of same amino acid per gram of egg protein)

Vitamins

Vitamin	*Remarks*
Folic acid is useful in the treatment of	**Tropical sprue**
Deficiency of folate may be because of	**Phenytoin, primidone, phenobarbitone, pyrimethamine, methotrexate, cotrimoxazole**
Vitamin B_2 may be destroyed by	**UV light**
Vitamin D	**Does not cross placenta**
Ocular effects of riboflavin deficiency	**Cataract, corneal vascularization**
Appearance of tongue in niacin deficiency	**Raw beef tongue**
Appearance of tongue in riboflavin deficiency	**Magenta red tongue**
Vitamin C is necessary for	**Wound healing**
Vitamin E is useful in	**Fibroadenosis & intermittent claudication**
Pyridoxine is useful in patients suffering from	**Bronchial asthma**
Vitamin A supplementation is needed in patient suffering from	**Measles**
Vitamin A excess may lead to	**Pseudo-tumour cerebri**
Vitamin C & D deficiency lead to	**Pseudo-paralysis**
Vitamin K causes	**Neonatal jaundice**
Vitamin K can cause	**Hemolysis**
Vitamin C is useful in	**Alkaptonuria**
Pyridoxine is useful in	**Homocystinuria**
Deficiency of pyridoxine may lead to	**Convulsions**
Vitamin C is useful in managing	**Met-hemoglobinemia**
Vitamin E is	**Anti-oxidant**
Vitamin B_{12} deficiency may occur with infestation of	**Diphyllobothrium latum**
Deficiency of vitamin B_{12} leads to increased excretion of	**Methyl-malonic acid**

Deficiency of vitamin folate leads to increased excretion of	**FIGLU**
Vitamin D is synthesized in	**Skin**
Vitamin B_2, B_{12} & vitamin K are synthesized in	**Gut (flora)**
Vitamin C & folic acid are	**Heat labile vitamins**
Vitamin B_{12} and D are present in	**Animal foods**
Vitamin C is	**White crystalline substance**
Vitamin B_{12} is	**Red crystalline substance**
Riboflavin is	**Yellow crystalline substance**
Main source of thiamine	**Cereals**
Richest source of vitamin A	**Cod-liver oil**
Vitamin D is stored in	**Fat**
Vitamin B_{12}, A, D, K and folate is stored in	**Liver**
Vitamin B_{12} is	**Erythrocyte maturation factor**
Folic acid is	**Pteroylglutamic acid**
Pantothenate is needed for	**Function of Coenzyme A**
Pyridoxine is needed in metabolism of	**Dopa & GABA**
Pyridoxine is needed for	**Transaminases**
Vitamin B_2 and K is needed for	**Electron transport (coenzyme Q)**
Vitamin K & riboflavin	**Heat stable & light sensitive**

VITAMIN

- Earliest sign of vitamin A deficiency: Conjunctival xerosis
- Daily requirement of vitamin A in children: 1,500 units
- Effect of fat on absorption of vitamin A: Increases
- Vitamin A deficiency is a child health problem if prevalence of night blindness in children's aged 6 months to 6 years is: 1%
- Vitamin which prevents lipid peroxidation: Vitamin E
- Vitamin which is required for gamma carboxylation: Vitamin K
- During pregnancy, IFA tablets contain (specific protection): 100 mg elemental iron & 500 microgram of FA (daily) [Amount is 1/5th for paediatric population (under RCH)]

Vitamin A prophylaxis

- Newborn: 50000 IU at birth
- Children below 12 months: 100000 IU at 9 Months with MMR and then after every 6 months
- Children more than 12 months: 200000 IU till 3 years of age
- Pregnant and lactating women: 5000 IU everyday

EGG & MILK

- Highest biological value is: Egg
- Egg is poor in: Carbohydrate, Vitamin C
- Energy yielded from egg: 70 Kcal
- Milk is a poor source of: Vitamin B, Iron
- Pasteurization of milk is: Precurrent disinfection
- Pasteurization kills: 90% of bacteria in milk, including heat resistant tubercle bacillus & Q fever (doesn't kill thermoduric bacteria, nor the bacterial spores)
- Tests for pasteurization of milk: Phosphatase test
- Methylene blue reduction test in milk is done to: Detection of micro-organism in the milk

CEREALS

- Jaggery has high concentration of: Iron
- Ragi, dates are rich source of: Calcium
- Pulses are deficient in: Methionine
- Cereals are deficient in: Lysine
- Maize is deficient in: Tryptophan/ Lysine

Food toxicity

- Neurolathyrism: BOAA- Lathyrus sativus (kesari dal)
- Aflatoxins: Hepatotoxicity- Aspergillus flavus, Aspergillus Parasiticus infection of groundnut, tapioaca, cereals
- Ergotism: Cereals and millets, infected by field fungus claviceps fusiformis

- Epidemic dropsy: Mustard oil adulterated with argemone oil. Toxins are benzophenanthridine alkaloids-sanguinarine and dihydrosanguinarine. Leg edema with diarrhea
- Endemic ascites: Panicum miliare- (gondhli) contaminated with weed seeds of vrotalaria (jhunjhunia)-ascites with jaundice
- Fusarium toxin: Rice, sorghum, Fusarium incarnatum

NPCB

- Under National Programme for Control of Blindness, vision screening for children is conducted by: School teachers
- WHO definition of blindness: Visual acuity of less than 3/60 in better eye with best possible correction (BEBPC)
- MC cause of blindness in India: Cataract
- Diseases included in global vision 2020:
  - o Cataract
  - o Refractive errors
  - o Childhood blindness
  - o Trachoma
  - o Onchocerciasis

SAFE strategy for trachoma

- S- Trichiasis Surgery
- A- Antibiotic Treatment
- F- Facial cleanliness
- E- Environmental improvement

PNEUMOCONIOSIS

- Bagassosis: Inhalation of sugar cane dust
- Thermoactinomyces causes: Bagassosis
- Farmers lung is caused by: Micropolyspora faeni
- Byssinosis: Textile industry
- Monday fever is associated with: Byssinosis
- Snow storm appearance is seen in: Silicosis

WASTE MANAGEMENT

- Yellow colour: Human anatomical waste (treated by incineration, deep burial)
- Black colour: Discarded medicine, Plastic wrappers etc. (Treated by chemical treatment & disposal in secured land-fills)

Color coding & Waste category

- Yellow: Human anatomical waste
- Red: Microbiology and biotechnology waste
- White translucent: Waste sharps
- Black: Discarded medicines, incineration ash

Chlorination

Mechanism	Disinfection is mainly by HOCl (hypochlorous acid and to small extent by hypochlorite ions)
pH	Chlorine best acts at pH of 7
Break-point chlorination	Point at which chlorine demand is met with
Residual chlorine required for proper disinfection	0.5 mg/ L
Contact period required with free chlorine levels	1 hour
Free chlorine levels are estimated with	Ortho-toluidine test

INSTRUMENTS

- Kata thermometer: Assess cooling power of air & air velocity
- Sling psychrometer: Humidity
- Venturimeter: Measuring bed strength in slow sand filter

COMMITTEES

- Chaddah committee:
  - o PHC at block level
  - o Concept of multipurpose worker
- Kartar Singh committee: MPHW
- Bhore committee: PHC/ primary health centre concept

PRIMARY HEALTH CARE SYSTEM

- 1 village health guide caters to a population of: 1000
- Population covered by PHC in hilly area is: 20, 000
- 1 subcentre caters to a population of: 5,000
- Recommended population for 1 PHC & subcentre for tribal area: 20,000 3,000 respectively
- A trained birth dai caters to a population of: 1000
- As per RCH, first referral unit is: CHC
- Under NTCP (National TB control programme), PHC is said to be PHC-R if: Microscopy + Radiology facility exist

Suggested norms

- Primary centre: 1/ 30000 population in general areas, 1/ 20000 population tribal, hilly and backward areas
- Subcentre: 1/5000 in general areas, 1./ 3000 in tribal, hilly and backward areas
- Community centre: 1/80000 to 1.2 lakhs population
- Dai: 1 per village
- Anganwadi worker: 1 per 1000 population
- Village health guide: 1/ 1000 population or village

BIOSTATISTICS

- Central tendency is given by: Mean, mode, median
- Most commonly used statistical average: Mean
- Normal/ Bell curve is:
    - o A graph representing the density function of the normal probability distribution
    - o Smooth
    - o Bell shaped
    - o Symmetrical curve
    - o Normal standard deviation has variance = 1
- 2SD = 95% of values
- Chi Square test:
    - o Used to compare non-continuous data in 2 groups/ association between 2 variables
    - o Both samples should be mutually exclusive
- True positive (sensitivity): A positive result in the presence of the disease
- True negative (Specificity): A negative test in the absence of the disease

Statistic variables

- Variance = SD^2= Sum of squares/ n-1
- Coefficient of variation= SDX 100/ mean
- Standard error of mean= SD/ Square root of 'n'

Characteristic of data

- Nominal: Cannot be quantified, but divided into qualitative categories, e.g. male- female
- Ordinal: Data can be arranged in a meaningful order, but difference between the value is not constant, e.g. ranking in a class
- Discrete: Variables which can take place only certain values but not between them, e.g. number of children immunized in a village
- Interval: Data can be arranged in meaningful order and the difference between them is meaningful
- Continuous: Variables can take any value, e.g. weight
- Median: Middle observation when the data is arranged in an ascending or descending order
- Mean: Average value of an observation
- Mode: Most commonly occurring value

Area under normal distribution curve

- Mean + 1 SD: 68.3 percent
- Mean + 2 SD: 95.4 percent
- Mean + 3 SD: 99.7 percent

Skewing

- Positive skewing: Mean > median
- Negative skewing: Median > mode

SAMPLING

- Simple random sampling: Sample is drawn in such a way that each unit has an equal chance of being drawn in a sample

- Stratified random sampling: People are divided into certain groups & then some are picked randomly from sub groups
- Cluster sampling: Basically used for assessing immunization status of children under immunization (Error rate is low)
- Work sampling: Systemic observations & recording of activities of one or more individuals carried out at different intervals

HEALTH LEGISLATIONS

- Medical qualifications awarded by institutions outside India & registered by MCI are registered in part II of 3rd schedule of Indian Medical Council Act: 1956
- Information technology act: 2000
- Transplantation of human organs act: 1994

Factory: An establishment employing

- 10 or more workers where power is used
- 20 or more where power is not used
- A minimum of 500 cubic feet of space has been prescribed for each worker
- Prohibits employment of children below 14 years
- Maximum of 48 hours working hours per week, not exceeding 9 hours per day, with rest for atleast ½ hour after 5 hours of continuous work
- Total number of hours in a week (including overtime) shall not exceed 60 hours.

HEADQUARTERS OF HEALTH AGENCIES

- UNICEF: New York, USA
- UNESCO: Paris
- FAO: Rome, Italy

Organization & Location

- ILO, WHO, IRC: Geneva
- UNICEF, UN: New York
- FAO: Rome

UNICEF'S GOBI- FFF program

- Growth monitoring
- Oral rehydration
- Breast feeding
- Immunization
- Female education
- Family spacing
- Food supplements

DEMOGRAPHY

Demographic cycle

- First stage- high stationary: High birth rate and a high death rate which cancel each other and the population remain stationary
- Second stage-early expanding: Death rate begins to decline while birth rate remains unchanged
- Third stage-late expanding: Death rate decline still further and the birth rate tends to fall, population continues to grow as births exceed deaths
- Fourth stage-low stationary: This stage is characterized by low birth and low death rate the population becomes stationary

Population growth

- Stationary population: No growth
- Slow growth: < 0.5
- Moderate growth: 0.5-1
- Rapid growth: 1-1.5
- Very rapid growth: 1.5-2
- Explosive growth: > 2

CALCULATION BASED QUESTIONS

1. **In a case-control study, 300 women aged 20-45 years suffering from breast cancer were compared with age-matched 300 women without breast cancer. It was observed that 120 women among cases and 60 women among controls were obese. The odds ratio of developing breast cancer among obese women is:**

A. 9/5 B. 11/5

C. 8/3 D. 11/3

Odd's ratio:

Obesity (Exposure)	***Cases***	***Controls***
Yes	120 (a)	60 (b)
No	180 (c)	240 (d)
Total	300 (a+c)	300 (b+d)

Odd's ratio (Cross product ratio): ad/ bc

120 × 240/ 60 × 180 = 8/3

Answer: C i.e., 8/3

2. **In a family of six (2 parents and 4 children), the youngest child catches measles infection. The parents are immune to the infection. On 3rd and 5th day of the infection of the first child, the two other children also suffer from measles. The secondary attack rate (SAR) of measles is:**

A. 33.3 % B. 40 %

C. 50 % D. 66.6 %

SAR: Number of exposed persons developing the disease × 100/ Total number of exposed/ susceptible persons.

In this case, 2 children had developed the disease out of the total number of exposed/ susceptible 3 children. The one child, who have the disease would not be counted in numerator or denominator. Parents are immune so they are not susceptible. So, SAR would be: 2 × 100/ 3

Answer: D i.e., 66.6 %

3. **What is the relative risk of developing pulmonary embolism in users of oral contraceptives as per the information given below?**

Women using OCs	***Pulmonary embolism: Yes***	***Pulmonary embolism: No***	***Total***
Yes	120 (a)	80 (b)	200 (a+b)
No	10 (c)	70 (d)	80 (c+d)
Total	130	150	280

A. 0.48 B. 4.80

C. 2.40 D. 0.24

Incidence among exposed: a / a + b = 120/ 200 = 600

Incidence among non-exposed: c/ c + d = 10/ 80 = 125

Relative risk: Incidence among exposed/ Incidence among non-exposed = 600/ 125 = 4.80

Answer: B i.e., 4.80

4. **In a population of 5000, there are 19% eligible couples. To achieve a couple protection rate (CPR) of 60%, how many of these should be covered for family planning services:**

A. 530 B. 550

C. 570 D. 590

In this MCQ, 19% (eligible couple) of total population (5000) is 950. 60% (Couple protection rate) of the total eligible couples (950) comes out to be 570.

Answer: C i.e., 570

5. **An adult weigh 73 kgs and has a height of 1.75 meters. For the purpose of classification of overweight and obesity as per WHO recommendation, this person will be classified as:**

A. Underweight B. Normal

C. Pre-obese D. Overweight

BMI = Weight in kilograms/ (height in meter)^2 = 73/ (1.75)^2 =23.85. Normal BMI is 18.5 to 24.9

Answer: B i.e., Normal

6. **A village 'X' has a population of 5000 with a birth rate of 25 per thousand. In any given month, how many pregnancies should be registered with the ANM of this village:**

A. 66 B. 67

C. 68 D. 69

Birth rate = 25/1000 population

Population = 5000

Therefore, expected number of live births = Birth rate × Population/ 1000 = (25 × 5000)/1000 = 125 births

Correction factor (pregnancy wastage) = 10% of expected number of live births = 10% of 125 (i.e. [10/100] × 125) = 13

As a thumb rule, in any given month, approximately half the number of pregnancies estimated above should be in ANMs records.

Therefore, total no. of expected pregnancies in a year = 125 + 13 = 138

The ANM should have about 69 pregnancies registered with her

Answer: D i.e., 69

7. What is the relative risk of developing tuberculosis among tobacco users as per the information given below?

Tobacco user	*Tuberculosis*		*Total*
	Yes	*No*	
Yes	40	80	120
No	10	70	80
Total	50	150	200

A. 0.48 B. 1.33

C. 2.67 D. 3.90

Relative risk/ risk ratio is the ratio of incidence of the disease among exposed and the incidence of the disease among unexposed (RR=IE/ IO)

IE is calculated as number of subjects developing the disease out of the total exposed.

IE=40/120 = 0.333

IO is calculated as number of subjects developing the disease out of the total un-exposed.

IO=10/80 = 0.125

RR = 0.333/0.125 = 2.664

Answer: C i.e., 2.67

8. What is the attributable risk of tobacco for developing tuberculosis as per the information given below?

Tobacco users	*Tuberculosis*		*Total*
	Present	*Absent*	
Yes	40	80	120
No	10	70	80
Total	50	150	200

A. 50.5% B. 62.5%

C. 70.6% D. 80.6%

Attributable risk/ AR is the ratio of risk difference/ RD and the incidence of the disease among exposed, often expressed as percentage.

AR = RD/IE

RD = IE - IO

IE (Incidence in exposed) is calculated as number of subjects developing the disease out of the total exposed.

IE=40/120 = 0.333

IO (Incidence in unexposed) is calculated as number of subjects developing the disease out of the total unexposed.

IO=10/80 = 0.125

RD = IE – IO = 0.208

AR = 0.208/ 0.333 = 62.46%

Answer: B i.e., 62.5%

9. What is the sensitivity of EEG for detecting brain tumours as per the information given below?

	Brain tumour	
EEG result	*Absent*	*Present*
Positive	54,000	36
Negative	3,06,000	4
	3,60,000	40

A. 90% B. 85%

C. 0.07% D. 99.99%

Sensitivity is the ability of a test to correctly identify those having the disease, i.e., true positives (% of the disease persons, showing the test result positive)

Sensitivity = a × 100/ a+c

Where a is number of patients showing positive test in the presence of disease and c is number of patients showing test negative in the presence of disease (so a+c is the total number of the subjects with disease).

Sensitivity = 36000/40 = 90%

Answer: A i.e., 90%

10. A cohort study was conducted among 200 men aged 20–30 years in Rampur village. Out of 200, 120 men were tobacco users and rest 80 didn't take any form of tobacco. At the end of one year, 40 men among tobacco users and 10 men among non-tobacco users developed tuberculosis. The incidence of tuberculosis among tobacco users is:

A. 12.5 per 100 men/ year

B. 25.0 per 100 men / year

C. 30.0 per 100 men/ year

D. 33.3 per 100 men/ year

Incidence rate of the disease among exposed =

Number of persons developing the disease after exposure (a) × 1000/ Total number of persons exposed/ at risk (a+b)

Incidence among tobacco users = 40 × 1000/ 120 = 33.3 per 100 men/ year

Answer: D i.e., 33.3 per 100 men/ year

CHAPTER 9

ENT

RAPID REVISION NOTES

Dimensions

Structure	*Dimensions*
External auditory meatus/ EAM	**24 mm**
Cartilaginous portion of EAM	**8 mm (outer 1/3rd)**
Bony portion of EAM	**16 mm (inner 2/3rd)**
Eustachian/ pharyngo-tympanic tube/ ET	**36 mm**
Cartilaginous portion of ET	**24 mm (inner 2/3rd)**
Bony portion of ET	**12 mm (outer 1/3rd)**
Vocal cords/ VC	**17-21 mm**
Membranous part of VC	**Anterior 2/3rd**
Cartilaginous part of VC	**Posterior 1/3rd**

EXTERNAL EAR

- Nerve supply of external ear: Auriculotemporal nerve & Vagus
- Length of external auditory canal:
  - o 24 mm;
  - o Outer third: Cartilaginous
  - o Inner two-thirds: Bony
- Cauliflower ear: Perichondritis of external ear (Boxers & wrestlers)
- Special features of malignant otitis externa:
  - o Infection with P. aeruginosa
  - o Elderly diabetics with poor metabolic control &
  - o Granulation tissue found

Boundaries of Suprameatal triangle/ Surface marking for mastoid antrum/MacEwen's triangle

- Anterior: Posterosuperior border of bony external auditory canal along with the Suprameatal spine of Henle
- Superiorly: Supramastoid crest
- Posteriorly: Vertical line drawn tangential to the posterior margin of the external auditory canal

TYMPANIC MEMBRANE

- Parts of tympanic membrane: 2 parts:
  - o Pars tensa &
  - o Pars flaccida (Shrapnell's membrane)
- Location of cone of light: Antero-inferior
- Nerve supply of tympanic membrane:
  - o Auriculotemporal nerve
  - o Auricular branch of vagus

- Normal appearance of tympanic membrane: Pearly white
- Functional surface area of tympanic membrane: 55 m^2

MIDDLE EAR

- Attic/ Epitympanum is:
  - o Part superior to the level of tympanic membrane
  - o Prussak's space lies in the epitympanum
- Narrowest part of middle ear: Mesotympanum
- Location of mesotympanum: Directly medial to the tympanic membrane
- Location of tegmen/ roof of the tympanum: Opposite the middle cranial fossa
- Hyperacusis is prevented by: Stapedius

INNER EAR

- Location of inner ear: Petrous part of temporal bone
- Nerve which gets injured in inner ear (transverse fractures of temporal bone): Facial nerve
- Bony labyrinth is: Cancellous bone
- Location of organ of Corti: Organ of Corti (with its hair cells) rests on Basilar membrane
- Contents of perilymph:
  - o Resemble ECF
  - o Low K^+ & high Na^+
- Angular acceleration is sensed by: Semi-circular canal

Acceleration & part of ear stimulated

- Angular acceleration: Semicircular canal
- Linear acceleration: Utricles and saccules
- Horizontal linear acceleration: Saccules
- Vertical linear acceleration: Saccules
- Gravity: Utricles and saccules
- Position of head in space: Utricle and saccules

Nerve supply

Structure	*Nerve supply*
Middle ear	Tympanic branch of IX cranial nerve
Tympanic membrane	Auriculotemporal nerve, auricular branch of vagus
Pinna	Auriculotemporal nerve, auricular branch of vagus
Larynx above the vocal cords	Internal branch of superior laryngeal nerve
Larynx below the vocal cords	Recurrent laryngeal nerve
Nose	V cranial nerve (sensory)

EUSTACHIAN TUBE

- Development of eustachian tube: 1st pharyngeal pouch
- Special feature of eustachian tube: Opens during swallowing (Tensor palati)

Management of some common conditions

Conditions	*Management*
Maggots in ear	Chloroform vapour application, later removal
Otomycosis	2% salicylic acid in alcohol
Acute & chronic otitis externa	Gentamycin & corticosteroid
Diffuse otitis externa	Irrigation with normal saline mop
Furuncle of external ear	Ichthammol glycerine

OTITIS EXTERNA

- Diffuse otitis externa is also known as: Singapore ear/ Tropical ear/ swimmers' ear/ Telephonists' ear
- Commonest causative agent of otitis externa is: Staphylococcus aureus
- Investigation of choice in malignant otitis externa is: Gallium CT scan

OTITIS MEDIA & COMPLICATIONS

- Mastoid reservoir phenomenon is associated with: Acute suppurative otitis media (ASOM)

- Special features of serous otitis media/ secretory otitis media/ glue ear:
    - o Marginal perforation
    - o B shaped tympanogram
    - o Medical treatment ineffective
    - o Myringotomy with Ventilation tube insertion
- Location of perforation in CSOM:
    - o Safe CSOM: Central
    - o Unsafe CSOM: Marginal
- Complications of CSOM:
    - o Mastoiditis (MC complication of CSOM)
    - o Brain abscess (MC cause of brain abscess is CSOM)
    - o Bezolds abscess (Sternocleidomastoid)
    - o Gradenigo's syndrome: (Retro-orbital pain, photophobia & lacrimation, V & VI (ipsilateral) cranial nerve involvement) and otitis media
- Special features of cholesteatoma/ epidermolysis / keratoma:
    - o Basically a bony erosion
    - o Usually found in apex of petrous temporal bone
    - o Attic/ posterior-superior marginal region is usually involved
    - o Modified radical mastoidectomy is done (spares the tympanic membrane & ossicles)
- Pathognomonic sign of lateral sinus thrombosis (LST):
    - o Tenderness & edema over mastoid process (Griesinger's sign)
    - o Tobey-Ayer test is done for LST
- MC procedure done for CSOM: Modified radical mastoidectomy
- Radical mastoidectomy is done for: Attico-antral cholesteatoma

ASOM

- Cartwheel appearance: Radially placed dilated blood vessels on the surface of tympanic membrane
- Lighthouse sign: Pulsatile discharge of the exudates under pressure, Synchronized with pulse

Abscess related to ear

- Bezold's abscess: Deep to sternocleidomastoid
- Luc's abscess: Roof of bony canal, subtemporal
- Citelli's abscess: Digastric triangle, posterior belly of digastric

Terms related with lateral sinus thrombosis

- Griesinger's sign: Thrombosis of mastoid emissary vein, Edema over posterior part of mastoid
- Tobey-Ayer test/ Queckenstedt's test: Compression of vein on the thrombosed side produces no effect, while on healthy side it leads to rapid rise in CSF pressure

OTOSCLEROSIS

- Otosclerosis begins in: Fossula ante-fenestram
- MC site of otosclerosis: Oval window
- MC bone affected in otosclerosis: Stapes
- Presenting features of otosclerosis:
    - o Positive family history
    - o Reversible conductive deafness
    - o Paracusis Willisii (ability to hear better in noisy environment)
- Appearance of tympanic membrane in otosclerosis: Flamingo pink tympanic membrane
- Audiometric finding of otosclerosis: Carhart's notch at 2000 Hz
- Stapedectomy (Surgical procedure of choice)
- Sodium fluoride

MENIERE'S DISEASE

- Also known as Endolymphatic hydrops/ Ear glaucoma
- Triad of Meniere's disease:
    - o Hearing loss (low frequency sensorineural)
    - o Tinnitus (non-pulsatile) &
    - o Recurrent prostrating vertigo
- Pathologic change in the inner ear in Meniere's disease: Generalized dilatation of the membranous labyrinth

BELL'S PALSY

- Features:
  - o Unilateral facial palsy
  - o Lower motor neuron lesion
  - o Acute onset
  - o Increased predisposition in DM

CHEMODECTOMA

- Chemodectoma/ Non-chromaffin Paraganglioma's are seen at:
  - o Area of Jacobson's nerve in the tympanic plexus on the promontory of middle ear (Glomus tympanicus tumour)
  - o Glomus jugulare body in the jugular bulb of IJV (Glomus jugulare tumour)
- Special features of glomus tumour:
  - o MC type is squamous cell Ca
  - o Multicentric with lymphatic metastasis
- Treatment:
  - o Modified radical mastectomy
  - o Excision of petrous temporal bone (Surgical procedures)

ACOUSTIC NEUROMA/ VESTIBULAR SCHWANNOMA

- They arise from: Vestibular division of the eight nerve
- MC involved structure: Superior vestibular nerve
- Earliest symptom: Deafness (Retrocochlear type)
- Other features:
  - o V cranial nerve involvement
  - o Loss of corneal reflex
- Most sensitive & specific test: Gadolinium enhanced MRI (head)

OTOTOXIC DRUGS

- Aminoglycosides:
  - o Gentamycin
  - o Kanamycin
  - o Neomycin
- Loop diuretics:
  - o Furosemide
  - o Ethacrynic acid

DEAFNESS (SYNDROMES)

- Pendred syndrome:
  - o Deafness
  - o Goitre
- Ushers syndrome:
  - o Deafness
  - o Mental retardation
  - o Seizures
  - o Retinitis pigmentosa
  - o Cataracts
- Alport's syndrome:
  - o Progressive sensorineural loss
  - o Progressive severe glomerulonephritis

Hearing loss

- Mild deafness: Hearing loss between 20-30 db
- Moderate deafness: Hearing loss between 30-60 db
- Severe deafness: Hearing loss above 60 db

LAB ASSESSMENT OF HEARING

- Otoacoustic emissions (OAE):
  - o Their presence shows that outer hair cells of the organ of corti are intact
  - o Can be used to distinguish sensory from neural hearing loss
- Brainstem auditory evoked responses (BAER's):
  - o Useful in differentiating the site of sensori-neural hearing loss

TESTS RELATED TO EAR

- Tobey Ayer test: Lateral sinus thrombosis
- Hallpike test: Vestibular function
- Recruitment test: Meniere's disease
- Caloric test: Vestibular function

Rinne test

- Atleast 15 db of hearing loss should be present for it to become negative
- Positive: Normal and sensorineural deafness
- Negative: Conductive deafness

Weber test

- Atleast 5 db of hearing loss should be present for it to become lateralized
- Normal: Equal on both sides
- Conductive deafness: Lateralised to the affected ear
- Sensorineural deafness: Sound is Lateralised to the better ear

MC ORGANISM

- Malignant otitis externa: P. aeruginosa
- Perichondritis: P. aeruginosa
- Hemorrhagic otitis externa: Influenza
- Bullous myringitis: Influenza virus
- Ramsay Hunt syndrome: Herpes Zoster virus
- Furuncle: Staph. aureus
- Otomycosis:
  - o Aspergillus niger
  - o Candida

Arterial supply

Structure	*Arterial supply*
Middle ear	Middle meningeal artery, maxillary artery, ascending pharyngeal artery, stylomastoid branch of posterior auricular artery
Inner ear	Internal auditory artery
Larynx	Superior thyroid artery, inferior thyroid artery, cricothyroid artery
Tonsil	Tonsillar branch of facial artery
Little area/ Kiesselbach's plexus	Sphenopalatine artery, greater palatine artery, superior labial branch of facial artery

NOSE

- Arterial supply to nasal mucosa: Branches of external carotid artery
- Functions of nasal cavity:
  - o Warming
  - o Filtration &
  - o Moistening of air
- Opening of nasolacrimal duct: Inferior meatus
- Openings in middle meatus:
  - o Maxillary sinus
  - o Anterior ethmoidal sinus
  - o Naso-frontal ducts
- Opening in spheno-ethmoid recess: Sphenoid sinus

Dangerous area of face

- Lower part of external nose and upper lip
- Infection may spread to the cavernous sinus through the inferior ophthalmic veins via the anterior facial vein

Dangerous area of nose

- Also olfactory area may infect the meninges along the pia mater and arachnoid mater sheath of the olfactory nerve passing through the cribriform plate of the ethmoid causing meningitis, encephalitis and brain abscess

Opening in the lateral wall of nose

- Spheno-ethmoidal recess: Opening of sphenoid sinus
- Superior meatus: Opening of posterior ethmoidal sinus
- Middle meatus: Frontal sinus, Maxillary sinus, Anterior ethmoidal sinus, Middle ethmoidal sinus
- Inferior meatus: Nasolacrimal duct

Paranasal sinuses

Sinus	*Remarks*
Maxillary & ethmoidal sinuses	Common site for angiomas, inverted papillomas & ossifying fibromas
Frontal sinus	Common site for osteoma
Ethmoidal sinus	Common site for adenocarcinoma
Frontal sinus	Rudimentary sinus at birth
Frontal sinusitis	Can cause osteomyelitis in adults
Maxillary sinusitis	Can cause osteomyelitis in children
Frontal sinusitis is associated with	Extra-dural abscess
Ethmoid sinusitis is associated with	Orbital lesions
Ethmoid sinus	Commonest site for polyp
Maxillary sinus	Commonest site for malignancy
Frontal sinus	Commonest sinus for mucocele
Maxillary sinus	Commonest site for sinusitis

SINUSITIS

- Mucopurulent pus in middle meatus suggests: Maxillary sinusitis
- Periodicity is a feature of: Frontal sinusitis
- Sinusitis not seen at birth: Frontal sinusitis
- Definitive diagnosis of sinusitis: Sinoscopy
- FESS (Functional Endoscopic Sinus Surgery):
  - o Nasal polyps
  - o Mucocele

Management of epistaxis

Site/ condition	*Method*
Bleeding above the middle turbinate	**Clip the anterior ethmoidal artery**
Bleeding from below the middle turbinate	**Clip the maxillary artery and branch**
If clotting factors are decreased	**No pack, cautery is best (cautery is the treatment of choice EXCEPT in children)**
In children's	**Petroleum jelly application**

EPISTAXIS

- MC site:
  - o Kiesselbach's plexus (plexus of vessels);
  - o In Littles area (Antero-inferior part of nasal septum)
- Arteries contributing to Little area:
  - o Sphenopalatine artery
  - o Greater palatine artery
  - o Superior labial artery
  - o Anterior ethmoidal artery
- Recurrent epistaxis is seen in:
  - o Deviated nasal septum
  - o Atrophic rhinitis
  - o Maxillary Ca
- MC cause of epistaxis in pubescent male: Angiofibroma
- MC cause of epistaxis in children: Trauma
- Commonest cause of epistaxis in elderly is hypertension

MISCELLANEOUS (NOSE)

- Pale, edematous nasal mucosa indicates: Nasal allergy
- Depressed nasal bridge:
  - o Trauma/ Abscess
  - o Syphilis
- Parosmia: Perception of bad smell
- Young's operation is done in: Atrophic rhinitis
- Histological feature of rhinoscleroma: Mikulicz cells (Foamy histiocytes)
- Condition presenting as black eschars in nasal cavity, particularly in poorly controlled DM, transplantation, heamtologic malignancy, on long term desferrioxamine therapy: Mucormycosis

- Jarjawey fracture: Oblique fracture of nasal septum
- Apple jelly nodules on nasal septum: Lupus vulgaris
- Features of CSF rhinorrhea: Fracture of cribriform plate of ethmoid/ Naso-ethmoid fracture, Beta 2 transferrins levels are high

Antrochoanal polyp

- From maxillary sinus
- Usually single
- Seen in children and adults
- Due to infection
- Extends backwards
- Recurrence unlikely

Ethmoidal polyp

- Ethmoidal sinus
- Multiple and bilateral
- After puberty
- Allergy and infection
- Extends forwards
- Recurrence likely

ORAL CAVITY

- Ludwig's angina:
  - o Edema floor of mouth
  - o Involves submandibular & Sublingual spaces
- Ranula:
  - o Thin walled
  - o Retention cyst
  - o Sublingual
- MC malignant tumour of adult male: Oral cancer
- Pre-malignant conditions (for oral cancer):
  - o Leukoplakia
  - o Erythroplakia
  - o Oral submucosal fibrosis
- Treatment:
  - o Surgery (treatment of choice)
  - o Radiosensitive

PHARYNX

- Nasopharynx:
  - o Oval shaped
  - o Opening of eustachian tube

Waldeyer's ring

- Palatine tonsil
- Nasopharyngeal tonsil
- Tubal tonsils
- Lingual tonsils
- Lateral pharyngeal bands
- Pharyngeal nodules

JUVENILE NASOPHARYNGEAL ANGIOFIBROMA

- Features:
  - o Benign
  - o Vascular neoplasm (Biopsy contra-indicated)
  - o Millers sign
- MC site: Posterior part of nasal cavity (close to spheno-palatine foramen)
- Investigation of choice: Contrast enhanced CT scan
- Treatment of choice: Surgery; (they are responsive to radiotherapy)

Management of tumors

Type	*Management*
Angiofibroma	**Surgery**
Angiofibroma with bone destruction	**Radiation**
Nasopharyngeal Ca and lymphoma	**Radiation including neck lymph nodes**
Squamous cell Ca face	**Radiotherapy**
Squamous cell Ca with cartilage involvement	**Surgery**

NASOPHARYNGEAL CARCINOMA

- MC age group affected: Bimodal
- MC site: Lateral wall of nasopharynx (Fossa of Rosenmuller)
- Associated with:
  - o EBV infection
  - o Serous otitis media
- Trotter's triad:
  - o Conductive deafness
  - o Palatal paralysis
  - o Temporo-parietal neuralgia

PERITONSILLAR ABSCESS/ QUINSY

- MC organism: Streptococcus
- Timing of surgery: 6 weeks after appearance

LARYNX

- Primary function of larynx: Protection of the lower airways
- Abductor of vocal cord: Posterior crico-arytenoid
- Adductor of vocal cord:
  - o Lateral crico-arytenoid
  - o Transverse crico-arytenoid
- Epithelial lining of larynx: Stratified squamous
- Nerve supply of cricothyroid: External laryngeal nerve

LARYNGOMALACIA

- MC cause of stridor in newborn
- Omega shaped epiglottitis
- Reassurance (NO active treatment)

Singer's nodes/ Vocal nodules

- In persons who misuse or overuse their voice
- Excision by microlaryngoscopy

VOCAL CORD PARALYSIS

- Maximum stridor is seen with:
  - o Bilateral
  - o Incomplete Vocal cord palsy
- Most dangerous vocal cord palsy:
  - o Bilateral
  - o Abductor palsy
- MC cause of vocal cord palsy: Total thyroidectomy
- Bilateral recurrent laryngeal nerve palsy occurs in:
  - o Thyroid malignancy
  - o Thyroidectomy
- Thyroplasty type I is: Medialization of vocal cords

EPIGLOTTITS

- MC causative organism for epiglottitis: H. influenzae type B
- MC cause of death in epiglottitis: Complete airway obstruction

MALIGNANT NEOPLASM OF LARYNX

- Premalignant conditions:
  - o Keratosis
  - o Papilloma etc.
- MC type: Squamous cell Ca
- Supraglottic Ca:
  - o Pain is the MC manifestation
  - o Early lymphatic spread
- Glottic Ca:
  - o Hoarseness is the earliest & MC manifestation,
  - o Best prognosis
  - o No lymphadenopathy
- Post-cricoid Ca: Metastasis to both sides of the neck is common
- Verrucous Ca is treated by: Endoscopic surgery

Management of laryngeal carcinoma

Type	*Management*
Transglottic Ca	Total laryngectomy and radical neck dissection (if lymph nodes are involved)
Subglottic Ca	Radiation (surgery in recurrence)

MISCELLANOEUS (LARYNX)

- Features of laryngeal TB:
  - o Mammillated appearance
  - o Turban epiglottitis
- Laryngitis sicca: Laryngitis atrophica (Caused by Klebsiella ozaenae)
- Quincke's disease: Edema of uvula
- Reinke's edema: Edema of vocal cords
- Kiss ulcer of larynx/ Contact ulcer of larynx: Vocal abuse

TRACHEOSTOMY

- Tracheostomy tube:
  - o Double tube
  - o Made of titanium silver alloy
- Structures damaged in emergency tracheostomy:
  - o Isthmus of thyroid
  - o Inferior thyroid vein
  - o Thyroid ima artery
- Common complication of tracheostomy: Tracheal stenosis (Mitomycin is used for this complication)

CLINICAL PRESENTATIONS

- Parapharyngeal abscess:
  - o Post-dental extraction
  - o Swelling in posterior 1/3rd of sternocleidomastoid
  - o Medial shift of tonsil
- Angiofibroma:
  - o 13 years old male
  - o Swelling in cheek
  - o Recurrent epistaxis

X-rays in ENT

Sinus	*Best viewed in*
Maxillary sinus	**Occipito-mental**
Frontal & ethmoidal sinus	**Occipito-frontal**
Frontal & sphenoid	**Straight lateral**
Ethmoid sinus	**Oblique**
Sphenoid sinus	**Sub-mento-vertical**
Petrous cells	**Stenver's or Towne's view**
To confirm fluid	**Tilted films**

CLINICAL QUESTIONS

1. **A known case of asthma presented to the ENT OPD with the complaints of chronic rhinorrhoea and nasal polyps. After evaluation, a diagnosis of Samter's triad was made. Which drug should be AVOIDED in such a patient?**

A. Aspirin B. Co-amoxi-clav

C. Penicillin D. Cotrimoxazole

Samter's triad is the triad of nasal polyps, asthma and aspirin intolerance.

Answer: A i.e., Aspirin

2. **A 3 years old child presented to the Emergency department with difficulty in breathing. Chest X-ray was done and it showed hyperinflation of right side, left side being normal. True statement related to this clinical picture:**

A. Use of flexible bronchoscope is indicated in management

B. If there is decreased air entry on right side, it suggests foreign body

C. Ball valve effect is the mechanism responsible for hyperinflation of right lung

D. Clinical diagnosis is of croup is made

Clinical presentation is indicative of bronchial foreign body.

Children less than 5% of age constitute more than 50% of the patients.

They have the tendency to put the things in their mouth, which can go either in the food passages or air passages.

Right bronchus is the most common site of FBs (foreign bodies) because it is wider and more in line with the tracheal lumen.

A FB may either totally obstruct a lobar/ segmental bronchus (atelectasis), or produce a check valve obstruction (obstructive emphysema) which allows only ingress of air.

Atelectasis is due to complete step valve obstruction.

It can affect lung or its segment.

Poor air entry is found on auscultation of the lower lobe on the back of the thorax.

X-ray chest PA and lateral views especially at the end of inspiration and expiration show atelectasis and obstructive emphysema, and provide indirect evidence of radiolucent FB.

Rigid bronchoscopy under GA is the standard procedure for FB removal.

Answer: B i.e., If there is decreased air entry on right side, it suggests foreign body

3. **A patient with damage to basilar membrane presented with high frequency hearing loss. Most likely site of lesion:**

A. Stria vascularis B. Helicotrema

C. Oval window D. Modiolus

Fibers near the upper end of the cochlea (i.e., helicotrema) resonate to lower frequency sound.

Those near the oval window respond to higher frequencies.

Answer: C i.e., Oval window

4. **Which is the most pulsatile condition found in the ear, which bleeds on touch?**

A. CSOM

B. Chronic adhesive otitis media

C. Acute otitis media

D. Glomus tumour

Clinical presentation is suggestive of glomus tumour.

On increasing the ear canal pressure with Siegel's speculum, glomus tumour pulsates vigorously and then blanches. Reverse happens with release of pressure (Brown's sign).

Answer: D i.e., Glomus tumour

5. **A patient with history of head injury developed unilateral conducting hearing loss. On examination, tympanic membrane is normal and mobile. The cause for deafness could be:**

A. Collection of fluid in the middle ear

B. Osteoma

C. Dislocation of the incudostapedial joint

D. ASOM

Clinical presentation is suggestive of dislocation of the incudo-stapedial joint.

Conductive Hearing Loss/ CHL with normal TM can be seen in temporal bone fracture, congenital fixity of ossicles, otosclerosis, congenital cholesteatoma or glomus tumour.

Answer: C i.e., Dislocation of the incudostapedial joint

6. **A child with otitis media, not responding to ampicillin presents with bulging membrane with dull look. Treatment of choice is:**

A. Ciprofloxacin B. Mastoidectomy

C. Myringotomy D. Grommet insertion

Indications of myringotomy in ASOM: (i) Bulging eardrum (ii) Acute excruciating pain (iii) Unresponsiveness to antibiotics (iv) Complications like facial paralysis, labyrinthitis or meningitis with bulging tympanic membrane.

Answer: C i.e., Myringotomy

7. **A patient presented with high fever & signs of raised intracranial tension. There is past history of CSOM (chronic suppurative otitis media). Likely diagnosis is:**

A. Brain abscess

B. Pyogenic meningitis

C. Acute subarachnoid hemorrhage

D. Acute osteomyelitis of the skull

Clinical presentation is suggestive of brain abscess.

Fifty percent cases of brain abscesses in adults and 25% in children are otogenic.

In adults, cholesteatoma and in children AOM are the most common causes.

Cerebral abscess occurs more frequently than cerebellar abscess.

Answer: A i.e., Brain abscess

8. **A patient is having scanty, foul-smelling discharge from the ear and hearing loss. Treatment of choice in such a case:**

A. Radical mastoidectomy

B. Modified radical mastoidectomy

C. Suction clearance

D. Cautery with trichloroacetic acid

Clinical presentation is suggestive of CSOM

Modified radical mastoidectomy eradicates diseases from the attic and mastoid and exteriorizes both into EAC by removal of the posterior meatal and lateral attic walls.

The remnant of tympanic membrane, functioning ossicles and the reversible mucosa and function of the Eustachian tube, which are necessary to reconstruct hearing mechanism, are preserved.

Answer: B i.e., Modified radical mastoidectomy

9. **Unilateral nasal obstruction with blood-stained discharge in a child is commonly due to:**

A. Foreign body B. Choanal atresia

C. Polyps D. Fungal infection

Clinical presentation is suggestive of nasal foreign body

Causes of unilateral blood-stained discharge include forgotten foreign body nose, rhinolith and sequestra, nasal diphtheria, nasal myiasis (maggots), acute & chronic unilateral sinusitis and malignancy of nose and paranasal sinuses

Answer: A i.e., Foreign body

10. **A patient who had undergone tooth extraction for dental caries, presents with swelling in posterior part of middle 1/3rd of sternomastoid & tonsil is pushed medially. The diagnosis is:**

A. Retropharyngeal abscess

B. Parapharyngeal abscess

C. Ludwig's angina

D. Vincent's angina

Clinical presentation is suggestive of parapharyngeal abscess.

The parapharyngeal abscess collects medial to the medial pterygoid muscle.

The otogenic parapharyngeal abscess is caused by petrositis.

In other instances, it occurs due to caries/ extraction of molar tooth.

Patient develops trismus, fever and swelling that pushes the tonsil medially and spreads laterally posterior to sternocleidomastoid.

Answer: B i.e., Parapharyngeal abscess

11. **A child presents with unilateral, foul smelling nasal discharge. Most probable cause could be:**

A. Acute sinusitis B. Foreign body

C. Rhinolith D. Nasal synechiae

Clinical presentation is suggestive of nasal foreign body.

A unilateral foul smelling purulent nasal discharge in a child is mostly due to forgotten foreign body nose.

Answer: B i.e., Foreign body

12. **A 31 years old female patient complains of bilateral impairment of hearing for the past 5 years. On examination, tympanic membrane is normal and audiogram shows a bilateral conductive deafness. Acoustic reflexes are absent. All constitute part of treatment EXCEPT:**

A. Hearing aid B. Stapedectomy

C. Sodium fluoride D. Gentamycin

Clinical presentation is suggestive of otosclerosis.

In aminoglycoside antibiotics group, streptomycin, gentamycin and tobramycin are primarily vestibulotoxic.

So, patients present with dizziness/ vertigo.

In large doses, they can damage the cochlea also.

So, gentamycin should never be used in patients with hearing loss.

Answer: D i.e., Gentamycin

13. **Adult patient presented with headache, epiphora and nasal obstruction, but there was NO fever. Condition could be:**

A. Meningitis

B. Foreign body obstruction

C. Cavernous sinus thrombosis

D. Carcinoma of maxillary sinus

Clinical presentation is suggestive of carcinoma of maxillary sinus.

Late features of maxillary carcinoma appear when tumour spreads and destroys the bony confines and involves surrounding structures.

Medial spread towards nasal cavity result in nasal obstruction, discharge and epistaxis.

Superior spread towards orbit result in facial paresthesia/ anesthesia, proptosis, diplopia, ocular pain and epiphora.

Answer: D i.e., Carcinoma of maxillary sinus

14. **Child presented with ear pain & markedly congested tympanic membrane. Diagnosis is:**

A. ASOM B. CSOM

C. Serous otitis media D. Otosclerosis

Clinical presentation is suggestive of ASOM (acute suppurative otitis media)

In stage of pre-suppuration, patient present with marked throbbing ear pain, which can awake the child from sleep in night.

On examination, pars tensa is congested and bulging out with cart-wheel appearance (leash of blood vessels along the handle of malleus and at the periphery of tympanic membrane) and loss of light reflex.

Answer: A i.e., ASOM

15. **An infant with a past history of ear infection is suspected to have meningitis. Organism commonly responsible for such a presentation would be:**

A. Mycobacterium

B. Moraxella catarrhalis

C. Pseudomonas

D. Streptococcus pneumoniae

Meningitis is the MC (most common) intracranial complication of SOM (suppurative otitis media).

In infants and children, meningitis is often the complication of AOM (acute otitis media), while in adults it occurs due to cholesteatoma.

The one-third cases of meningitis are otogenic in origin.

Major pathogens are Hemophilus influenza and Streptococcus pneumoniae.

Answer: D i.e., Streptococcus pneumoniae

CHAPTER 10

OPHTHALMOLOGY

RAPID REVISION NOTES

Cataracts

Type	*Feature*
Nuclear cataract	Brown/ black cataract (Brunescent cataracts)
Incipient cataract	Wedge with base to periphery
Cupuliform cataract	Senile cataract seen in posterior part
Posterior cortical cataract in choroiditis	Polychromatic lusture; bread-crumb appearance in slit lamp
Morgagnian cataract	Senile cataract
Heat cataract	Infra-red rays
Senile cataract	May be produced by UV rays
Progressive congenital cataract	Rubella
Coralliform cataract	Spindle shaped
Coronary cataract	Club shaped
Zonular cataract	Riders are seen
Coerulea cataract	Blue dots are seen

CATARACTS

- Snowflake cataract: DM
- Rossette cataract: Trauma
- Christmas tree pattern: Myotonic dystrophy
- Sunflower cataract: Wilsons disease
- Oil drop cataract: Galactosemia

IMPORTANT VALUES

- Diameter of optic nerve: 1.5 mm
- Anteroposterior length of eyeball: 24 mm
- Depth of anterior chamber: 2-3 mm
- Volume of vitreous: 4 ml
- Volume of orbit: 30 cc

Normal values

- Refractory index of emmetropic eye = 60 D
- Normal intraocular pressure is 10-22 mm Hg

EXTRAOCULAR MUSCLES

- Intorters of the eye:
  - o Superior oblique &
  - o Superior rectus
- Actions of superior oblique:
  - o Abduction

- o Inortion &
- o Depression

- Nerve supply of superior oblique: Trochlear (4th cranial nerve)
- Levator palpebrae superioris is supplied by: 3rd cranial nerve (oculomotor)
- Muscle attached to posterior tarsal margin: Muller's muscle

PUPIL

- Argyll Robertson pupil (ARP):
  - o Small pupils
  - o Irregular in shape
  - o No reaction to light
  - o Accommodation reflex present (ARP)
- Marcus's Gunn pupil (pupillary escape):
  - o Affected pupil may paradoxically dilate, when light source is swung from eye to eye (normally constricts)
  - o Defect anterior to optic chiasma

Pupil

- Adie's pupil: Due to degeneration of ciliary ganglion. Dilated pupil. Tonic reaction to light and accommodation. Associated with hyporeflexia (Holmes-Adie pupil)
- Marcus-Gunn pupil: Normal sized pupil. Relative afferent pupillary defect. Cause optic nerve/retinal disease

Corneal ulcer

Ulcer	*Condition/ cause*
Keratitis without ulcer	Interstitial keratitis, disciform keratitis
Ulcer without perforation	Fascicular ulcer
Ulcers where steroid are contraindicated	Phlyctenular ulcer
Ulcer with virus demonstrable in anterior chamber	Herpes
Dendritic ulcer	Herpes simplex

CORNEA

- Epithelium: Non-keratinized stratified squamous
- The substantia propria of cornea of the cornea is mostly composed of: Collagen
- Cornea can absorb oxygen from: Air (directly)
- Nutrients can diffuse into cornea from: Aqueous humour
- Medial longitudinal fasciculus (MLF) is important for: Conjugate gaze
- A lesion in MLF results in: Inability to medially rotate (adduct) the ipsilateral eye on attempted lateral gaze (Intranuclear ophthalmoplegia)

Organisms penetrating intact cornea

- N. gonorrhea
- N. meningitides
- C. diphtheria
- Acanthamoeba
- Listeria monocytogenes

Layers of cornea

- Epithelium - Stratified squamous epithelium
- Bowman's membrane - Condensed collagen fibrils
- Stroma / substantia propia - Collagen fibrils
- Descemet's membrane / posterior elastic lamina
- Endothelium – Single layer

Causes of neurotrophic keratopathy

- Herpes zoster
- Herpes simplex
- Fifth nerve damage
- Diabetes
- Leprosy

EMBRYOLOGY

- Structures derived from mesoderm:
  - o Corneal stroma & endothelium
  - o Only smooth muscles of iris
  - o All muscles (EXCEPT iris muscle)

- Structures derived from surface ectoderm:
  - o Conjunctival epithelium
  - o Lens
- Structures derived from neuroectoderm:
  - o Epithelium of iris & ciliary body
  - o Muscles of iris (constrictor & dilator pupillae)

Avascular ocular structures

- Vitreous
- Cornea
- Lens

DEVELOPMENT

- Eye of newborn:
  - o Hypermetropic
  - o 2-3D
- Critical period of development of fixation reflex: 2-4 months

ANGLES OF EYE

- Visual angle: Angle subtended by object at nodal point of lens
- Alpha angle: Between visual axis & optical axis
- Kappa angle: Between pupillary axis & visual axis

Instruments in ophthalmology

Instrument	*Use*
Ishihara chart	**Colour vision**
Retinoscope	**Refractive errors**
Placido's disc	**Assess the surface of cornea**
Gonioscope	**Measure the angle of anterior chamber**
Tonometer	**Ocular pressure**
Slit-lamp	**Examine different planes in eyes**
Ophthalmoscope	**Visualize retina**
Exophthalmometer	**Proptosis**
Perimeter	**Field of vision**

OPHTHALMOLOGICAL TEST

- Direct ophthalmoscopy:
  - o Image is virtual & erect
  - o Magnified 15 times
- Indirect ophthalmoscopy:
  - o Image is real & inverted
  - o Magnified 5 times
  - o It is done for examination of periphery of retina (upto ora serrata)
- Keratometry: Measures curvature of cornea
- Electronystatogram: Graph of movement of eye
- Anomoloscope: Detects colour blindness
- Retinoscopy: Objective assessment of refractive state of eye
- Gonioscopy: Measures angle of anterior chamber
- Tonometry:
  - o Measures intraocular pressure
  - o Best is applanation tonometry
- Swinging flash test: Tests pupil
- Snellen chart test: Vision
- Ishihara plates, Hardy Rand Rattler plates: Color vision
- Landolt's rings: Visual acuity in illiterates, children
- Macular function tests:
  - o Card board test (2 point discrimination test)
  - o Amsler grid test
  - o Maddox rod test etc.

Image in ophthalmoscopy

Direct ophthalmoscopy	*Indirect ophthalmoscopy*
Erect	Inverted
Virtual	Real
15 times magnification	5 times magnification
Visualize slightly beyond equator	Upto ora serrata
Not useful in hazy media	Helpful
Stereopsis absent	Present
Distance of 15 mm from eye	At an arm's distance

Colour blindness

- Protanopia: Defective red colour perception
- Deuteranopia: Defective green colour perception
- Tritanopia: Defective blue colour perception

Hirschberg test (Used to roughly estimate the angle of deviation in strabismus)

- Edge of pupil: 15 degree
- Mid cornea: 30 degree
- Corneal margin: 45 degree
- Sclera: 60 degree
- 1 mm from papillary centre: 7 degree
- Nasal limbus: -35 degree

The plan followed in the management of squint (in order)

- Refraction
- Orthoptic exercise
- Operative correction
- Prism for remaining error after operation

LID

- MC type of lid Ca: Squamous cell Ca
- Adhesion of margins of 2 eyelid is known as: Ankyloblepharon
- Recurrent chalazion may predispose to: Sebaceous cell Ca
- Features of congenital chronic dacryocystitis:
  - o Epiphora (abnormal overflow of tears);
  - o Regurgitation of pus
  - o Conjunctivo-cysto-rhinostomy is one of the procedures done

Conditions & affected glands

- Chalazion: Chronic inflammation of meibomian gland
- Hordeolum externum: Suppurative inflammation of glands of Zeiss
- Hordeolum internum: Suppurative inflammation of meibomian glands

Optic pathway lesions

Site of lesion	*Defect*	*Pupil*
Cortex	Macula spared	Pupil spared
Temporal lobe	Homonymous quadrantanopia	-
Subcortex	Quadrantanopia	-
Optic tract posterior part	Homonymous hemianopia	Wernicke's hemianopic
Optic chiasma	Bitemporal hemianopia	-
Optic nerve	Total visual loss on same side	Direct reflex- absent; consensual reflex- present

VISUAL FIELD DEFECTS

- Homonymous hemianopia: Lesions of optic tract (incongruous defects)
- Homonymous quadrantanopia: Lesion of temporal lobe (superior)
- Bitemporal hemianopia: Lesions of optic chiasm

VISUAL PATHWAY

- Optic pathway: Receptors: Rods & cones (retina)
- Thalamic nucleus for vision: Lateral geniculate body
- Light reflex: Excess Light → retina → optic nerve → optic chiasma → optic tract Some fibres from optic tract → Reach pretectal nucleus (part of superior colliculus) → Each pretectal nucleus sends fibres to Edinger Westphal nucleus (EW), part of 3rd cranial nerve → Finally constriction of pupil (sphincter pupillae)
- Corneal reflex: Light touching of the cornea/ conjunctiva, results in blinking of the eyelids
- Most sensitive part of eye: Fovea (contains photo-receptors)

CRANIAL NERVES

- 3rd cranial nerve:
  - o Supplies all extra-ocular muscle EXCEPT superior oblique & lateral rectus

- o Complete paralysis results in external ophthalmoplegia (Inability to move the eye upward, inward & downward)
- o Drooping of the upper eyelids due to paralysis of levator palpebrae superioris (ptosis)
- o Pupillary sparing is a feature of DM

- 4th cranial nerve:
    - o Weakness/ paralysis of superior oblique muscle
    - o Which normally moves the eye downwards & inwards
- 6th cranial nerve:
    - o Weakness/ paralysis of lateral rectus
    - o Which normally rotates the eye laterally
- Horner's syndrome:
    - o Ptosis (partial)
    - o Enophthalmos
    - o Miosis
    - o Anhidrosis
    - o Loss of ciliospinal reflex
    - o Treated by Fasanella Servat operation
- Weber's syndrome:
    - o Ipsilateral 3rd nerve palsy
    - o Contralateral hemiparesis

Laws of ocular motility

- Herring's law: Yoke antagonist muscles and yoke agonist muscles receive Equal innervation
- Sherrington's law of reciprocal innervation: Increased innervation of contacting agonist muscle is accompanied by simultaneous decreased innervation of its antagonist.

PTOSIS

- Ptosis is drooping of Upper eyelid
- Tylosis is Hypertrophy & drooping of eyelid
- Feature of eye with ptosis in 3rd nerve palsy: Larger, or normal pupil
- Feature of ptosis in Marcus Gunn Jaw winking syndrome: Non-retractable ptosis may get corrected with chewing action
- Surgical procedure for ptosis: Blaskovics operation

Jaw winking of Marcus Gunn

- Due to aberrant regeneration of nerve fibres
- Spasm of one Levator palpebrae occurs on movement of jaw
- Seen in congenital Ptosis.

MYOPIA

- Rays of light are focused in front of retina
- Size of eyeball is big
- Complications of myopia:
    - o Lattice & snail degeneration
    - o Peripheral retinal degeneration
- Surgical procedure:
    - o Radial keratotomy (small degree)
    - o Soft lens
    - o LASIK

Pre-requisites for LASIK (Laser assisted in situ keratomileusis)

- Age should be more than 21 years
- Stable refractory error
- Corneal thinning disorder should be ruled out
- It can correct myopia of range -6 to 30 diopters

Acanthamoeba infection

- Contact lens wearers who use distilled water and salt tablets instead of commercial saline solution
- Corneal scrapings are stained with calcofluor white dye/ potassium hydroxide mount/ lactophenol cotton blue
- Treated with polymethylene biguanide or chlorhexidine with propamidine

Staphyloma

- Anterior: Ectasia of pseudocornea

- Intercalary: Localized bulge in limbal area lined by iris root
- Ciliary: 2-3 mm away from limbus, lined by ciliary body
- Equatorial: Choroidal incarceration at the equator
- Posterior: Lined by choroids behind the equator

PRESBYOPIA

- Physiological insufficiency of accommodation
- Loss of power of accommodation
- Due to loss of elasticity of lens capsule
- Treatment is by convex lens

ASTIGMATISM

- Spherical aberration
- Due to irregular curvature of cornea

NYSTAGMUS

- Down beat nystagmus is seen in:
  - o Cerebellar/ brain stem lesions
  - o Multiple sclerosis
  - o Alcohol
  - o Anticonvulsants
  - o Lithium toxicity
- Rotatory nystagmus: Miner's nystagmus

Terms with "ANISO"

- Aniseikonia: Difference in image size
- Anisometropia: Difference in refraction of two eyes

CONJUNCTIVA

- Haemorrhagic conjunctivitis:
  - o Enterovirus
  - o Adenovirus
  - o Coxsackie virus
- Phlyctenular conjunctivitis: TB
- Giant papillary conjunctivitis: Contact lens
- Angular conjunctivitis: Moraxella

Conditions affecting conjunctiva

- Ophthalmia nodosa/ Caterpillar hair conjunctivitis:
  - o Granulomatous inflammation of conjunctiva
  - o Leading to formation of nodule on the bulbar conjunctiva in response to irritation caused by the retained hair of caterpillar
- Pinguecula: Yellowish white patch on the bulbar conjunctiva near the limbus
- Pterygium: Folds of conjunctiva encroaching upon the cornea

PHYLECTENULAR CONJUNCTIVITIS

- Type IV hypersensitivity reaction
- MC allergic manifestation is Koeppe's nodule

SPRING CATARRH

- Horner trantas spots on bulbar conjunctiva
- Cobble stone appearance of palpebral conjunctiva
- Papillary hypertrophy
- Type I hypersensitivity
- Maxwell Lyon sign:
  - o Stringy
  - o Ropy discharge

Vernal keratoconjunctivitis / spring catarrh

- Recurrent bilateral external ocular inflammation
- Seasonal – Summer
- Cobblestone/ pavement stone - Hard, flat topped papillae in upper tarsal conjunctiva and
- Tranta's spots - Discrete whitish raised dots along the limbus

TRACHOMA

- Characterized by the presence of:
  - o Limbal follicles/ Herbert's pits (formed on cornea, near limbus)

  - o Arlt's line (conjunctival scarring in sulcus subtarsalis)
  - o Pannus (infiltration of cornea with vascularization)
- SAFE strategy
  - o Surgery
  - o Antibiotics
  - o Facial cleanliness
  - o Environmental improvement
- DOC:
  - o Tetracycline (local)
  - o Azithromycin (Oral)

Trachoma

- Caused by Chlamydia trachomatis serotypes A, Ba, and C, D and K
- The organism produces:
  - o Intracytoplasmic inclusion bodies called H.P. bodies (Halberstaedter Prowazeke bodies)
  - o Arlt's line- linear scars present in sulcus subtarsalis
  - o Herbert follicles- typical follicles present in the limbal area
  - o Herbert pits- circular pitted scars left after healing of Herbert follicles

Diagnostic criteria for trachoma (At least 2 of following)

- Follicles on upper tarsal conjunctiva
- Limbal follicles or Herbert's pits
- Typical conjunctival scarring
- Vascular pannus most marked in the superior limbus

WHO Classification (1987): Meant to be used by field Workers

- TF (Trachomatous Inflammation Follicular): > 5 follicles
- (> 0.5 mm diameter) on upper tarsal conjunctiva
- TI (Trachomatous Inflammation Intense): Inflammation and papillary hypertrophy Obscuring > ½ of tarsal vessels
- TT (Trachomatous Trichiasis): At least 1 trichiatic cilia rubbing on the globe or evidence of its recent removal
- TS (Trachomatous Scarring): Obvious trachomatous scarring of upper tarsal conjunctiva
- CO(Corneal Opacity): Trachomatous corneal opacity at least a part of which extends over the pupil

Mac Callan's classification of trachoma based on conjunctival characteristics

- Stage 1: Incipient trachoma; Immature follicles on superior palpebral conjunctiva
- Stage 2: Established trachoma; Mature follicles on superior palpebral conjunctiva
- Stage 3: Cicatrizing trachoma; Follicles, scales, scarring on superior Tarsus
- Stage 4: Healed trachoma; No follicles, extensive conjunctival Scarring

Sequelae of trachoma

- Distortion of lids
- Entropion
- Trichiasis
- Ectropion (hypertrophy of conjunctiva)
- Herbert's pits
- Ptosis (tylosis and infiltration of LPS)
- Madarosis
- Posterior symblepharon
- Parenchymatous xerosis
- Defective lid closure, lid deformity and deficient tear film, corneal Damage. Cicatrization involving lacrimal drainage and dacryolith formation, epiphora, Glaucoma (perilimbal fibrosis and infiltration of the outflow channels)
- Secondary Infection: H. aegyptius (commonest)

PTERYGIUM

- Elastotic degeneration with proliferation of vascularized granulation tissue
- Stocker's line is seen

CONGENITAL GLAUCOMA

- Boys affected more
- Buphthalmos (big eyes)
- Ox eyes
- Large cornea
- Presents as photophobia
- Cornea:
  - o Hazy frosted glass cornea with
  - o Haab's striae
- Managed by: Combined trabeculotomy & trabeculectomy
- Hereditary glaucoma is due to: Optineurin abnormality

Causes of cloudy cornea at birth

- Glaucoma
- Trauma
- Intrauterine infections
- Mucopolysaccharidoses
- Mucolipidosis

PRIMARY OPEN ANGLE GLAUCOMA

- Mostly asymptomatic OR
- Progressive painless loss of vision
- Genes implicated in pathogenesis:
  - o Optineurin gene &
  - o MYOC gene
- Early visual field defect:
  - o Isopter contraction
  - o Barring of blind spot
- 1st line of treatment: Timolol (beta blocker)
- Surgical procedure: Argon LASER trabeculoplasty

Order of less visual field in glaucoma

- First: Isopter contraction
- Second: Baring of blind spot
- Third: Wing shaped paracentral scotoma (first clinically significant)
- Second last: Loss of temporal island
- Last: Macular fires lost

Epidemic dropsy glaucoma/ Bengal glaucoma

- Characterized by diarrhea, edema legs, myocarditis
- Visual field changes resemble those of chronic simple glaucoma

ANGLE CLOSURE GLAUCOMA

- Predisposing factor: Shallow anterior chamber
- May present as:
  - o Painful, red eye with
  - o Headache, nausea, vomiting
- Pupil is:
  - o Semi-dilated
  - o Vertically oval &
  - o Fixed
- Surgical procedure:
  - o LASER iridotomy
  - o Surgical iridectomy

Sudden painful loss of vision

- Acute congestive glaucoma
- Acute iridocyclitis
- Injuries

Causes of tunnel vision

- Glaucoma
- Retinitis pigmentosa
- High myopia
- High powered glasses
- CRAO with sparing of cilioretinal artery
- Luetic chorioretinitis

Sudden painless loss of vision

- Central retinal artery occlusion
- Vitreous hemorrhage
- Retinal detachment

- Central retinal vein occlusion
- Central serous retinopathy
- Optic neuritis

Gradual painless loss of vision

- Pterygium encroaching on papillary area
- Corneal degeneration
- Corneal dystrophies
- Senile cataract
- Optic atrophy
- Diabetic retinopathy
- Refractive errors

Gradual painful loss of vision

- Chronic iridocyclitis
- Corneal ulceration
- Chronic simple glaucoma

Transient loss of vision/ amaurosis fugax

- Migraine
- Carotid artery disease
- Raynaud's disease

NEOVASCULAR GLAUCOMA

- Usually associated with neovascularization of iris (rubeosis iridis)
- Associated with: CRAO
- Treated by: Pan retinal photocoagulation

KERATOCONUS

- Protrusion of central part of cornea with thinning
- Corneal nerves are visible
- Associated features:
  - o Munson's sign
  - o Fleischer sign

LENS

- Respiratory coefficient of lens: 1
- Equatorial diameter of lens: 9 mm
- Maximum refractive power is in: Centre of lens
- Lens derives its nutrition from:
  - o Aqueous humour
  - o Perilimbal capillaries &
  - o Oxygen in air
- Lens is thicker anteriorly

Ectopia lentis

- Marfan's syndrome: Most common cause of inheritable EL; Bilateral Upward and temporal displacement
- Homocystinuria: Second most common cause; Downward nasal displacement
- Weill-Marchesani syndrome: Forward displacement

Other conditions causing ectopia lentis

- Sulfite oxidase deficiency
- Hyperlysinemia
- Ehlers-Danlos syndrome
- Refsum's disease
- Sturge –Weber syndrome
- Pierre Robin syndrome

CATARACT

- Systemic causes of cataract:
  - o HTN
  - o Smoking
  - o DM
- MC cataract in adults: Cortical cataract
- Complicated cataract: Characteristic sign is polychromatic lustre
- Posterior hyperplastic primary vitreous cataract:
  - o Unilateral (always) &

- o Associated with poor visual prognosis
- Lamellar cataract: Associated with
  - o Malnutrition &
  - o Hypoparathyroidism
- After cataract: Nd: YAG LASER capsulotomy is done

Laser & uses

- ND-YAG: After cataract
- Excimer laser: LASIK, keratotomy
- Frequency doubled ND-YAG, Argon-green, diode, krypton: Retinal photocoagulation

Special types of cataract

- Christmas tree: Myotonic dystrophy
- Sunflower: Wilson's disease
- Rosette: Concussion trauma
- Oil drop: Galactosemia
- Snowflake/ snowstorm: Diabetes mellitus
- Polychromatic luster: Complicated cataract
- Blue dot: Cortical developmental cataract
- Glassblower's: Infrared radiation
- Anterior subcapsular: Anti-cholinesterase
- Posterior subcapsular: Radiation/ steroids
- Shield cataract: Atopic dermatitis
- Spoke like cataract: Mannosidosis
- Propeller cataract: Fabry's disease

Stages of maturation of cortical senile cataract

- Stage of lamellar separation by fluid
- Stage of incipient cataract
- Immature senile cataract
- Mature senile cataract
- Hypermature senile cataract

Second sight

- In nuclear cataract, refractive of lens increases so the light rays become more convergent and patient becomes more myopic. So his near vision improves and presbyopia is corrected

PAPILLOEDEMA

- Seen in raised intracranial tension (intracranial infections like cavernous sinus thrombosis, cerebral abscess)
- Clinical features:
  - o Headache, nausea
  - o Projectile vomiting
- Visual field changes:
  - o Enlargement of the blind spot
  - o Progressive contraction of the visual field
- Disc findings:
  - o Blurring of the margins of optic disc
  - o Hyperemia of disc
  - o Elevation of the disc (mushroom/ dome shaped)

Foster Kennedy syndrome

- Tumor of anterior cranial fossa
- Ipsilateral papilloedema
- Contralateral optic atrophy

Differences

Feature	*Papilloedema*	*Papillitis*
Signs of raised intracranial pressure	Present	Absent
Vitreal opacities	Absent	Present
Swelling of optic disc	2-6D	2-3D
Blind spot	Increased	Not increased
Pain	Absent	Present
Central vision	Unaffected	Greatly depressed

PAPILLITIS/ OPTIC NEURITIS

- Pseudopapillitis is seen in: Hypermetropia
- Features: Relative afferent pupillary defect (Marcus Gunn pupil)
- Complete afferent pupillary defect: Optic nerve lesion

Differences

Features	*Papillitis*	*Pseudo-papillitis*
Cause	Inflammatory	Hypermetropia
Vitreal opacities	Present	Absent
Pain	Present	Absent
Central vison	Depressed	Normal
Swelling of disc	2-3D	Never more than 2D

UVEAL TRACT

- Scleritis is: Associated with connective tissue disorder like RA
- Feature of iridocyclitis: Cells & flare in aqueous

Iridocyclitis

- Keratic precipitates - Proteinaceous cellular deposits at the back of cornea
  - o Mutton fat KP - Occur in granulomatous iridocyclitis, composed of epithelioid cells and macrophages. Large, thick and fluffy
  - o Granular KP - Small and medium, of non-granulomatous origin, composed of lymphocytes
  - o Red KP - Along with lymphocytes, erythrocytes also take part in composition, seen in hemorrhagic uveitis
  - o Old KP - Healed uveitis; shrunken, lightly pigmented and crenated

ACUTE ANTERIOR UVEITIS

- Associated with:
  - o Juvenile rheumatoid arthritis &
  - o Ankylosing spondylitis
- Miotic pupil
- Treatment:
  - o Steroids (DOC) followed by
  - o Mydriatics
- Steroids reduces inflammation & scarring;
- Dilation of the pupil by atropine:
  - o Reduces pain &
  - o Prevents synechiae formation
- Posterior uveitis is associated with:
  - o Sarcoidosis
  - o Vogt-Koyanagi-Harada syndrome (disease of melanocyte containing tissue)
  - o Behçet's syndrome

SYMPATHETIC OPHTHALMITIS/ SO

- Ciliary body is injured,
- Seen after penetrating injury in ciliary region (dangerous region)
- 1st sign of SO: Keratic precipitates/ Retrolental flare
- May present as: Difficulty in reading from one eye after 3-4 weeks of injury to other eye

OCULAR MALIGNANCY

- MC intra-ocular malignancy in children: Retinoblastoma
- MC tumour of lacrimal gland: Benign mixed tumour

RETINOBLASTOMA/ Rb

- May be bilateral in 30-40% cases (particularly familial ones)
- Most cases of familial retinoblastoma are bilateral
- Knudson's hypothesis is related to Rb
- MC manifestation of Rb: Leukocoria/ Amaurotic cat's eye reflex
- Most common presenting feature of retinoblastoma is Leucocoria
- Trilateral retinoblastoma: Bilateral retinoblastoma with midline intracranial tumour
- Amaurotic cat's eye reflex: yellowish white, non-reacting, pupil in retinoblastoma and pseudoglioma
- Treatment of diffuse Rb: Enucleation (removal of eyeball with portion of optic nerve from orbit)
- Treatment of small Rb: Brachytherapy
- Treatment of bilateral Rb & metastatic disease: Chemotherapy

- Rhabdomyosarcoma is the most common primary orbital malignant tumor and most common soft tissue tumor malignancy in children

Retinoblastoma Treatment

- Small tumors: Photocoagulation; Transpupillary thermotherapy with laser or cryotherapy
- Medium tumors: Brachytherapy; External beam radiotherapy with cobalt Chemotherapy
- Large tumors: Enucleation; Chemoreduction
- Enucleation is most widely practiced modality of treatment in unilateral sporadic disease and in the more affected eye in bilateral disease

Causes of leucocoria

- Retinoblastoma
- Congenital cataract
- Coloboma choroids
- Retinopathy of prematurity
- Persistent hyperplastic primary vitreous
- Toxocara endophthalmitis
- Coat's disease

RETINAL DETACHMENT/ RD

- Rhegmatogenous RD: Formation of hole in retina/ retinal tear
- Associated with:
  - o Myopia
  - o Trauma
  - o Cataract surgery
  - o HTN
  - o Eales disease
- Investigation of choice: Indirect ophthalmoscopy
- Primary aim of RD surgery: Closure of break/ tear

RETINITIS PIGMENTOSA

- Feature: Loss of visual acuity
- Microscopy: Irregular black deposits of clumped pigment in the peripheral retina (Bone spicules)

Fundus

- Candle wax spots: Retinopathy of sarcoidosis
- Salt and pepper fundus: Congenital syphilis
- Watered silk appearance of fundus: Hypermetropia

Refsum's syndrome

- Retinitis pigmentosa
- Peripheral neuropathy
- Cerebellar ataxia

Fundus appearance

Disease	*Appearance*
Congenital syphilis	**Pepper & salt appearance**
Phenothiazine	**Pigmentary retinopathy**
Chloroquine	**Bull's eye retinopathy**
Retinitis pigmentosa	**Tessellated/ tigroid fundus, bony corpuscles like lesions**
Partial central retinal artery obstruction	**Cattle truck appearance**
Central retinal artery obstruction, Niemann Pick disease, Tay-Sachs disease	**Cherry red spot**

DIABETIC RETINOPATHY

- Fundus examination in DM:
  - o NIDDM: As early as possible
  - o IDDM: 5 years after diagnosis of DM
- Incidence of diabetic retinopathy increases with disease duration

Grading of hypertensive retinopathy

- Grade 1: Mild generalized arteriolar attenuation.
- Grade 2: Grading of hypertensive retinopathy- Marked generalized Narrowing and focal attenuation of arterioles, with deflection of veins at the arteriovenous junction
- Grade 3: Grade 2 plus copper wiring of arterioles, Banking of veins, distal to A-V crossing. Flame shaped hemorrhages, cotton wool spots and hard exudates

- Grade 4: Grade 3 plus silver wiring of arterioles and papilloedema

Signs of hypertensive retinopathy

- Salu's sign: Arteriovenous nipping
- Bonnet's sign: Dilated vein distal to A-V crossing
- Gunn's sign: Tapering of vein on either side of crossing, Right angle deflection of vein
- Elschnig's spots: Ischemic Choroidal infarcts

Retinal changes in sickle cell

- Sea fan neovascularisation
- Black sun bursts
- Salmon patch haemorrhage
- Angioid streaks

Causes of cherry red spot in macula are:

- CRAO
- Tay –Sach's disease
- Niemann-Pick disease
- Gaucher's disease
- Sandhoff's disease
- Sialidosis

HIV & OCULAR MANIFESTATIONS

- MC abnormal finding on fundoscopic examination: Cotton wool spots
- Most devastating consequences of HIV infection on eye: CMV retinitis

EYE IN THYROID DISEASES

- Muscle MC involved in thyroid ophthalmopathy: Inferior rectus

Hyperthyroidism

- Lid lag (Von Grafe's sign)
- Poor convergence (Mobius sign)
- External ophthalmoplegia
- Large extraocular muscles

TEARS

- Tears are produced in newborn after: 4 weeks
- Layers in tear film: 3 layers
- Mucin deficiency is seen in:
  - o Steven Johnson syndrome
  - o Trachoma
  - o Burns
  - o Pemphigoid
  - o Vitamin A deficiency

BLINDNESS

- MC cause of ocular morbidity in India: Refractive error
- MC cause of blindness in children in India: Vitamin A deficiency
- MC cause of blindness in adults in India: Cataract

Causes of night blindness

- Vitamin A deficiency
- Retinitis pigmentosa
- Myopia
- Peripheral cortical cataract
- Oguchi disease
- Goldmann-Favre disease
- Central nuclear cataract
- Central corneal opacities
- Central vitreous opacities

Blindness

- Economic blindness: Vision less than 6/60
- Social blindness: Inability to move around. Vision less than 3/60

SURGERY

- Evisceration: Done in panophthalmitis, (Frill's excision is done for panophthalmitis)
- Enucleation is done in (C/I in panophthalmitis):
  - o Retinoblastoma (children)

- o Malignant melanoma (adults)
- o Endophthalmitis &
- o Phthisis bulbi

TRAUMA TO ORBIT

- Features of trauma to eye:
    - o Vossius ring (concussion of lens)
    - o Commotio retinae/ Berlin's edema (concussion injury)
    - o D shaped pupil (iridodialysis)

MYDRIATICS

- Shortest & quickly acting mydriatic: Tropicamide
- Mydriatic with no cycloplegia: Phenylephrine
- Mydriatic used as an ointment in children: Atropine
- MC complication of topical steroid: Glaucoma

Drugs

- Tropicamide: Shortest and quickest acting
- Phenylephrine: Only mydriatic
- Cyclopentolate: Only cycloplegic

TERMS & ASSOCIATED CONDITIONS

- Bulls eye maculopathy: Chloroquine
- Whorled keratopathy: Amiodarone
- Arcus senilis: Old age
- Schwalbes ring: Descemet membrane
- KF rings: Wilson disease
- Angioid streaks: Pseudoxanthoma elasticum
- Ring scotoma: Retinitis pigmentosa
- Scintillating scotoma: Migraine
- Dalen Fuch's nodule: Sympathetic ophthalmitis
- Epibulbar dermoid's: Goldenhar's syndrome
- Roth spots: Bacterial endocarditis
- Sago grains, Arlt's line: Trachoma
- Fleischer ring: Keratoconus
- Candle wax spots: Sarcoidosis
- Macular toxicity: Gentamycin

KEYWORDS & CONDITIONS

- Recurrent attacks of conjunctivitis, Intense itching, Ropy discharge: Vernal conjunctivitis
- Lady, Severe sudden onset of pain, sacroiliitis: Anterior uveitis
- Neonate, Lacrimation, photophobia, Large & hazy cornea: Congenital glaucoma
- Normal anterior chamber & hazy cornea in one eye & Shallow anterior chamber & miotic pupil in fellow eye: Acute anterior uveitis

Conditions & causative agent

Lesion	*Caused by*
Panophthalmitis	**Pneumococci**
Macular degeneration	**Toxoplasmosis**
Subacute infective retinitis (septic retinitis of Roth)	**Bacterial endocarditis, puerperal septicemia**
Disseminated choroiditis	**Often obscure syphilis**
Anterior choroiditis	**Syphilis**
Interstitial keratitis	**Treponema pallidum (secondary syphilis)**
Secondary infection in phlyctenular keratitis	**Staphylococcus**
Epidemic keratoconjunctivitis	**Adenovirus 3, 7, 8, 19**
Disciform keratitis	**Vaccinia, herpes**
Marginal ulcer	**Moraxella, H. aegyptius**
Mycotic hypopyon ulcer	**Aspergillus**
Ulcus serpens (hypopyon ulcer)	**Pneumococci**
Ophthalmia neonatorum	**Gonococci, Chlamydia**
Angular conjunctivitis	**Moraxella**
Purulent conjunctivitis	**gonococcus**

CLINICAL QUESTIONS

1. **Microscopy of corneal ulcer showed branching septate hyphae. The probable diagnosis is:**

   A. Candida B. Mucormycosis

   C. Aspergillus D. Histoplasma

   Clinical presentation is suggestive of Aspergillus.

   Aspergillus and many other species have septate hyphae.

   Answer: C i.e., Aspergillus

2. **A 28 years old male complains of glare in both eyes. Examination of cornea showed whorl like opacities of epithelium. There is a past history of Amiodarone therapy. Most likely diagnosis is:**

   A. Arcus senilis

   B. Band shaped keratopathy

   C. Cornea verticillata

   D. Terrain's marginal degeneration

   Clinical presentation is suggestive of cornea verticillata

   Cornea verticillata, also called Fleischer vortex, Vortex keratopathy or Whorl keratopathy, is a condition characterised by corneal deposits at the level of the basal epithelium forming a faint golden-brown whorl pattern.

   It is seen in Fabry disease or in case of prolonged amiodarone intake.

   Answer: C i.e., Cornea verticillata

3. **Lesions of the visual cortex with homonymous hemianopia may be seen in occlusion of:**

   A. Basilar artery

   B. Middle cerebral artery

   C. Posterior cerebral artery

   D. Anterior cerebral artery

   Clinical presentation is suggestive of posterior cerebral artery occlusion.

   Vascular and neoplastic (malignant or benign tumours) lesions from the optic tract, to visual cortex can cause a contralateral homonymous hemianopsia.

   Injury to the right side of the brain will affect the left visual fields of each eye.

   The more posterior the cerebral lesion, the more symmetric (congruous) the homonymous hemianopsia will be.

   For example, a person who has a lesion of the right optic tract will no longer see objects.

   Homonymous hemianopsia secondary to posterior cerebral artery occlusion – may result in syndromes of memory impairment, opposite visual field loss (homonymous hemianopsia), and sometimes hemisensory deficits

   The PCA supplies the occipital lobe and the medial portion of the temporal lobe.

   Answer: C i.e., Posterior cerebral artery

4. **A person has inability to look downward and laterally. The nerve injured is:**

   A. Oculomotor B. Trochlear

   C. Abducent D. Trigeminal

   Clinical presentation is suggestive of trochlear nerve palsy.

   Trochlear nerve supplies superior oblique muscle.

   The primary (main) action of the superior oblique muscle is intorsion (internal rotation), the secondary action is depression (primarily in the adducted position) and the tertiary action is abduction (lateral rotation).

   Answer: B i.e., Trochlear

5. **Visual field defect in pituitary tumour with suprasellar extension is:**

   A. Bitemporal hemianopia

   B. Binasal hemianopia

   C. Homonymous hemianopia

   D. Pie in the sky vision

   Clinical presentation is suggestive of bitemporal hemianopia.

   Bitemporal hemianopsia (bitemporal heteronymous hemianopsia or bitemporal hemianopia) is a type of partial blindness where vision is missing in the outer half of both the right and left visual field.

It is usually associated with lesions of the optic chiasm, the area where the nasal fibers of optic nerves from the right and left eyes cross near the pituitary gland.

Answer: A i.e., Bitemporal hemianopia

6. **Which condition represents fat like nodules, bilaterally on nasal side of conjunctiva?**

A. Pterygium   B. Pinguecula

C. Chalazion   D. Hordeolum

Clinical presentation is suggestive of pinguecula.

Pinguecula is seen as a yellow-white deposit on the conjunctiva adjacent to the limbus (the junction between the cornea and sclera).

It is to be distinguished clinically from pterygium, which is a wedge-shaped area of fibrosis that appears to grow into the cornea.

It usually does not cause any symptoms.

It is most prevalent in tropical climates and is in direct correlation with UV exposure.

Answer: B i.e., Pinguecula

CHAPTER 11

MEDICINE

RAPID REVISION NOTES

Important test

Test	*Condition*
Hess test	**Capillary fragility**
CPK-MB	**Myocardial infarction**
Mitsuda test, Dharmendra test	**Leprosy**
Increased paraprotein level with destruction of bone in X-rays	**Multiple myeloma**
TRAP (tartrate resistant acid phosphatase) in RBC	**Hairy cell leukemia**
Raised gastrin levels	**Zollinger Ellison syndrome**
Goldman's fluorescent stain	**Toxoplasmosis**
8 hour I/V cortisol test	**Addison's disease**
Direct assay of epinephrine & nor-epinephrine	**Pheochromocytoma with paroxysmal hypertension**
Low plasma cortisol	**Addison disease**
Raised TSH	**Primary hypothyroidism**
Weil Felix reaction	**Rickettsial infection**
Dick test	**Scarlet fever**
Schick test, elek's test	**Diphtheria**
Tzanck test	**Acantholysis (pemphigus)**
Ito test	**Chancroid**
Kveim test	**Sarcoidosis**
Fincham's test	**Differentiating coloured halos of cataract from glaucoma**
Frie' s test	**LGV**
Guthrie test	**Phenylketonuria**
Schilling test	**B12 deficiency**
Schiller test	**Carcinoma cervix**
Rothera test, Gerhardt test	**Ketone bodies in urine**

Important condition & test done

Condition	*Test done/ finding*
Intravascular hemolysis	Low haptoglobin, hemoglobinuria present
Adrenogenital syndrome	Increased urinary 17-ketosteroid excretion
Late congenital syphilis	Fluorescent treponemal antibody test (IgM FTAb)
Pharyngeal pouch, hypopharynx tumour	Barium swallow

LUNG CARCINOMA

- MC to produce hypercalcemia: Squamous cell Ca
- MC type of lung Ca: Adeno Ca
- Lung Ca with worst prognosis: Small cell Ca

- Best prognosis among lung Ca: Squamous cell Ca
- Lung Ca most responsive to radiotherapy: Small cell Ca
- 2nd MC lung Ca: Squamous cell Ca
- MC metastasizing to opposite lung: Adeno Ca
- MC cavitating lung Ca: Squamous cell Ca
- Lung Ca most sensitive to chemotherapy: Small cell Ca
- MC type in non-smokers: Adeno Ca
- MC in peripheral location: Adeno Ca
- MC in young patient: Adeno Ca
- MC in females: Adeno Ca

SPOTS

- Koplik spots: Measles
- Roth spots: SABE
- Bitot's spots: Vitamin A deficiency
- Herald spot: Pityriasis rosea

HYPOKALEMIA

- Associated with:
  - o Diuretics
    - ♦ Thiazide
    - ♦ Bumetanide
    - ♦ Furosemide
    - ♦ Ethacrynic acid
  - o Theophylline intoxication
  - o Cortisol
  - o Villous adenoma of colon etc.
- ECG changes of hypokalemia:
  - o ST segment depression
  - o Increased U wave amplitude etc.

HYPERKALEMIA

- Serum potassium more than 5.5 mEq/L
- Pseudohyperkalemia: Hemolysis of blood sample or the release of potassium from RBC, WBC & platelets
- Hyperkalemia is associated with:
  - o Digitalis intoxication
  - o Beta blockers
  - o Acute intravascular hemolysis
  - o Acute oliguric states
    - ♦ Severe crush injury
    - ♦ Burns
    - ♦ Adrenal insufficiency
- ECG changes:
  - o Shortening of QT interval
  - o PR interval prolongation
  - o Tall, peaked T wave
- Acute emergency treatment:
  - o Calcium gluconate
  - o Sodium bicarbonate
  - o Insulin etc.

ECG changes in hyper and hypokalemia

Hypokalemia	*Hyperkalemia*
ST segment depressed	Peaked tall T waves
Flat or inverted T waves	Sine- wave, P wave decreased
U waves	Widening of QRs complex
PR prolonged	PR interval prolonged Ventricular asystole /ventricular fibrillation

HYPOMAGNESEMIA

- Associated with:
  - o Inadequate intake
  - o Alcohol
  - o Impairment of gut/ renal absorption
  - o Oftenly with hypocalcemia & hypophosphataemia
- EMG studies: Myopathic potentials

HYPERMAGNESEMIA

- Associated with: Magnesium containing medications in renal failure (antacids, laxatives etc.)

Calcium, phosphorous & alkaline phosphatase

Condition	*Ca*	*P*	*AP*
Osteoporosis	Normal	Normal	Normal
Rickets	Low	Low	High
Osteomalacia	Low	Low	High
Paget's disease	Normal	Normal	High
Hypo-parathyroidism	Low	High	Normal
Hyper-parathyroidism	High	Low	High
Multiple myeloma	High	-	Normal
Bone metastasis	High	-	High

HYPOCALCEMIA

- Idiopathic hypoparathyroidism is associated with:
  - o Genetic syndrome of hypoparathyroidism
  - o Addison's disease &
  - o Mucocutancous candidiasis
- Pseudohypoparathyroidism: No deficiency of parathormone, but target organ (bone & kidney) are unresponsive to its action
- Chvostek's sign: Contraction of facial muscles, elicited by light tapping of the facial nerve
- ECG changes: Prolongation of QT interval

HYPERCALCEMIA

- Associated with:
  - o Sarcoidosis
  - o Primary hyperparathyroidism
  - o Milk alkali syndrome
  - o Myeloma
  - o Lithium therapy
- Treatment:
  - o Furosemide
  - o Pamidronate
  - o Gallium nitrate
  - o Plicamycin etc.

Classic triad of myeloma

- Marrow plasmacytosis > 10 Percent
- Lytic bone lesions
- Serum and /or urine M component

Remember

- Thiazides are used for treating hypercalciuria
- Tumour lysis causes hypocalcemia (NOT hypercalcemia)

METABOLIC DISORDERS

- Respiratory acidosis:
  - o Raised CO_2 &
  - o Raised HCO_3^- (reduced pH)
- Metabolic alkalosis:
  - o Raised HCO_3^-
  - o CO_2 unchanged (raised pH)
- Metabolic acidosis is seen in:
  - o Lactic acidosis
  - o Diabetic Ketoacidosis
  - o Renal tubular acidosis
  - o Ethylene glycol, etc.

ANION GAP

- Increased anion gap is seen in:
  - o Starvation
  - o Salicylate poisoning
  - o Renal failure etc.

BREATHING

- Paradoxical breathing is seen in: Diaphragmatic palsy
- Amphoric breathing: Pneumothorax
- Cavernous breathing: Cavity
- Tubular breathing: Consolidation

LUNG DISEASE

- Obstructive lung disease: Reduced FEV1/ FVC
- Restrictive lung disease
    - o Reduced FVC
    - o Raised FEV1/ FVC

RESPIRATORY FAILURE

- Type I:
    - o Parenchymal disease
    - o ARDS
    - o Pneumoniae
    - o Emphysema
- Type II:
    - o COPD
    - o Flail chest etc.

Acute respiratory failure

- Type 1:
    - o Severe hypoxemia refractory to oxygen
    - o Due to airspace filling - intrapulmonary shunting
- Type 2:
    - o Alveolar hypoventilation
    - o Increased $PaCO_2$
- Type 3: Perioperative
- Type 4:
    - o Circulatory shock
    - o Acute respiratory failure

Pneumocystis carinii pneumoniae

- Prophylaxis is given in HIV positive patients with CD4 count of less than 200
- Single double – strength tablet of sulphamethoxazole-trimethoprim is given daily.

Mycobacterium avium intracellulare

- Treatment of choice - Clarithromycin + ethambutol + rifabutin

ASTHMA

- Increased leukotrienes
- Hyper-responsive airways
- Constriction of small airways
- Curschmann's spirals seen
- FEV1 improves maximum with bronchodilator therapy

Bronchial Asthma

- Creola bodies: Desquamated epithelial cells
- Curschmann spirals: Bronchial mucous casts

Sarcoidosis

- Pseudo tuberculosis/ Osteitis tuberculosa/ Multiplex cystoids/ Jungling disease/ Scheuermann's disease
- Biopsy evidence of mononuclear cell granulomatous inflammatory process is mandatory for definitive diagnosis of sarcoidosis
- Lung is the most common site to biopsied

Shrinking lung syndrome

- Seen in SLE
- Diaphragmatic dysfunction with loss of lung volume

EMPHYSEMA & CHRONIC BRONCHITIS

- Smoking is an important predisposing factor
- Alpha1 antitrypsin deficiency is associated with: Panacinar emphysema
- Breathlessness is a characteristic feature
- Diurnal variation in peak expiratory flow rate is seen

BRONCHIECTASIS

- Nodular bronchiectasis is seen in infection with: Mycobacterium avium
- Chest x-ray shows: Tram track lines
- MC site: Left lower lobe
- Clubbing is seen
- Investigation of choice: HRCT scan

REMEMBER

- Bronchiectasis does NOT predispose to lung Ca

KARTAGENER SYNDROME

- Situs inversus
- Bronchiectasis & sinusitis
- Infertility

CYSTIC FIBROSIS

- Autosomal recessive
- Results due to mutation in a gene on chromosome 7
- Predisposes to chronic infection by Staph. aureus & pseudomonas
- Cavitation is oftenly seen with staphylococcal infections

PLEURAL EFFUSION

- Exudative pleural effusion is seen in:
  - RA
  - Bronchogenic Ca etc.
- Blood stained pleural effusion:
  - Pulmonary infarction
  - Metastatic Ca etc.
- Low glucose in pleural fluid:
  - RA
  - Empyema
- Increased amylase in pleural fluid:
  - Pancreatitis
  - Esophageal perforation
- Cholesterol in pleural fluid:
  - RA
  - TB
  - Hypothyroidism

MYCOPLASMA PNEUMONIAE

- Causes atypical pneumonia in younger patients
- Chest radiography: Bilateral consolidation
- Serology is helpful in diagnosis
- Treatment: Erythromycin

HYPERSENSITIVE PNEUMONITIS

- Farmers lung: C
  - Caused by micro-poly-sporafaeni;
  - Associated with moldy hay
- Bagassosis:
  - Caused by Thermoactinomycetes sacchrii;
  - Associated with: Sugar cane dust

PULMONARY TB

- Acid fastness of mycobacterium TB is due to: Mycolic acid & cell wall
- Assmans focus: Infraclavicular lesion of chronic pulmonary TB

PRIMARY PULMONARY TB

- Peripheral lesion
- Accompanied by hilar/ paratracheal lymphadenopathy
- Ghon's focus (healed primary pulmonary TB)
- Associated with:
  - Fibrocaseous lesion/ phlyctenular conjunctivitis
  - Unilateral lymphadenopathy usually

POST PRIMARY TB

- Popcorn calcification
- Hemorrhagic pleural effusion &
- Cavitation can occur

PNEUMOCYSTIS CARINII

- Opportunistic pathogen
- Fungus causing pneumonia in AIDS
- Damage of type I pneumocytes
- Hypertrophy of type II pneumocytes

- Interstitial pneumonitis
- Seen with immunologic deficiencies:
  - o Defects in cell mediated immunity
  - o Hematologic malignancies
- X-ray of P. carinii pneumonia shows:
  - o Bilateral diffuse infiltrates in perihilar region
  - o Eosinophilic infiltrates
- P. carinii pneumonia in adults, mainly presents as: Alveolar predominant (interstitial in children)
- Treatment: Co-trimoxazole

SMALL CELL Ca LUNG/ OAT CELL Ca

- MC Ca causing superior vena caval syndrome
- Causes paraneoplastic syndrome
  - o Cushing syndrome
  - o SIADH
- Treated by chemotherapy

Paraneoplastic syndromes in lung cancer

Small cell Ca	*Adenocarcinoma*	*Squamous cell Ca*
Eaton-Lambert Syndrome Cushing's syndrome Acromegaly SIADH	Clubbing	Hypercalcemia

Management lung Carcinoma

- Treatment of small cell carcinoma: Chemotherapy
- Treatment of squamous cell Carcinoma and adenocarcinoma: Radiotherapy and surgery
- Best response to chemotherapy and radiotherapy is shown by small cell carcinoma, but it has worst prognosis.

Bronchial carcinoids

- No known relationship to cigarette smoking
- Neuroendocrine differentiation of Kulchitsky cells of bronchial mucosa
- Carcinoid syndrome:
  - o Episodic flushing, diarrhea, bronchospasm, cyanosis
  - o Due to release of vasoactive amines like serotonin, from carcinoid tumours
- Pancoast tumor is a type of squamous cell carcinoma
- Clara cells are seen in bronchoalveolar carcinoma
- Most common site of metastasis from lung carcinoma is adrenal glands

PULMONARY EMBOLISM

- MC & earliest manifestation: Dyspnea
- ECG findings: S1Q3T3
- Signs seen on Chest X-ray:
  - o Hampton's sign
  - o West marks sign
- Plasma D-dimer ELISA level is elevated (> 90%)
- Most specific test: Pulmonary angiography
- Wells grading is done

PNEUMOTHORAX

- Presentation: Sudden dyspnea following cough & chest pain
- Exclusively in smokers
- Rupture of subpleural bleb is a common cause of primary spontaneous pneumothorax
- Intrapleural pressure is equal to atmospheric pressure in open pneumothorax

ARDS/ DIFFUSE ALVEOLAR DAMAGE/ SHOCK LUNG

- Hypoxia
- Hypercapnia
- Acute onset of respiratory failure
- Ground glass appearance
- Air bronchogram sign is positive

- Associated with:
    - o Pancreatitis
    - o Trauma
    - o Multiple blood transfusions etc.

PULSE

- Pulsus bisferiens (collapsing & slow rising): Aortic stenosis with aortic regurgitation
- Water hammer pulse: Aortic regurgitation
- Pulsus paradoxus:
    - o Asthma
    - o Pericarditis
    - o Cardiac tamponade

Pulse	*Description*	*Seen in*
Anacrotic	Slow rising, twice Beating, both in systole	AS
Pulsus bisferiens	Rapid rising, twice Beating, both in systole	Idiopathic Hypertrophic subaortic stenosis with mild AR
Dicrotic pulse	Twice beating, 1in Systole, 1 in diastole	Decreased peripheral resistance and diastolic pressure like typhoid CCF, cardiac tamponade, open heart surgery
Pulsus parvus et tardus	Slow rising	AS
Pulsus alternans	Strong and weak Beats alternately	Left ventricular failure, toxic myocarditis, Paroxysmal tachycardia, Following a premature beat
Pulsus paradoxus	Systemic blood Pressure falls more than 10 mm Hg on inspiration	Superior vena obstruction, COPD, pericardial effusion, severe CCF, Constrictive Pericarditis
Pulsus bigeminus	Coupling of pulses	Alternate premature beat, AV block, pericardial effusion, SA node block with ventricular escape
Water hammer Pulse	Increased stroke volume	Fever, pregnancy, alcoholism, anemia, Beriberi, Cor-pulmonale, cirrhosis, Paget's disease, AV fistula, thyrotoxicosis, AR, PDA, rupture sinus of Valsalva , bradycardia, systolic hypertension

JVP

- 'a' wave is due to: Atrial systole
- 'c' wave is due to: Isometric contraction phase causing bulging of AV valves into atrium

Jugular Venous Pulsation

Normal waves with their causes

Waves	*Causes*
A	**A**trial contraction
C	Ventricular **C**ontraction
V	Inflow from **V**enacavae
X	Atrial rela**X**ation
Y	Atrial empt**X**ing

Abnormal waves with causes

Waves	*Causes*
Large 'a'	Tricuspid stenosis / Pulmonary stenosis/ pulmonary hypertension
Absent 'a'	Atrial fibrillation
Cannon 'a'	Complete heart block
c-v waves	Tricuspid regurgitation
Deep y descent	Chronic constrictive pericarditis
Raised JVP	Right ventricular failure
Kussmaul's sign	Constrictive pericarditis, Constrictive Cardiomyopathy, Pericardial effusion, Severe right hear failure
Deep x descent	Acute cardiac tamponade
Prominent v ware	Tricuspid regurgitation
Accentuated x descent	Constrictive pericarditis
Reversed x descent	Tricuspid regurgitation

HHEART SOUNDS

- Soft S1: Mitral stenosis (long standing, calcified) etc.
- Loud S1: Mitral stenosis (prolonged flow through AV valve) etc.
- Wide split S2:
  - o ASD
  - o Pulmonary stenosis etc.
- Reverse splitting of S2:
  - o Left bundle branch block
  - o Aortic stenosis etc.
- S3 is heard in:
  - o Children
  - o Hyperdynamic states etc.
- Causes of S4:
  - o Hypertension
  - o HOCM etc.

Heart sounds

Loud S1	Mitral stenosis
Soft S1	Mitral regurgitation, mitral stenosis
Reversed splitting of S2	LBBB

ECG

- P wave is due to: Atrial depolarization
- QRS complex is due to: Ventricular depolarization
- Duration of QRS complex: 0.08-0.10 seconds

WOLFF PARKINSON WHITE/ WPW SYNDROME

- ECG changes:
  - o Short PR interval
  - o Wide QRS complex etc.
- Management:
  - o Procainamide
  - o Radiofrequency ablation

ARRHYTHMIA & DOC

- Ventricular arrhythmia: Lidocaine
- Paroxysmal supraventricular tachycardia: Adenosine
- WPWS: Procainamide

A-V Block

- 1st degree: PR interval > 200 msec, every P is followed by QRS
- 2nd degree: Progressive increase in PR till P is not
- Mobitz's type I: transmitted. Block is usually in the His-Purkinje system
- 3rd degree: Atria and ventricles beat independently

Arrhythmias	*Drug of choice*
Atrial extrasystole	Quinidine
PSVT	Adenosine/Verapamil
Atrial flutter	Cardioversion/ Verapamil
Ventricular extrasystole	Lidocaine
Ventricular tachycardia	Lidocaine/ cardioversion
Ventricular fibrillation	Defibrillation, Lidocaine
Wolff Parkinson White syndrome	Cardioversion / Amiodarone

Torsades de pointes

- Ventricular tachycardia characterized by polymorphic QRS complexes that change in amplitude and cycle length
- Magnesium sulphate is the drug of choice

RHEUMATIC HEART DISEASE

- Major criteria:
  - o Subcutaneous nodule
  - o Erythema marginatum
  - o Sydenham's chorea
  - o Carditis &
  - o Migratory polyarthritis
- Associated terms:
  - o Aschoff bodies
  - o Anitschkow cells/ caterpillar cells

- o Pancarditis
- o McCallum patch (subendocardial)

Jone's criteria for rheumatic fever

Major criteria	*Minor criteria*
Carditis	Fever
Sydenham's	Arthralgia
Subcutaneous nodules	Prolonged PR interval
Erythema marginatum Migratory polyarthritis	Elevated acute phase reactants

Essential criteria

- Evidence of recent group A streptococcal infection
- Positive throat culture of rapid antigen detection test
- Elevated or increasing streptococcal antibody test

Gamna-Gandy bodies

- Are foci of fibrosis containing iron and calcium
- Seen in sickle cell anemia, CML, cirrhosis with portal hypertension

MITRAL STENOSIS/ MS

- Features:
  - o Atrial fibrillation
  - o Hemoptysis
  - o Pulmonary hypertension
  - o Hoarseness of voice
- Most important differential diagnosis: Left atrial myxoma
- Investigation of choice for MS: Echocardiography
- Mitral valve area less than 0.6 cm is incompatible with life

AORTIC STENOSIS

- Features:
  - o Sustained heaving apex
  - o Angina
  - o Sudden death
- Degenerative calcification is a cause of AS
- Exercise testing is C/I in AS

AORTIC REGURGITATION/ AR

- Murmur heard: Mid diastolic Austin Flint murmur (severe AR)
- AR may be seen in:
  - o Rheumatic fever
  - o Aortic dissection etc.

Signs in aortic regurgitation

Sign	*Explanation*
Watsons sign/ Water hammer pulse	Bounding peripheral pulses
Corrigan's pulse	Rapid upstroke and collapse of the carotid artery pulse
de Musset's sign	Head nodding in time with the heart beat
Quincke's sign	Pulsation of the capillary bed in the nail
Duroziez's sign	Systolic and diastolic murmurs described as 'pistol shots' heard over the femoral artery when it is gradually compressed
Traube's sign	A double sound heard over the femoral artery when it is compressed distally
Lighthouse sign	Blanching and flushing of forehead
Landolfi's sign	Alternating constriction and dilatation of pupil
Becker's sign	Pulsations of retinal vessels
Muller's sign	Pulsations of uvula
Mayen's sign	Diastolic drop of BP > mm Hg with arm raised
Rosenbach's sign	Pulsatile liver
Gerhardt's sign	Enlarged spleen
Hill's sign	A≥ 20 mm Hg difference in Popliteal and brachial systolic cuff pressures, seen in chronic severe Al
Lincoln sign	Pulsatile popliteal
Sherman sigh	Dorsalis pedis pulse is quickly located and unexpectedly prominent in age > 75 yr

MITRAL VALVE PROLAPSE/ FLOPPY VALVE SYNDROME

- Myxomatous degeneration
- More common in: Females
- Murmur: Mid systolic murmur
- Sudden death can be there (rare complication)

Mitral valve prolapse/Barlow's syndrome/floppy valve syndrome

- Commoner in females
- Mostly asymptomatic
- Non-ejection systolic click
- Echocardiography is the investigation of choice

HOCM

- ECHO may show mitral regurgitation
- Murmur of HOCM: Ejection systolic murmur
- Sudden death may be a complication
- Avoid digoxin

Murmur	*Characteristics*
Murmur of AR	High pitched, blowing, decrescendo, diastolic, best heard in third intercostals space along left sternal border.
Austin Flint murmur	Soft, low pitched ejection murmur (seen in AR)
Mill wheel murmur	Air embolism
Lerman scratch	Grating systolic sound, heard over sternum in second space seen in thyrotoxicosis
Graham Steel murmur	Pulmonary regurgitation
Seagull murmur	Seen in rheumatic fever, due to turbulence of low around swollen valves.

Continuous murmurs

- Patent ductus arteriosus
- Coronary fistula
- Ruptured aneurysm of sinus of Valsalva
- Aortic septal defect
- Anomalous left coronary artery
- Mammary soufflé
- Intercostal arteriovenous fistula
- Cervical venous hum
- Bronchial collateral circulation

Conditions & their effects on murmur

- Standing increases murmur of MVP, HOCM
- Sustained handgrip accentuates murmur of MR, AR, HOCM

INFECTIVE ENDOCARDITIS/ IE

- MC cause of sub acute IE: Strept. viridans
- MC cause in I/V drug abusers: Staph. aureus (esp. with acute presentation)
- Endocarditis with destruction of underlying myocardium: Libman-sack's endocarditis
- Osler's nodes: Painful, pea-sized nodules in pulp of fingers
- Janeway's lesions: Non-tender lesions in soles/palm
- Spots in retina: Roth's spot
- Condition with low risk of IE: ASD

Lesion seen in infective endocarditis

- Osler's nodes: Painful tender pea-sized erythematous nodules in the pulp of fingers and soles in patients of infective endocarditis
- Janeway's lesions: Small maculopapular erythematous or hemorrhagic emboli to distal digital arteries, commonly seen in palm and soles
- Roth's spots: Oval, retinal hemorrhages with a clear pale center
- Splinter hemorrhages: Linear, subungual dark red streaks commonly seen in fingers.

ATHEROSCLEROSIS

- Risk factors:
  - o Low HDL
  - o Raised apolipoprotein A
  - o Smoking etc.
- Amino acid associated with atherosclerosis: Homocysteine

- Organism associated with coronary atherosclerosis:
  - o H. pylori
  - o Chlamydia etc.

MYOCARDIAL INFARCTION

- ECG change in hyperacute phase: ST elevation
- ECG changes in anterolateral infarct:
  - o V4-6
  - o I
  - o aVL (left main stem)

MARKERS IN MI

- In stable angina, enzyme levels are: Normal
- Enzyme to raise at the earliest: Myoglobin; followed by CK-MB
- Sensitive marker for MI: Troponin T

CK

- Rises at 4-8 hours
- Peaks at 16-24 hours &
- Returns to normal at 3-4 days

Troponin T

- Begins to rise at 4-6 hours
- Peaks at 12-24 hours &
- Returns to normal at 7-10 days

Contraindication to thrombolytic therapy

Absolute	*Relative*
Past history of cerebro-vascular hemorrhage	Current use of anticoagulants
Any cerebrovascular event in past one year Suspicion of aortic dissection Active internal bleeding	Recent invasive or surgical the procedure or prolonged cardiopulmonary resuscitation Known bleeding diathesis Pregnancy A hemorrhagic ophthalmic condition Active peptic ulcer disease Adequately controlled severe hypertension

Enzyme Markers in MI

Creatinine phosphokinase	Appears within 2-4 hours, peaks by 24 hours, returns to normal by 3 days.	Very sensitive, less specific
Lactate dehydrogenase	Seen within 24 hours, peaks by 4-5 days, returns to normal in days.	Not specific
Troponin T/ I	Rises within 4-8 hours, Peaks in 10 days	MC used Very sensitive and specific

Troponin is elevated in

- Myocardial infarction
- Pulmonary embolism
- Congestive heart failure

DIGOXIN TOXICITY

- Precipitating factors:
  - o Hypokalemia (classically)
  - o Hypomagnesemia
  - o Hypercalcemia
  - o Hypernatremia etc.
- Features:
  - o Yellow green vision
  - o Arrhythmia etc.
- Management
  - o Withdrawal of digoxin
  - o Potassium supplement
  - o Correct arrhythmia etc.

CARDIAC TAMPONADE

- Features:
  - o Pulsus paradoxus
  - o Electrical alterans
  - o Raised JVP
  - o ‘x’ descent is prominent

- Chest X-ray findings: Big globular heart
- Beck's triad:
  - o Hypotension
  - o Silent heart &
  - o Raised JVP

Principle features of cardiac tamponade

- Elevation of intracardiac pressure
- Limitation of ventricular
- Limitation of ventricular filling
- Reduction of cardiac output

CONSTRICTIVE PERICARDITIS

- Features:
  - o Right heart failure occurs
  - o Raised JVP
  - o Prominent 'x' descent
  - o Kussmaul sign seen

ANEMIA

Conditions associated with hypochromic microcytic anemia/ HcMcA are:

- Thalassemia (normal level of free erythrocyte proto-porphyrin)
- Iron deficiency anemia:
  - o Increased TIBC
  - o Increased red cell distribution width
  - o Decreased ferritin
  - o Decreased MCV
  - o Decreased MCH
- Sideroblastic anemia
- Lead toxicity
- Anemia of chronic diseases:
  - o HcMcA may or may not be seen
  - o Increased serum ferritin
  - o Decreased serum iron levels &
  - o Decreased total iron binding capacity/ TIBC
- HcMcA with decreased serum iron & increased TIBC suggests: Iron deficiency anemia
- HcMcA with decreased serum iron & decreased TIBC suggests: Anemia of chronic diseases
- Conditions associated with normocytic, normochromic anemia are:
  - o Sickle cell anemia
  - o Fanconi anemia
  - o Hereditary spherocytosis
- Haemochromatosis: Elevated serum ferritin, elevated serum iron & elevated percent transferrin saturation

IRON DEFICIENCY ANEMIA (IDA)

- Commonest cause of anemia in India
- Increased iron absorption is seen in: Iron deficiency anemia, pregnancy, hypoxia, acidic pH of stomach, ferrous iron salts
- Causes of IDA: Hookworms, celiac sprue, carcinoma colon
- Features diagnostic of IDA: Decreased serum ferritin, increased TIBC
- Earliest sign of IDA: Decrease in serum ferritin
- Most sensitive & specific test for diagnosing IDA: Serum ferritin levels
- Hypochromia may be preceded by microcytosis

MEGALOBLASTIC ANEMIA

- Causes:
  - o Orotic aciduria
  - o Liver disease
  - o Fish tapeworm infestation etc.
  - o Drugs:
    - ♦ Folate antagonists
    - ♦ Phenytoin etc.
- Hematological findings:
  - o Multisegmented nuclei
  - o Anisocytosis (increased variation in size of RBC)

- o Poikilocytosis (abnormal shaped RBC)
- o Pancytopenia etc.
- Associated with: SACD of spinal cord
- Tongue in vitamin B12 deficiency:
  - o Macroglossia
  - o Atrophic glossitis etc.

HEMOLYTIC ANEMIA

- Features:
  - o Increased reticulocyte count
  - o Increased serum LDH level
  - o Decreased serum haptoglobin level etc.

SICKLE CELL ANEMIA

- Pathology: Replacement of glutamate by valine at 6 beta chain of HbA
- MC symptom (acute presentation): Bone pain
- Other features:
  - o Cardiomegaly
  - o Fish mouth vertebra etc.
- Hematological findings:
  - o Hemosiderinuria
  - o Leukocytosis
  - o Target cells
- Thrombotic crisis/ painful crisis/ vaso-occlusive crisis is precipitated by:
  - o Infection
  - o Dehydration
  - o Deoxygenation
- Aplastic crisis is caused by infection with: Parvovirus

Hyperbaric oxygen used in the treatment of

- CO poisoning
- Gas gangrene
- Radiation induced tissue injury
- Diabetic leg ulcers
- Very severe blood loss, anemia
- Decompression sickness

HEREDITARY SPHEROCYTOSIS

- Assessed by: Raised osmotic fragility of the RBC
- Basic pathology:
  - o Defect in ankyrin (50%) (Binds protein 3 & spectrin)
  - o Mutation in protein 3 &
  - o Mutations of spectrin
  - o Paladini defect
- Management: Splenectomy

PAROXYSMAL NOCTURNAL HEMOGLOBINURIA

- Stem cell defect, leading to hemolysis
- Features:
  - o Hemoglobinuria (dark coloured urine in morning)
  - o Thrombosis (Budd Chiari syndrome)
  - o LAP score &
  - o Hypercellular marrow
- Tests for PNH:
  - o HAM test
  - o Analysis of GPI linked proteins (diagnostic test)

Hemolytic transfusion reactions

- Most common symptom is sensation of heat and pain along the vein into which the blood is being transfused, flushing on face, lumbar pain
- Oliguria and hemoglobinuria is seen
- In anesthetized patients - Abnormal bleeding and continued hypertension despite adequate replacement are seen

Concentrations of abnormal hemoglobin-complexes producing cyanosis

- Sulph Hb: 0.5 percent
- Meth Hb: 1.5 percent
- Deoxy Hb: 5 percent

POLYCYTHEMIA RUBRA VERA

- Hyperviscosity (thrombosis)
- Bleeding
- Normal erythropoietin levels &
- Raised LAP score
- Prognosis: May progress to acute leukemia
- Tumours associated with polycythemia:
  - o Hypernephroma
  - o Hepatoma

Age at diagnosis is the most important prognostic factor in AML

- ALL- peak incidence is before 10 years
- AML- after 65 years

THROMBOCYTOPENIA

- Causes of severe thrombocytopenia:
  - o ITP
  - o DIC
  - o TTP
- Test used for ITP: Hess/ tourniquet test

Bernard-Soulier syndrome

- Platelet function disorder characterized by deficiency of glycoprotein Ib (von Willebrand's factor receptor)
- Thrombocytopenia with giant platelets

Glanzmann thrombasthenia

- Deficiency of glycoprotein IIb and III a (fibrinogen receptor Platelet count is normal

HAEMOPHILIA

- Features
  - o Decreased VIII level
  - o Raised PTT

VON WILLEBRAND DISEASE

- MC inherited bleeding disorder
- Features
  - o Prolonged bleeding time
  - o Normal PT
- Management: Cryoprecipitate

ANTIPHOSPHOLIPID SYNDROME

- Features:
  - o Venous/ arterial thrombosis (NO bleeding)
  - o Recurrent fetal loss (2nd trimester abortions)
  - o Prolonged APTT

COMPLICATIONS OF BLOOD TRANSFUSION

- Hyperkalemia
- Citrate toxicity
- Hypothermia
- ARDS

TTP

- Pentad of TTP:
  - o Fever
  - o Thrombocytopenia
  - o Microangiopathic hemolytic anemia
  - o Neurological symptoms &
  - o Renal failure

HODGKIN'S LYMPHOMA

- EBV may be causative in some cases
- Malignant cell is: Reed sternberg cell
- RS cells are positive for:
  - o CD 15
  - o CD 30 (EXCEPT lymphocytic predominant)
- CNS involvement is uncommon
- Cerebellar degeneration is seen
- MC type: Nodular sclerosis
- MC type in India: Mixed cellularity

- Histogenitically different subtype: Lymphocytic predominant (negative for CD15, CD30; positive for CD20)
- Features of lymphocytic predominant:
  - o Popcorn cells
  - o Best prognosis
- Regimes used:
  - o ABVD
  - o MOPP

Hodgkin's disease

Most common type	Nodular sclerosis
Best prognosis	Lymphocytic predominance
Popcorn cells are seen in	Lymphocytic predominance
Lacunar cells seen in	Nodular sclerosis
Reed-Sternberg cells	Seen in all varieties, maximum in mixed cellularity

Order of involvement nodes in Hodgkin's disease

- Cervical, mediastinal, para-aortic

Epstein- Barr virus (Associated with)

- Infectious mononucleosis
- Thymoma
- Burkitt's lymphoma
- CNS lymphoma
- Hodgkin's disease
- NHL
- B cell lymphoma
- T cell lymphoma
- Oral hairy leukoplakia
- Tonsillar carcinoma
- Angioimmunoblastic lymphoma

HAIRY CELL LEUKEMIA

- Rare malignant proliferation of B cells
- DOC: Cladribine
- Pentostatin & interferon alpha are also used

POLYARTERITIS NODOSA

- Features:
  - o Necrotizing vasculitis of small & medium sized muscular arteries
  - o Intimal proliferation
  - o Preceded by H/O of asthma

KAWASAKI DISEASE

- Also known as mucocutaneous node disease
- Diagnostic criteria includes:
  - o Swelling/ erythema of the hand's & feet's
  - o Swollen lymph node in the neck of at least 15 mm etc.
- Standard treatment: I/V immunoglobulin

TEMPORAL ARTERITIS

- MC in: Females
- Features:
  - o Severe headache
  - o Visual disturbances etc.
- Clinical diagnosis should be verified by: Temporal artery biopsy (as prolonged steroid therapy is indicated)

SLE

- Musculoskeletal finding: Non-erosive arthritis
- Renal manifestations:
  - o Papillary necrosis
  - o Wire loop lesions
- MC cause of death: Renal involvement
- Haematologic manifestations:
  - o Autoimmune hemolytic anemia
  - o Cold antibodies
  - o Mild thrombocytopenia
  - o Pancytopenia etc.

- Pulmonary system findings:
    - o Cavitation
    - o Pulmonary fibrosis
    - o Shrinking lung syndrome
    - o Polyserositis
- Specific antibody for SLE:
    - o Anti-ds DNA
    - o Anti-Sm

Cold AIHA	*Warm AIHA*
IgM	IgG
Mycoplasma infection	Lymphomas
Mononucleosis	SLE
Idiopathic Paroxysmal cold hemoglobinuria	Methyldopa

SCLERODERMA

- Associated with:
    - o Raynaud's phenomenon
    - o Anti-centromere antibody
    - o Sclerodactyly
    - o Peptic esophagitis with ulceration & stricture etc.

Therapeutic nuclear magnetic resonance

- I 131: Thyroid cancer, Graves disease
- I 131MIBI: Pheochromocytomas, Neuroblastomas
- Yttrium-90 – Octreotide: Carcinoma with Somatostatin receptors
- P- 32, Sr- 87: Bone metastasis, pain palliation, Rheumatoid arthritis
- I 131, I 125 lipiodol: Hepatic carcinoma
- Au-198: Pleural/Pericardial effusion

BEHCET'S SYNDROME

- Also known as oculo-genital syndrome
- Associated with:
    - o HLA B5
    - o Recurrent DVT

HLA association of diseases

- HLA A3: Hemochromatosis
- HLA B5/ B51: Behçet's syndrome
- HLA B27: Ankylosing spondylitis, Reiter's syndrome, Reactive arthritis, Psoriatic arthritis, JRA
- HLA DR2: Narcolepsy, Multiple Sclerosis
- HLA DR3: Celiac disease, Sjögren's syndrome, Dermatitis herpetiformis, Chronic active hepatitis, Adrenal insufficiency
- HLA B8/HLA DR3: Grave's disease, Myasthenia gravis
- HLA DR4/ DW4: Rheumatoid arthritis
- HLA DR2/DR3/DR4: IDDM
- HLA DQ2/ HLA B8: Gluten sensitive enteropathy
- HLA BW47: Inherited error of metabolism

HENOCH SCHONLEIN PURPURA

- Features:
    - o Arthralgia
    - o Abdominal pain &
    - o Glomerulonephritis
- MC cause of death: Renal failure
- Lab findings:
    - o Normal platelet count
    - o Serum complements are normal
    - o Elevated IgA levels

Immune thrombocytopenic purpura

- Therapy includes steroids, intravenous immunoglobulins, anti-D immunoglobulin and splenectomy

TOXIC MYOPATHIES

- Drugs/ chemical induced muscle damage
- Chloroquine causes: Vacuolar myopathy
- Excess alcohol causes:
    - o Muscle weakness
    - o Rhabdomyolysis
- Steroid myopathy involves: Pelvis

POLYMYOSITIS

- No involvement of extraocular & facial muscles
- No cutaneous manifestations
- Proximal limb muscles are involved
- Pharyngeal muscles are involved
- Pain is a feature
- Raised CPK

Polymyositis

- Ocular muscles are not involved

Dermatomyositis

- Classical rash - Heliotrope rash in butterfly distribution
- Gottron rash
- Erythema of the knuckles with a raised violaceous scaly eruption seen in dermatomyositis

Appearance of rash

Condition	*Appearing time (in days)*
Chicken pox	**1**
Scarlet fever	**2**
Rubella	**2**
Small pox	**3**
Measles	**4**
Typhus	**5**
Typhoid	**6-8 days**

Pyrexia of unknown origin

- In 1961, Petersdorf and Beeson suggested the following criteria
- Fever higher than 38.3^{0}C (101^{0}F) on several occasions, persisting without diagnosis for at least 3 weeks.
- At least 1 week's investigation in hospital
- Tuberculosis is the commonest cause of PUO

Cause of fever

Type	*Seen in/ cause*
Metal fume fever	**Zinc poisoning**
Pel-ebstein fever	**Brucellosis & Hodgkin's disease**
Double rise of temperature in a day	**Kala-azar**
Pontiac fever	**Legionella**
Scarlet fever	**Streptococci**
Oroya fever	**Bartonella**
Glandular fever	**Ebstein Barr virus**
Lassa fever	**Arena virus**

Hereditary angioedema

- Deficiency of C1 inhibitor
- Autosomal dominant

DUCHENNE MUSCULAR DYSTROPHY

- Inheritance: X linked recessive
- Defect lies in:
  - o Dystrophin gene
  - o Sarcolemmal protein defect
- Features: Pseudohypertrophy of muscles
- Gowers sign: Patient, while standing, tries to climb on himself

MYOTONIC DYSTROPHY

- Location of gene: Chromosome 19q
- Features:
  - o High incidence of cataracts
  - o Premature balding
  - o Testicular atrophy

MYASTHENIA GRAVIS

- Decreased myoneural junction
- Features:
  - o Dysarthria
  - o Dysphagia
  - o Proximal muscle weakness
  - o Sensory modalities & deep tendon reflexes are NORMAL
- MC used cholinergic drugs: Pyridostigmine/ neostigmine

- Surgical procedure (should be done in all cases): Thymectomy

Myasthenia gravis

- Extraocular muscles are most commonly affected first
- Pupils are never affected
- Associated with thymoma
- Edrophonium, a quick and short acting anticholinesterase is used for diagnosis

Lambert- Eaton neuromuscular syndrome

- Associated with malignancy in only 50 percent
- Most commonly associated with small cell carcinoma
- Neoplasm induced IgG antibody against the voltage gated calcium channels in the terminus of the motor neuron

MENETRIER'S DISEASE

- Characterized by large, tortuous gastric mucosal folds
- Protein losing enteropathy
- Increased risk of adenoCa

H. PYLORI

- More prevalent in developing countries
- Urel is: pH gated urea channel in H. pylori
- Associated condition:
  - o Gastritis
  - o Gastric Ca
  - o Peptic ulcer disease &
  - o Gastric lymphoma
- Extra gastric diseases:
  - o Coronary atherosclerosis
  - o Iron deficiency anemia
- Test for documenting eradication: Urea breath test
- Test for epidemiology: Serology

DUODENAL ULCER

- More associated with H. pylori
- Usually < 1 cm in diameter
- 1st portion of duodenum

ULCERS

- MC site of Cushing's ulcer: Distal duodenum
- MC site of peptic ulcer: 1st part of duodenum
- Curling's ulcer: Stress ulcer after burns
- MC complication of peptic ulcer: Hemorrhage

WHIPPLE DISEASE

- Specific test: Biopsy
- Caused by: Tropheryma whipplei
- CNS involvement:
  - o Dementia
  - o Seizures etc.

CELIAC DISEASE

- Sensitivity to protein gluten
- Associated with: Myasthenia gravis
- Diagnosed by: Immunology & jejunal biopsy
- Findings on jejunal biopsy:
  - o Villous atrophy
  - o Crypt hyperplasia
  - o Thickness of mucosa unaltered

Important diagnostic features

Condition	*Features*
Wernicke's encephalopathy	Bilaterally symmetrical ophthalmolegia (most valuable sign)
Spring catarrh	Itching
Chronic dacryocystitis	Epiphora
Glomus jugulare tumour	Pulsating tinnitus
Temporal obe abscess	Homonymous hemianopia
Extra-medullary tumour of spinal cord	Nerve root pain
Secondary's/ metastasis to spine	Back-pain

Osteomalacia	Looser's zone
Scurvy	Swollen spongy gums (scurvy buds)
Acoustic neuroma	Unilateral deafness
Vesical (urinary bladder) calculus	Frequency of micturition
Neuroblastoma	Abdominal mass in infant
Renal calculus	Intermittent dull ache in loin area
TB of kidney	Increased frequency
Varicose veins	Tired, aching pain in calf (late in day)
Biliary cirrhosis	Itching
Ulcerative colitis	Diarrhea
Zenker's diverticulum	Dysphagia
Appendicitis	Pain followed by vomiting followed by fever (Murphy's traid)
Acute crohn's disease	Like appendicitis
Chronic crohn's disease	Pain
Achalasia cardia	Intermittent dysphagia
Carcinoma esophagus	Progressive dysphagia
Urticaria	Itching
Scleroderma	Raynaud's phenomenon
CML	Chronic ill health & lassitude
CLL	Painless, discrete lymphadenopathy
Anemia	Pallor
Tetanus	Trismu's first
Brucellosis	Sweating

ULCERATIVE COLITIS

- Associated terms:
  - o Toxic megacolon
  - o Pseudopolyps etc.

CROHN'S DISEASE

- Associated terms:
  - o Skip lesions
  - o Creeping fat
  - o Anti-saccharomyces cerevisiae antibody etc.

- Mainstay of therapy for inflammatory bowel disease: 5 amino salicylic acid

Ulcerative colitis	*Crohn's disease*
Cigarette smoking is protective	Cigarette smoking causes disease
Commonest symptom is bloody Diarrhea and abdominal pain	Commonest symptom is non bloody diarrhoea, abdominal pain
No cobblestoning of mucosa	Cobblestoning of mucosa +
Rectum is always involved	Rectum is spared
Continuous lesions	Skip lesions
No recurrence after surgery	Recurs after surgery
Antibiotics not effective	Antibiotics are effective
Toxic megacolon is seen	Not seen
Lead pipe appearance	String sign on barium meal
pANCA present	ASCA present

Causes of Pseudomembranous colitis

- Clostridium difficile
- Ischemic colitis
- Volvulus
- Staphylococcus
- Shigella
- Candida

HEPATITIS

- Reverse transcriptase of HBV is coded by: P gene
- Hepatitis spreading by feco-oral route: HAV, HEV
- First viral marker to appear after HBV infection: HBsAg
- Indicator of intrahepatic viral replication/ presence of which marker indicates high infectivity: HbeAg, HBV DNA
- Recent infection of HBV is indicated by: IgM anti-HBcAg
- HBV is associated with: Polyarteritis Nodosa
- Agents used treating for HBV:
  - o Interferon

- o Lamivudine
- o Adefovir
- MC cause of sporadic hepatitis in adults: HEV
- Worst prognosis in pregnancy: HEV
- Treatment of HCV: Interferon + ribavirin
- Most prone to chronicity: HCV
- Conditions associated with HCV:
  - o Cryoglobulinemia
  - o Glomerulonephritis
  - o Arthritis etc.

Liver

- 5' nucleotidase-determines whether raised alkaline phosphatase is hepatic in origin.
- Gamma glutary1 transpeptidase/ GGT - Increased in cholestasis, Increased in patients of alcohol abuse.
- Auxiliary liver transplant: Transplanted liver provides temporary support till the native liver recovers.

Purtscher's retinopathy

- Complication of acute pancreatitis
- Sudden and severe loss of vision
- Due to occlusion of posterior retinal artery with aggregated granulocytes
- Fundoscopic appearance of cotton wool spots and hemorrhages confined to an area of optic disc and macula

Grading of hepatic encephalopathy

Grade	*Clinical features*
Subclinical	Impaired psychomotor testing
1	Asterixis
2	Disorientation
3	Stupor
4	Deep coma

WILSON DISEASE

- Inheritance: Autosomal recessive
- Diagnostic criteria:
  - o S. Ceruloplasmin level < 20 mg/dl + KF rings OR
  - o S. Ceruloplasmin level < 20 mg/dl + concentration of Cu in liver biopsy sample > 250 microgram/ gram dry weight
- Urinary excretion of Cu in most symptomatic patients: > 100 microgram Cu/ day
- Features:
  - o Hepatic dysfunction
  - o Eye changes (KF rings in descemet's membrane of cornea; they do not interfere with vision)
  - o Neurologic manifestations (NO sensory changes)
- Drug used in penicillamine sensitive patients: Trientine
- Drug for maintenance therapy: Zinc acetate/ gluconate

HEMOCHROMATOSIS

- Autosomal dominant
- Associated with:
  - o DM
  - o Arthropathy (MCP joints)
  - o Chondrocalcinosis
  - o Pseudogout (CPP deposition)
  - o Cardiac involvement (Congestive heart failure)
- Treatment:
  - o Phlebotomy (treatment of choice)
  - o Venesection
  - o Desferrioxamine

URINARY CASTS

- Tom Horsfall protein: Normal (from tubules)
- RBC casts: Glomerulonephritis
- Dysmorphic RBC's: Glomerular pathology
- WBC cast: Pyelonephritis
- Coarse granular cast: Acute tubular necrosis

PRE-RENAL UREMIA

- Urine sodium: <20 mmol/ L (>30 in ATN)

- Fractional sodium excretion: <1% (>1% in ATN)
- Fractional urea excretion: <35% (>35% in ATN)
- Specific gravity: >1020 (<1010 in ATN)

CHRONIC RENAL FAILURE

- Broad cast in urine
- Hyper/ hypo natremia
- Hyper/ hypo kalemia
- Membranoproliferative GN
- Restless leg syndrome etc.

DIABETIC NEPHROPATHY

- IDDM presentation: Usually <25 years
- HLA link of NIDDM: No links
- Ketoacidosis commoner in: IDDM
- Dawn phenomenon: Glucose level rise in early morning
- Somogyi effect: Rebound hyperglycemia may appear after 1-24 hours after moderate to severe hypoglycemia
- Leading cause of end stage renal disease/ ESRD: Diabetic nephropathy
- Absence of chest pain in DM patients is: Silent ischemia (due to neuropathy)
- Parameter used to monitor DM control: HbA1c
- Early test for DM nephropathy: Persistent albuminuria (>300 mg/d or >200 mcg/ min) soon at least 2 occasions, 3-6 months apart
- Kimmelstiel Wilson nodule: Characteristic histological feature of DM nephropathy

Terms

- Somogyi effect: Overnight hyperglycemia after hypoglycemia due to counter regulatory hormones. Management – decrease insulin dose
- Dawn phenomenon: Early morning hyperglycemia. Management – increase dose or delay it
- Honeymoon period: Seen in type I diabetes, Drastic decrease in insulin requirement followed by rise due to temporary recovery of beta cells
- Brittle diabetes: Seen in type I diabetes, Rapid changes in blood glucose level, from hypoglycemia to ketoacidosis

NEPHROTIC SYNDROME

- Severe proteinuria
- Increased fibrinogen
- Platelet activation
- Decreased HDL etc.

MINIMAL CHANGE DISEASE

- Causes:
  - o Idiopathic
  - o HIV
  - o Hodgkin's disease etc.
- Responds well to: Steroids
- Deposition of: IgA
- Electron microscopy findings: Fusion of foot process
- Changes on light microscopy: No change

RPGN/ CRESCENTIC GN

- Features:
  - o Rapid onset (often presents as ARF)
  - o Crescent formation
- Causes:
  - o ANCA positive vasculitis
  - o Infective endocarditis

HYPERTENSION & KIDNEY

- Benign HTN: Hyaline arteriosclerosis
- Malignant HTN: Fibrinoid necrosis
- Renin dependent HTN: Renovascular HTN
- MC cause of paroxysmal HTN: Pheochromocytoma

Classical triad of pyonephrosis

- Anemia
- Fever
- Loin swelling

Causes of papillary necrosis

- Analgesic abuse
- Diabetes mellitus
- Infant in shock
- Pyelonephritis
- Obstruction
- Sickle cell disease
- Ethanol

Dietl's crisis

- Intermittent unilateral hydronephrosis after an attack of renal colic
- Followed hours later by passage of urine
- Disappearance of swelling and relief of pain

Bartter's syndrome

- Hypertrophy and hyperplasia of Juxtaglomerular cell
- Hypokalemic alkalosis and hyperaldosteronism

POLYCYSTIC KIDNEY DISEASE

- Adult PKD is: Autosomal dominant
- Chromosome involved in type I adult polycystic kidney disease, involves: 16
- Chromosome involved in type II adult polycystic kidney disease, involves: 4
- MC associated with:
  - o Colonic diverticula
  - o Hepatic cysts
  - o Splenic cysts

RENAL ARTERY STENOSIS

- MC cause of RAS in middle age & elderly: Atheromatous plaque (at the origin of renal artery)
- In younger female, stenosis is due to: Fibromuscular dysplasia
- Most sensitive & specific modality for diagnosing RAS: Magnetic resonance angiography/ MRA

HYPERTHYROIDISM

- CVS features of hyperthyroidism:
  - o Wide pulse pressure
  - o Cardiomyopathy
  - o Tachycardia etc.

Diagnostic nuclear magnetic resonance

- I 131, I- 123: Thyroid
- Tc- 99m DTPA: Kidney glomerular function. Mucociliary clearance of lungs in pneumocystis carinii pneumoniae infection in AIDS
- HIDA: Liver function and biliary clearance
- Tc- 99m MAA: Lung perfusion
- Tc- 99m DMSA: Kidney cortical scarring
- Tc- 99m MIBI: Thyroid carcinoma
- Cr-51: RBC scan
- Thallium: Myocardial infarction
- Tc- 99m pertechnetate: Hot spots
- I 131 hippuran: Kidney
- Xe- 133: Lung ventilation scan
- Tc 99 m MDP: Bone tumors and infections
- Gallium- 67, Iridium – 111: Leucocyte scan
- Strontium: Fracture neck femur
- Gallium 67: Sarcoidosis

SUBACUTE THYROIDITIS/ DeQUERVAIN'S THYROIDITIS/ GRANULOMATOUS THYROIDITIS/ GIANT CELL THYROIDITIS

- Features:
  - o Myopathy
  - o Diffuse goitre
  - o Myxedema
- Radio-iodide scan shows: Reduced uptake

HYPOTHYROIDISM

- Features:

- o Carpal tunnel syndrome
- o Subnormal body temperature
- o Increased sleep
- o Cold intolerance

- TSH level: Increased
- Drugs associated with hypothyroidism:
  - o Lithium
  - o Amiodarone etc.
- MC cause of congenital hypothyroidism: Thyroid agenesis
- Treatment of childhood hypothyroidism: Levothyroxine

PRIMARY HYPERPARATHYROIDISM

- MC cause: Solitary adenoma (80%)
- Features:
  - o Bones (brown tumour)
  - o Stones (renal calculi)
  - o Abdominal groans (peptic ulcer) &
  - o Psychic moans (depression)
- Blood chemistry:
  - o Raised Ca
  - o Low phosphate &
  - o Normal alkaline phosphatase

MEA/ MEN

MEA I (Werner's)	Parathyroid gland- chief cell hyperplasia hyperparathyroidism, Pancreas – islet cell tumour, Zollinger- Ellison syndrome, Pituitary- anterior acromegaly, Cushing's syndrome
MEA II a	Parathyroid gland- pheochromocytoma Thyroid- medullar carcinoma
MEA II b	Parathyroid gland –chief cell hyperplasia Hyperparathyroidism, Adrenal gland- Phaeochromocytoma, Neurofibromatosis Thyroid – Medullary carcinoma

Thyroid

- Jod Basedow thyrotoxicosis: Large doses of iodine given to hyperplastic endemic goiter which is iodine-avid may produce temporary hyperthyroidism and occasionally persistent hyperthyroidism
- Wolf- Chaikoff effect: In normal individuals large doses of iodine act directly on the thyroid to produce a mild and transient inhibition of organic binding of iodide and hence of hormone synthesis

SIADH

- Dilutional hyponatremia
- Treatment: Water reduction, demeclocycline

Primary hyperparathyroidism

- Bones, groans, stones and psychic moans

CONN'S SYNDROME

- Basic pathology: Hyperaldosteronism
- Features:
  - o Hypertension
  - o Decreased K+
  - o Polyuria
  - o Polydipsia &
  - o Proximal myopathy

ADDISON'S DISEASE

- Pathology: Primary adrenocortical insufficiency
- Metabolic effects:
  - o Hyperkalemia
  - o Hyponatremia &
  - o Hypoglycemia
  - o Increased pigmentation (EXCEPT in secondary adrenal insufficiency due to pituitary failure)
- Definitive investigation: Short ACTH test
- Drug associated with addisonian like features: Busulfan

ALZHIEMER'S DISEASE

- MC cause of dementia in elderly: Alzhiemer's disease
- Presenile dementia occurs before the age of: 60 years
- Useful screening test for dementia: Mini mental status examination
- Maximum score in mini mental status examination: 30

PROGRESSIVE MULTIFOCAL LEUCOENCEPHALOPATHY

- Caused by: JC virus
- Affects: White matter
- Prognosis: Fatal within a year
- MC features: Visual defects (45%)
- Diagnosis:
  - o Positive CSF PCR for JC virus DNA
  - o Typical MRI lesions &
  - o Clinical findings

CREUTZFELDT JACKOBSON DISEASE

- Caused by: Prion (infectious proteins)
- Neurodegenerative disease
- Rapid progression is common &
- Can be transmitted by corneal implants

GUILLAIN BARRE SYNDROME

- Ascending type of motor paralysis
- Arreflexia
- Flaccidity
- Albumino-cytological dissociation
- Treatment:
  - o Plasmapheresis &
  - o Immunoglobulin

Landry-Guillain - Barre syndrome

- Acute inflammatory demyelinating polyradiculopathy
- History of preceding viral infection
- Ascending weakness
- Albumino-cytological dissociation present
- Treatment includes steroids, plasma exchange, intra-venous immunoglobulin.

Miller – Fisher variant of Guillian - Barre syndrome

- External ophthalmoplegia
- Ataxia
- Areflexia

Wallenberg's syndrome/ Lateral medullary syndrome

- Due to PICA infarct
- Ipsilateral loss of pain and temperature over the face
- Ipsilateral 9th, 10th, and 11th cranial nerve palsy
- Ipsilateral Horner's syndrome
- Ipsilateral cerebellar signs
- Ipsilateral vestibular signs
- Contralateral loss of pain and temperature over the limbs

Jackson's syndrome/ Medial medullary syndrome

- Ipsilateral twelfth nerve palsy
- Contralateral hemiplegic
- Contralateral loss of joint position sense and vibration

Millard-Gubler syndrome/ Ventral pontine syndrome

- Ipsilateral seventh nerve palsy
- Contralateral hemiplegia

Raymond – Foville syndrome

- Ipsilateral facial palsy
- Ipsilateral abducens palsy
- Contralateral hemiparesis

Weber's syndrome

- Ipsilateral third nerve palsy
- Contralateral hemiplegia

Bendict's syndrome

- Ipsilateral rubral tumor
- Contralateral hemiparesis

CNS causes of hemiplegia

- Thrombosis of unpaired anterior cerebral artery
- Superior sagittal sinus
- Parasagittal meningioma
- Cortical venous sinus thrombosis

FRIEDREICH'S ATXIA

- Inheritance: Autosomal recessive
- Earliest feature: Ataxia
- Structure affected earliest: Dorsal root ganglia
- Features: Absent knee jerk & extensor plantar response
- Cardiac involvement may be seen (cardiomyopathy)
- Involvement of: Pyramidal tract

CEREBELLAR LESION

- Manifestation:
  - o Ataxia/asynergia (inability to do movements smoothly & accurately)
  - o Hypotonia
  - o Intention tremor (NOT resting ones)
  - o Nystagmus etc.

MENINGITIS

- MC cause of neonatal meningitis: Gram negative bacilli
- MC cause of meningitis in adults: S. pneumonia

BACTERIAL MENINGITIS

- Purulent exudate
- Cloudy CSF
- Decreased glucose (<2.2 mmol/ L) &
- Increased protein concentration (>0.45 g/L)

VIRAL MENINGITIS

- MC caused by: Enterovirus (80-90%)
- Features:
  - o Lymphocytic pleocytosis
  - o Normal glucose level
  - o Normal/ mildly elevated pressure
- Test: CSF PCR test

ENCEPHALITIS

- MC cause of sporadic viral encephalitis: HSV
- Features:
  - o Hemorrhagic lesions &
  - o Temporal lobe involvement is common

NEUROSYPHILIS

- Tract involved: Dorsal column
- Features:
  - o Sensory loss
  - o Argyll Robertson pupil &
  - o Bladder dysfunction
- Associated term: Tabes dorsalis

Similar sounding terms

- Tabes dorsalis: Neurosyphilis affecting posterior column of spinal cord
- Tabes mesenterica: Tuberculous affection of mesenteric lymph nodes
- Tabes ergotica: A condition similar to Tabes dorsalis due to ergotism
- Friedrich's tabes: Friedrich's ataxia Lupus vulgaris: Skin TB
- Lupus pernio: A form of Sarcoidosis

Syphilitic aneurysm

- Most common site of syphilitic aneurysm is ascending and transverse portion of the arch of aorta
- It also leads to ventricular dilatation (Cor bovinum)

Brown- Sequard syndrome

- Ipsilateral lower motor neuron paralysis in the segment.
- Ipsilateral spastic paralysis below the level
- Ipsilateral band of cutaneous anesthesia at the level
- Ipsilateral band of posterior column sensation loss below the level
- Contralateral loss of pain and temperature sensation below the level
- Contralateral impaired tactile sensation below the level

Thalamic pain syndrome (Dejerine-Roussy syndrome)

- Affects contralateral side of the body
- Due to thalamic infarct in ventral posterolateral nucleus

Frontal disinhibition syndrome

- Loss of initiative, creativity and curiosity
- Pervasive emotional apathy
- Anomic aphasia is the single most common language disturbance seen in head trauma, metabolic encephalopathy and Alzheimer's disease
- Prolactin is increased after an episode of seizures

Déjà vu

- Déjà vu and jamais vu phenomenon are seen in partial seizures
- Déjà vu is seen in temporal lobe epilepsy, normal people, psychosis, hysteria
- Déjà vu feeling of familiarity with unfamiliar situations
- Jamais vu –felling of unfamiliarity with familiar situations.

West syndrome

- Epileptic encephalopathy
- Onset between 4-8 months of age
- Salaam attacks
- Hypsarrhythmia on EEG
- Treatment with ACTH or vigabatrin

NEUROPATHIC JOINT DISEASE

- MC cause of neuropathic joint disease: DM
- MC joint affected by DM: Tarsal joints
- Other associated conditions:
  - o Leprosy
  - o Syringomyelia
  - o Tabes dorsalis etc.
- Condition resembling Charcot's joint: CPPD deposition

PARKINSONISM

- Features:
  - o Tremor (at rest; worsens with emotional stress)
  - o Festinating gait
  - o Bradykinesia
  - o Decreased blinking etc.
- Symptoms of parkinsonism are due to: Loss of nerve cells in
  - o Substantia nigra
  - o Pars compacta & the
  - o Locus coeruleus (midbrain)
- Drugs causing parkinsonism:
  - o Methyl dopa
  - o Reserpine
  - o Thiazides
  - o Metoclopramide etc.

Gait	*Condition*
Circumduction	**Hemiplegia**
Scissoring gait	**Spastic paraplegia**
Festinating gait	**Parkinson's disease**
Wadding gait	**Muscular dystrophies**
Stamping gait	**Sensory ataxia**
Broad based gait	**Cerebellar disorders**
Broad based high stepping gait	**Posterior colum lesion**
Charlie Chaplin gait	**Tibial torsion, Homocystinuria**
Lurching gait	**Cerebellar ataxia**

SUBARACHNOID HEMORRHAGE

- Clinical presentation:

- o 60 years old patient with severe headache & neck stiffness of abrupt onset. She had never such a severe headache before. She may have photophobia & nausea
- Most aneurysm presents as: Sudden SAH
- Occipital & posterior cervical pain may indicate: Posterior/ anterior inferior cerebellar artery aneurysm (rare)
- Cause of clinical deterioration in a week following: Rebleed & vasospasm

Intracranial Aneurysm

- Most common site is between anterior cerebral and anterior communicating artery
- Intracranial aneurysms – rupture is likely if >7mm in diameter
- Progressively enlarging unruptured aneurysm most commonly involve oculomotor nerve
- Most common nerve to be involved with raised intracranial tension is the abducens nerve
- Most common site of hypertensive haemorrhage in brain is putamen
- Marchiafava–Bignami syndrome: Widespread demyelination of cerebral hemispheres due to chronic alcoholism

Craniopharyngioma

- It is called 90 percent tumour-
- 90 percent are calcified
- 90 percent are cystic
- 90 percent show enhancement

Brain secondary's

- Most common secondary's to brain are from:
  - o Carcinoma lung
  - o Carcinoma breast
  - o Carcinoma kidney

Cluster headache

- 1-3 short lived daily attacks, of unilateral, orbital or temporal pain of 4-8 weeks interval followed by pain free interval often of 1 year
- Associated with red, tearful eye, nasal stuffiness
- Commonly in males

PERIPHERAL NEUROPATHY

- Predominantly motor loss:
  - o Porphyria
  - o Lead poisoning
  - o Guillain Barre syndrome
  - o Inflammatory demyelination polyneuropathy etc.
- Predominantly sensory loss:
  - o DM
  - o Leprosy
  - o HIV etc.

AMYOTROPHIC LATERAL SCLEROSIS

- Affects:
  - o Anterior horn cells
  - o Corticospinal tracts
  - o Hyporeflexia may be seen

BRAIN TUMOUR

- MC brain tumours: Secondary's
- MC glial tumours: Astrocytoma
- MC intracranial tumour: Glioma
- MC posterior fossa tumour: Astrocytoma
- Conditions associated with brain tumour:
  - o Von Hippel Lindau syndrome
  - o Tuberous sclerosis etc.
- MC tumour associated with neurofibromatosis-I: Optic nerve glioma
- Feature of neurofibroblastoma-II: Bilateral acoustic neuroma
- Craniopharyngiomas are derived from: Rathke's pouch

Epilepsy

- Twilight sleep is seen in epilepsy

- Twilight sleep is the state of narrowing of field of consciousness for short duration followed by amnesia
- Jacksonian march - Seen in simple partial seizures, the abnormal motor activity begins in a limited area and then gradually spreads to involve larger areas
- Todd's paralysis - Type of post ictal focal neurological deficit seen in partial motor seizures
- Absence seizures - Typically, 3 Hz spike and wave pattern discharge is seen

Clinical triad of tuberous sclerosis

- Adenoma sebaceum
- Epilepsy
- Mental retardation

Wilm's tumor is associated with

- WAGR syndrome (Wilm's tumor, Aniridia, Genital abnormalities, mental Retardation)
- Denys- Drash syndrome
- Beckwith- Wiedemann syndrome

Charcot's triad (Seen in ascending cholangitis)

- Jaundice
- Abdominal pain
- Fever

Saint's triad

- Diverticulosis
- Gallstones
- Hiatus hernia

Reynold's pentad

- Jaundice
- Abdominal pain
- Fever
- Shock
- Confusion

CLINICAL PRESENTATIONS

- 66 years old male with back pain, anemia, raised ESR (85) & serum creatinine (3.2 mg%): Multiple myeloma
- Child with ascending flaccid paralysis, shows albumino-cytological dissociation of CSF studies: Guillain Barre syndrome
- A 26 years old male with pigmented macules over plam, sole & oral mucosa & pain in abdomen with anemia: Peutz-Jeghers syndrome
- 60 years old lady with severe unilateral headache & blindless with raised ESR. A thick cord like structure can be felt on lateral side: Temporal arteritis
- A 50-year old lady with hypertension & palpitation. CT scan showed suprarenal mass: Phaeochromocytoma
- A 4-year child has high BP. Her femoral pulses are weak as compared to radial & carotid pulses. Chest X-rays shows rib notching: Coarctation of aorta
- A 40-year patient with symptoms of hyperparathyroidism, pancreatic tumour, adrenal cortical hyperplasia, pituitary adenomas, islet cell tumour & cutaneous angiofibroma: MEN I
- A 48-year old man, smoker & alcoholic with shortness of breath & chest pain radiating to the back & interscapular region: Aortic dissection
- A patient is having chronic diarrhea. Biopsy showed villous atrophy. Anti-endomysial antibodies is positive: Gluten sensitive enteropathy
- A 8-year old girl with recurrent episodes of bleeding. APTT is prolonged but PT is normal: Von Willebrand disease
- A 42 years old male has hepatosplenomegaly, bilateral hilar lymphadenopathy & hypercalcemia: Sarcoidosis
- A patient is having dull retrosternal chest pain. Pulsus paradoxus & kussmaul sign is present. Raised JVP is seen. Heart sounds are muffled: Pericardial effusion

Disease associated with massive splenomegaly

- Chronic myelogenous leukemia
- Lymphomas
- Hairy cell leukemia
- Myelofibrosis with myeloid metaplasia
- Polycythemia vera
- Gaucher's disease

- Chronic lymphocytic leukemia
- Sarcoidosis
- Autoimmune hemolytic anemia
- Splenic hemangiomatosis
- Malaria
- Kala azar

Strawberry tongue

- Scarlet fever
- Kawasaki's disease
- Toxic shock syndrome

Diseases with their specific antibodies

- SLE: Anti ds DNA (specific) Anti Sm {Smith}
- Drug induced SLE: Anti Histone
- Systemic sclerosis: Anti DNA Topoisomerase {Scl 70}
- Scleroderma {CREST}: anti Centromere
- Sjogren's syndrome: SSA (Ro) SSB (La)
- Primary biliary cirrhosis: Anti Mitochondrial
- Inflammatory myopathy : Histidyl t- RNA synthetase
- Mixed connective tissue disorders: Anti Ribonucleo-protein
- Churg Strauss: Anti Ribonucleoprotein ANCA
- Multifocal motor neuropathy: Anti GM1
- Wegener's granulomatosis, Henoch-Schonlein purpura: c-ANCA
- Idiopathic crescentic nephritis, Ulcerative colitis, Microscopic polyangiitis, Polyarteritis nodosa: p-ANCA
- Crohn's disease: Anti-saccharomyces crevisiae (ASCA)
- Celiac sprue: Anti-endomysial and Anti-gliadin
- Psychosis/Depression due To CNS SLE: Anti-ribosomal –P

Vaccines recommended in HIV Positive patients

- Pneumococcal vaccine: Consider revaccination five years after initial dose.
- Hepatitis B vaccine: Administer to patients without serologic evidence of past or present Hepatitis B infection. Vaccinated patients after the third dose; non-responders should receive booster injections
- Hemophilus influenzae type B vaccine: Administer to asplenic patients and those with history of recurrent hemophilus infection
- Influenza vaccine: Administer to patients at high-risk for exposure to or morbidity from influenza. There is evidence that the vaccine may transiently promote HIV replication
- Tetanus toxoid: Td booster is recommended every 10 years
- Polio vaccine: IPV is administered

CRITERIA FOR AIDS –If two of the major with at least one of the minor signs are present

Major signs	*Minor signs*
Weight loss of more than 10 percent of body weight	Persistent cough for > 1 month
Chronic diarrhea for more than 1 month	Generalized pruritic dermatitis
Prolonged fever for more than 1 month	History of herpes zoster oropharyngeal candidiasis Chronic progressive or disseminated herpes simplex infection. Generalized lymphadenopathy

POEMS syndrome

- Polyneuropathy
- Organomegaly
- Endocrinopathy
- M protein band on electrophoresis with less than 5 percent plasma cells in bone marrow
- Skin hyperpigmentation

Glasgow Coma Scale

Remember EVM- 4-5-6

Eye opening

4 - Spontaneous

3 - On verbal stimuli

2 - On pain stimuli

1 - No response

Verbal response

5 - Oriented

4 - Confused

3 - Inappropriate

2 - Nonspecific sounds

1 - No response

Motor activity

6 - Follows command

5 - Localizes pain

4 - Withdraws to pain (pressure on nail bed, words if no response supraorbital pressure or suprasternal pressure)

3 - Flexion to pain

2 - Extension to pain

1 - None

Maximum score – 15

Minimum score – 3

Neurological derangement	*Score*
Severe	**≤ 8**
Moderate	**9 – 12**
Minor	**≥ 13**

Other scales used in ICU

- SOFA- Sequential Organ Failure Assessment Score
- SAPS II- Simplified Acute Physiology Score
- APACHE II/III – Acute Physiology and Chronic Health Evaluation
- Rancho Los Amigos cognitive scale

Conditions & related organism

Condition	*Causative organism*
Osteomyelitis in sickle cell anemia	**Salmonella**
Infections in immunosuppression	**Herpes simplex, CMV, aspergillus**
Vincent angina, cancrum oris	**Spirochetes vincentii & fusiform bacilli**
Myringitis bullosa (otitis external hemorrhagica)	**Hemolytic streptococci plus virus during influenza epidemic**
Endemic typhus/ Bejel	**Treponema pallidum**
Scleroma	**Klebsiella rhinoscleromatis**
Herpetiform genital ulcer	**LGV**
Acne	**Corynebacterium acnes**
Erythema multiforme major	**Mycoplasma**
Pulmonary alveolar proteinosis	**Nocardia**
Endemic hematuria	**Schistosoma hematobium**
Tropical hemoptysis	**Paragonimiasis westermani**
Tinea versicolor	**Malassezia furfur**
Fungus ball in lung cavity	**Aspergillosis**
Pericarditis	**Viral**
Myocarditis	**Coxsackie B**
Croup	**Para-influenza virus**
Malignant otitis externa	**Pseudomonas pyocyaneus**
Infection in burns	**Pseudomonas**
Meningitis in <2 months old	**E. coli, beta-hemolytic streptococci (streptococcus agalactaciae)**
UTI, peritonitis	**E. coli**
Viral pneumonia in adults	**Influenza**
Viral pneumonia in child	**Respiratory syncytial virus**
Bronchiolitis in children	**Respiratory syncytial virus**
Infection in cystic fibrosis	**Staphylococcus**
Toxic shock syndrome	**Staphylococcus**
Boil, carbuncle	**Staphylococcus**

CLINICAL QUESTIONS

1. **A 40 years old male is admitted with acute inferior wall myocardial infarction. Half an hour later his B.P. is 80/50 mm Hg and heart rate is 40/minute with sinus rhythm. The most appropriate step in the management of this patient would be:**

A. Administration of normal saline 300 ml over 15 minutes

B. Immediate insertion of temporary pacemaker

C. Intravenous administration of atropine sulfate

D. Intravenous administration of iso-prenaline 50µg/ minute

Bradycardia is defined as any rhythm disorder with a heart rate less than 60 beats per minute. There are 3 medications that are used in the Bradycardia ACLS Algorithm. They are atropine, dopamine (infusion), and epinephrine (infusion).

Answer: C i.e., Intravenous administration of atropine sulfate

2. **A patient of cirrhosis develops oliguria and worsening azotemia. Urinary sediment is normal. Urinary sodium concentration is 5 mEq/L. The most likely cause could be:**

A. Interstitial nephritis

B. Acute tubular necrosis

C. Acute glomerulonephritis

D. Hepato-renal syndrome

Hepatorenal syndrome (often abbreviated HRS) is a life-threatening medical condition that consists of rapid deterioration in kidney functions in individuals with cirrhosis or fulminant liver failure. Type 2 HRS is slower in onset and progression. It is defined by an increase in serum creatinine level to >133 µmol/L (1.5 mg/dL) or a creatinine clearance of less than 40 mL/ min, and a urine sodium < 10 µmol/L

Answer: D i.e., Hepato-renal syndrome

3. **A 55 years old man, non-smoker presents with sudden onset of shortness of breath. On examination, pulse rate is 110/minute and B.P. 180/110 mm Hg. Patient is restless and anxious. Examination of chest shows bilateral rhonchi and crepitation. S3 gallop is heard on auscultation of precordium. There is no history of chronic bronchitis. The most likely diagnosis is:**

A. Bronchial asthma

B. Acute LVF

C. Pneumothorax

D. Acute exacerbation of COPD

Features of left ventricular failure include increased rate of breathing (tachypnea) and increased work of breathing (non-specific signs of respiratory distress); rales or crackles or crepitation's, heard initially in the lung bases, and when severe, throughout the lung fields suggest the development of pulmonary edema (fluid in the alveoli); cyanosis which suggests severe low blood oxygen, is a late sign of extremely severe pulmonary edema; laterally displaced apex beat (which occurs if the heart is enlarged) and a gallop rhythm (additional heart sounds) may be heard as a marker of increased blood flow or increased intra-cardiac pressure.

Answer: B i.e., Acute LVF

4. **A 60 years old patient presents with gradually increasing dysphagia to solids for 3 months with significant loss of weight. The most probable diagnosis is:**

A. Stricture oesophagus

B. Carcinoma oesophagus

C. Reflux oesophagitis

D. Neurogenic oesophagus

The first and the most common symptom of carcinoma esophagus is usually difficulty in swallowing, which is often experienced first with solid foods and later with softer foods and liquids. Pain while swallowing is less usual at first. Weight loss is often an initial symptom in cases of squamous-cell carcinoma, though not usually in cases of adenocarcinoma. Eventual weight loss due to reduced appetite and undernutrition is common.

Answer: B i.e., Carcinoma oesophagus

5. **In a patient with lacerated injury foot who is not actively immunised against tetanus, which one of the following is indicated for tetanus prophylaxis?**

   A. Penicillin

   B. Tetanus toxoid

   C. Tetanus immunoglobulin

   D. Triple vaccine

   Anti-tetanus immunoglobulin, also known as tetanus immune globulin (TIG) and tetanus antitoxin, is made up of antibodies against the tetanus toxin. It is used to prevent tetanus in those who have a wound that is at high risk and have not been fully vaccinated with tetanus toxoid. It is also used to treat tetanus along with antibiotics and muscle relaxants.

   Answer: C i.e., Tetanus immunoglobulin

6. **A 16 years old boy presents with exertional dyspnea, haemoptysis and occasionally paroxysmal nocturnal dyspnea. There was history of joint pains five years back. The most probable diagnosis is:**

   A. Aortic regurgitation B. Mitral stenosis

   C. Tricuspid stenosis D. Aortic stenosis

   Signs and symptoms of mitral stenosis include heart failure symptoms, such as dyspnea on exertion, orthopnea and paroxysmal nocturnal dyspnea (PND); palpitations; chest pain; hemoptysis and thromboembolism in later stages when the left atrial volume is increased (i.e., dilation). The latter leads to increase risk of atrial fibrillation, which increases the risk of blood stasis (motionless). This increases the risk of coagulation. History of joint pains five years back suggests the episode of acute rheumatic fever (migrating polyarthritis).

   Answer: B i.e., Mitral stenosis

7. **A patient presents with breathlessness and occasional dry cough. On physical examination, he is found to have bilateral basal crepitations. His pulmonary function tests reveal a decrease in total lung capacity and vital capacity (VC), with normal FEV1/FVC ratio. He is most likely suffering from:**

   A. Chronic bronchitis

   B. Idiopathic pulmonary fibrosis

   C. Cystic fibrosis

   D. Allergic bronchopulmonary aspergillosis

   Most common clinical features of idiopathic pulmonary fibrosis include age over 50 years; dry, non-productive cough on exertion; progressive exertional dyspnea (shortness of breath with exercise); dry, inspiratory bibasilar "velcro-like" crackles on auscultation (a crackling sound in the lungs during inhalation similar to Velcro being torn apart slowly, heard with a stethoscope) and clubbing of the digits, a disfigurement of the finger tips or toes. Abnormal pulmonary function test results, with evidence of restriction and impaired gas exchange. Spirometry classically reveals a reduction in the vital capacity (VC) with either a proportionate reduction in airflows, or increased airflows for the observed vital capacity. The latter finding reflects the increased lung stiffness (reduced lung compliance) associated with pulmonary fibrosis, which leads to increased lung elastic recoil.

   Answer: B i.e., Idiopathic pulmonary fibrosis

8. **A 45 years old hypertensive male patient presented to the casualty with 3 hours history of sudden onset severe headache associated with nausea and vomiting. On clinical examination, patient had right sided ptosis and neck stiffness. Rest of the neurological examination was normal. The most likely diagnosis in this case is:**

   A. Hypertensive brain damage

   B. Migraine

   C. Aneurysmal subarachnoid bleed

   D. Acute pyogenic meningitis

   Subarachnoid hemorrhage (SAH) is bleeding into the subarachnoid space—the area between the arachnoid membrane and the pia mater surrounding the brain. Symptoms may include a severe headache of rapid onset, vomiting, decreased level of consciousness, fever, and sometimes seizures. Neck stiffness or neck pain are also relatively common. In about a quarter of people a small bleed with resolving symptoms occurs within a month of a larger bleed. SAH may occur as a result of a head injury or spontaneously, usually from a ruptured cerebral aneurysm.

   Answer: C i.e., Aneurysmal subarachnoid bleed

9. **A 60 years old male with Marfan's syndrome comes to emergency department with severe generalized tearing pain localized to chest anteriorly and inter scapular region, sweating and weakness. On examination, his BP is 200/140 mm Hg. X ray chest shows widening of superior mediastinum. ECG shows sinus tachycardia. What is the most likely diagnosis?**

A. Acute pulmonary embolism

B. Dissection of aorta

C. Acute myocardial infraction

D. Acute pericarditis

Aortic dissection is more common in those with a history of high blood pressure, a number of connective tissues disorder that affect blood vessel wall strength such as Marfan's syndrome, a bicuspid aortic valve, and previous heart surgery.

Answer: B i.e., Dissection of aorta

10. **A patient underwent hip replacement surgery. On fourth post-operative day, he had dyspnoea, pleuritic pain and haemoptysis. Most likely diagnosis is:**

A. Pulmonary embolism

B. Pneumonia

C. Pulmonary oedema

D. Pericarditis

Symptoms of pulmonary embolism are typically sudden in onset and may include one or many of the following: dyspnea (shortness of breath), tachypnea (rapid breathing), chest pain of a "pleuritic" nature (worsened by breathing), cough and hemoptysis (coughing up blood). More severe cases can include signs such as cyanosis (blue discoloration, usually of the lips and fingers), collapse, and circulatory instability because of decreased blood flow through the lungs and into the left side of the heart. About 15% of all cases of sudden death are attributable to PE.

Answer: A i.e., Pulmonary embolism

11. **A 55 years old male with a history of chronic obstructive pulmonary disease was rushed to emergency department with increasing shortness of breath, fever and a productive cough with yellow green sputum. He has difficulty in communicating because of his inability to complete a sentence. Measurement of arterial blood gas shows pH 7.3, $PaCO_2$ 68 mmHg, HCO_3 28 mmol/L, and PaO_2 60 mmHg. How would you interpret this?**

A. Respiratory acidosis, uncompensated

B. Respiratory alkalosis, uncompensated

C. Respiratory acidosis, partially compensated

D. Respiratory alkalosis, partially compensated

Normal pH: 7.35 – 7.45; Normal $PaCO_2$: 4.7 – 6 & Normal HCO_3: 22 – 24. Respiratory acidosis means pH is less and $PaCO_2$ is more. Partial compensation means there is slight increase in HCO_3.

Answer: C i.e., Respiratory acidosis, partially compensated

12. **A 40 years old woman presents with hematuria, ecchymoses and menorrhagia of six months duration. What is the most likely diagnosis?**

A. Haemophilia A

B. Haemophilia B

C. Idiopathic thrombocytopaenic purpura

D. Henoch Schonlein purpura

Signs of idiopathic thrombocytopenic purpura/ ITP include the spontaneous formation of bruises (purpura) and petechiae (tiny bruises), especially on the extremities, bleeding from the nostrils and/or gums, and menorrhagia (excessive menstrual bleeding), any of which may occur if the platelet count is below 20,000 per μl. A very low count (<10,000 per μl) may result in the spontaneous formation of hematomas (blood masses) in the mouth or on other mucous membranes.

Answer: C i.e., Idiopathic thrombocytopaenic purpura

13. **A 45 years old female comes to you with dysphagia. She is found to have anaemia and koilonychia. Most likely diagnosis is:**

A. Plummer Vinson syndrome

B. Boerhaave syndrome

C. Carcinoma oesophagus

D. Reflux oesophagitis

Plummer–Vinson syndrome (PVS), also called Paterson–Brown–Kelly syndrome or sideropenic dysphagia, is a rare disease characterized by difficulty in swallowing, iron-deficiency anemia, glossitis, cheilosis and esophageal webs. Treatment with iron supplementation and mechanical widening of the esophagus generally provides an excellent outcome.

Answer: A i.e., Plummer Vinson Syndrome

14. **A patient develops skin necrosis 3 days after being started on warfarin for deep vein thrombosis. What is the most likely cause?**

A. Antiphospholipid antibody syndrome

B. Protein C deficiency

C. Disseminated intravascular coagulation

D. Thrombotic thrombocytopenic purpura

Protein C is vitamin K-dependent. Patients with Protein C deficiency are at an increased risk of developing skin necrosis while on warfarin. Protein C has a short half life (8 hour) compared with other vitamin K-dependent factors and therefore is rapidly depleted with warfarin initiation, resulting in a transient hypercoagulable state.

Answer: B i.e., Protein C deficiency

15. **A 15 years old boy is brought to emergency with two days history of headache, vomiting and altered sensorium. His BP is 70 mmHg systolic and he has ecchymoses on his skin. Most likely organism causing his condition is:**

A. Haemophilus influenzae

B. Listeria monocytogenes

C. Neisseria meningitidis

D. Streptococcus pneumoniae

Waterhouse-Friderichsen Syndrome can be caused by a number of different organisms. When caused by Neisseria meningitidis, WFS is considered the most severe form of meningococcal sepsis. The onset of the illness is nonspecific with fever, rigors, vomiting, and headache. Soon a rash appears; first macular, not much different from the rose spots of typhoid, and rapidly becoming petechial and purpuric with a dusky gray color. Low blood pressure (hypotension) develops and rapidly leads to septic shock. The cyanosis of extremities can be extreme and the patient is very prostrated or comatose. In this form of meningococcal disease, meningitis generally does not occur.

Answer: C i.e., Neisseria meningitidis

16. **A child presents with episode of hematuria soon after respiratory tract infection. What is the most likely diagnosis?**

A. IgA nephropathy

B. Wegener granulomatosis

C. Post streptococcal glomerulonephritis

D. Churg Strauss syndrome

The classic presentation (in 40–50% of the cases) of IgA nephropathy is episodic hematuria, which usually starts within a day or two of a non-specific upper respiratory tract infection (hence synpharyngitic), as opposed to post-streptococcal glomerulonephritis, which occurs some time (weeks) after initial infection. Less commonly gastrointestinal or urinary infection can be the inciting agent.

Answer: A i.e., IgA nephropathy

17. **Widespread concave ST segment elevation and PR depression in most leads except aVR lead favours the diagnosis of:**

A. Acute myocardial infarction

B. Pericarditis

C. Digoxin toxicity

D. Hypertrophic obstructive cardiomyopathy

The preferred initial diagnostic testing in a suspected case of pericarditis is the ECG, which may demonstrate a 12-lead electrocardiogram with diffuse, non-specific, concave ("saddle-shaped"), ST-segment elevations in all leads except aVR and V1 and PR-segment depression possible in any lead except aVR; sinus tachycardia, and low-voltage QRS complexes can also be seen if there is subsymptomatic levels of pericardial effusion. The PR depression is often seen early in the process as the thin atria are affected more easily than the ventricles by the inflammatory process of the pericardium.

Answer: B i.e., Pericarditis

18. **A known case of lepromatous leprosy was initiated on treatment. She developed painful erythematous papules with fever and lymphadenopathy. What is the likely reactional state?**

A. Type 1 lepra reaction B. Type 2 lepra reaction

C. Lucio's phenomenon D. Lupus pernio

Erythema nodosum (EN), also known as subacute migratory panniculitis of Vilanova and Piñol, is an inflammatory condition characterized by inflammation of the fat cells under the skin, resulting in tender red nodules or lumps that are usually seen on both shins. EN may also be due to excessive antibody production in lepromatous leprosy leading to deposition of immune complexes.

Answer: B i.e., Type 2 lepra reaction

19. **A 20 years old male walked into outpatient department with high-grade fever, cough and chest pain for one day. Chest X-ray showed consolidation of left upper zone. His respiratory rate is 22/minute, pulse rate 96/minute, BP systolic 120 mmHg and blood urea 18 mg/dl. What is his CURB score?**

A. 0 B. 1

C. 2 D. 3

CURB-65	
Symptom	***Points***
Confusion	1
BUN >7 mmol/l	1
Respiratory rate ≥30	1
SBP <90mmHg, DBP ≤60mmHg	1
Age ≥65	1

Answer: A i.e., 0

20. **A 55 years old patient on treatment for pulmonary tuberculosis with Rifampicin, Isoniazid, Pyrazinamide and Ethambutol complain of pain in large and small joints. Which one of the following investigations will you order?**

A. Serum creatinine B. Serum amylase

C. SGOT/SGPT D. Serum uric acid

Gout is a form of inflammatory arthritis characterized by recurrent attacks of a red, tender, hot, and swollen joint. Pain typically comes on rapidly in less than twelve hours. The joint at the base of big toe is affected in about half of cases. It may also result in tophi, kidney stones, or urate nephropathy.

Answer: D i.e., Serum uric acid

21. **A middle aged male known smoker presented with recurrent sinusitis, haemoptysis, haematuria, arthralgia and palpable purpura. What is the most likely diagnosis?**

A. Wegener granulomatosis

B. Goodpasture syndrome

C. Polyarteritis nodosa

D. Systemic lupus erythematosus

Initial signs of Wegener granulomatosis/ Granulomatosis with polyangiitis (GPA) are extremely variable, and diagnosis can be severely delayed due to the nonspecific nature of the symptoms. In general, rhinitis is the first sign in most people. ***.*** *Lungs signs include pulmonary nodules (referred to as "coin lesions"), infiltrates (often interpreted as pneumonia), cavitary lesions, pulmonary hemorrhage causing hemoptysis, and rarely bronchial stenosis. Kidney signs include rapidly progressive glomerulonephritis (75%), leading to chronic renal failure. Arthritis is also seen, with pain or swelling (60%), often initially diagnosed as rheumatoid arthritis. Skin signs include subcutaneous nodules (granulomas) on the elbow, purpura etc.*

Answer: A i.e., Wegener granulomatosis

22. **A patient presents with diarrhoea, steatorrhea and weight loss. Which of the following disease is LEAST possible?**

A. Whipple disease B. Tropical sprue

C. Celiac disease D. Menetrier disease

Individuals with the Menetrier disease present with upper abdominal pain (epigastric), at times accompanied by nausea, vomiting, loss of appetite, edema, and weight loss. A small amount of gastrointestinal bleeding may occur, which is typically due to superficial mucosal erosions; large volume bleeding is rare. 20% to 100% of patients, depending on time of presentation, develop a protein-losing gastropathy accompanied by low blood albumin and edema.

Answer: D i.e., Menetrier disease

23. A patient with long term implantable cardioverter defibrillator device developed neck and facial swelling, hoarseness of voice, nasal congestion, dysphagia and haemoptysis. The facial swelling increased on supine position. This patient most likely developed:

A. Cardiac tamponade

B. Intracardiac thrombosis

C. Superior vena cava obstruction

D. Pulmonary thromboembolism

Superior vena cava/ SVC syndrome occurs due to partial or complete obstruction of the SVC. One of the causes is deep venous thrombosis due to pacemaker/ defibrillator leads. Features of Superior vena cava syndrome include shortness of breath is the most common symptom, followed by face or arm swelling, difficulty breathing, headache, facial swelling, venous distention in the neck and distended veins in the upper chest and arms, upper limb edema. light headedness, cough and edema (swelling) of the neck, called the collar of Stokes

Answer: C i.e., Superior vena cava obstruction

24. A patient of AIDS developed ophthalmoplegia, ataxia and global confusion. He is likely to have the deficiency of:

A. Biotin

B. Niacin

C. Pyridoxine

D. Thiamine

Wernicke encephalopathy (WE) also Wernicke's encephalopathy is the presence of neurological symptoms caused by biochemical lesions of the central nervous system after exhaustion of B-vitamin reserves, in particular thiamine (vitamin B1). Classically, Wernicke encephalopathy is characterised by the triad – ophthalmoplegia, ataxia, and confusion. However, only 10% of patients exhibit all three features, and other symptoms may also be present.

Answer: D i.e., Thiamine

25. An elderly male presents with persistent productive cough with large volume purulent sputum production. He has had several episodes in the past. He also had digital clubbing. He is a case of:

A. Empyema

B. Bronchiectasis

C. Bronchopneumonia

D. Necrotising pneumonia

Some people with bronchiectasis may have a cough productive of frequent green/yellow mucus (sputum), up to 240 ml (8 oz) daily. Bronchiectasis may also present with coughing up blood (hemoptysis) in the absence of sputum, called "dry bronchiectasis". Sputum production may also occur without coloration. People with bronchiectasis may have bad breath indicative of active infection. Frequent bronchial infections and breathlessness are two possible indicators of bronchiectasis. Crepitations and expiratory rhonchi may be heard on auscultation. Nail clubbing is rare.

Answer: B i.e., Bronchiectasis

26. A chemical factory worker has acute onset dyspnoea with fever, chills, and malaise, following a few hours of exposure to a new chemical. These symptoms resolve in four to five days after removal from exposure. He is likely to have:

A. Hypersensitivity pneumonitis

B. Atypical pneumonia

C. Cryptogenic organising pneumonia

D. Non-specific interstitial pneumonia

Hypersensitivity pneumonitis (HP; also called allergic alveolitis, bagpipe lung, or extrinsic allergic alveolitis, EAA) is an inflammation of the alveoli within the lung caused by hypersensitivity to inhaled organic dusts. Sufferers are commonly exposed to the dust by their occupation or hobbies. In the acute form of HP, symptoms may develop 4–6 hours following heavy exposure to the provoking antigen. Symptoms include fever, chills, malaise, cough, chest tightness, dyspnea, rash, swelling and headache. Symptoms resolve within 12 hours to several days upon cessation of exposure.

Answer: A i.e., Hypersensitivity pneumonitis

27. A 25 years old man presents with nausea, vomiting and diarrhoea with crampy abdominal pain. He gives history of consumption of rice preparation in his last meal. What is the likely organism causing the above complaints?

A. Clostridium perfringens

B. Bacillus cereus

C. Staphylococcus aureus

D. Campylobacter jejuni

The 'emetic' form of Bacillus foodborne illness is commonly caused by rice cooked for a time and temperature insufficient to kill any spores present, then improperly refrigerated. It can produce a toxin, cereulide, which is not inactivated by later reheating. This form leads to nausea and vomiting one to five hours after consumption. It can be difficult to distinguish from other short-term bacterial foodborne intoxications such as by staphylococcus aureus.

Answer: B i.e., Bacillus cereus

28. A 70 years old man reports to the emergency with acute chest pain. ECG shows inferior wall Myocardial Infarction (MI). He has recently been discharged 7 days back following thrombolysis with streptokinase for Acute Anterior wall MI. What will be the appropriate management?

A. Aspirin, Sublingual nitroglycerin, Clopidogrel, Primary PCI

B. Aspirin, Sublingual nitroglycerin, Clopidogrel, Streptokinase

C, Aspirin, Sublingual nitroglycerin, Clopidogrel, Heparin

D, Aspirin, Sublingual nitroglycerin, Clopidogrel, Beta blockers

Best management of such a case would be aspirin, sublingual nitroglycerin, Clopidogrel and primary PCI. For people who have already had a heart attack or stroke, taking aspirin daily for two years prevented 1 in 50 from having a cardiovascular problem (heart attack, stroke, or death), but also caused non-fatal bleeding problems to occur in 1 of 400 people. Improved myocardial oxygen demand vs oxygen delivery ratio (on administering sublingual nitroglycerine) leads to the following therapeutic effects during episodes of angina pectoris: subsiding of chest pain, decrease of blood pressure, increase of heart rate, and orthostatic hypotension. Clopidogrel is used to prevent heart attack and stroke in people who are at high risk of these events, including those with a history of myocardial infarction and other forms of acute coronary syndrome, stroke, and those with peripheral artery disease. Percutaneous coronary intervention/ PCI may be appropriate for patients with stable coronary artery disease if they meet certain criteria, such as having any coronary stenosis greater than 50 percent or having angina symptoms that are unresponsive to medical therapy.

Answer: A i.e., Aspirin, Sublingual nitroglycerin, Clopidogrel, Primary PCI

29. A 64 years old man presents with chest pain of 24 hours duration. His ECG reveals ST elevation, Anterior Wall Myocardial Infarction. The preferred treatment modality for him is:

A. Primary percutaneous coronary intervention

B. Thrombolysis with Alteplase

C. Thrombolysis with Streptokinase

D. Nitroglycerin infusion, Aspirin and Beta blockers

Management of anterior wall MI include aspirin is given straightaway in a dose of 325 mg to be chewed. It is the first line drug in the initial management of AMI and all other forms of ischemic heart disease. In acute MI with angina, congestive heart failure, persistent angina or hypertension, nitrates are given for the first 24-48 hours. Beta-blockers, when used in the early hours of infarction, they limit infarct size, reduce the incidence of ventricular arrhythmias, atrial fibrillation and cardiac arrest.

Answer: D i.e., Nitroglycerin infusion, Aspirin and Beta blockers

30. The treatment of choice for a 32 years old male patient of severe mitral stenosis (Rheumatic) with thickened and calcified valves on echocardiography is:

A. Balloon mitral valvuloplasty/ BMV

B. Mitral valve replacement/ MVR

C. Medical management only

D. Mitral valvotomy/ MV

MVR is an accepted procedure for patients who are not candidates for surgical commissurotomy or BMV. When there is associated MR or when the valve is rigid & calcified, MVR is indicated.

Answer: B i.e., Mitral valve replacement/ MVR

31. An adult with fever and right sided chest pain is found to have a moderate right sided pleural effusion. Chest X-Ray (PA view) also shows a moderate pleural effusion. A diagnostic thoracentesis reveals straw coloured exudates with 50 mg% of sugar and lymphocytic pleocytosis. ADA levels are borderline. What investigation would be most likely to confirm a diagnosis of tuberculosis?

A. Needle Biopsy of the Pleura

B. Pleural Fluid Xpert MTB/RIF assay

C. Pleural Fluid AFB smear

D. Pleural Fluid AFB-culture

Tubercle bacilli are difficult to demonstrate in serous effusion by conventional methods. Needle biopsy is helpful, but this is not required in the ordinary case.

Answer: A i.e., Needle Biopsy of the Pleura

32. A 26 years old woman presents with fever, arthralgia and erythema nodosum. Her chest X-ray reveals bilateral hilar lymphadenopathy. Her mantoux test is negative. The most likely diagnosis is:

A. Tuberculosis

B. Allergic bronchopulmonary aspergillosis

C. Sarcoidosis

D. Pulmonary thromboembolism

The commonest presentation of sarcoidosis is as bilateral hilar lymphadenopathy with associated fever & erythema nodosum.

Answer: C i.e., Sarcoidosis

33. A middle aged patient with chronic liver disease presents with pain abdomen and distension. He also has diarrhoea and fever since one day. On examination, he is hemodynamically stable with fever of 100 °F. There is jaundice, pallor, pedal edema and ascites. A diagnostic paracentesis is done. Ascitic fluid protein is 0.8 gm%, sugar 100 mg%, total count 500/mm^3 of which 85% are polymorphonuclear leaukocytes and 15% lymphocytes. Most likely diagnosis is:

A. Spontaneous bacterial peritonitis

B. Secondary bacterial peritonitis

C. Perforation peritonitis

D. T B peritonitis

Spontaneous bacterial peritonitis is diagnosed if the fluid contains neutrophils at greater than 250 cells per mm^3(equals a cell count of 250 x10^6/L) fluid in the absence of another reason for this (such as inflammation of one of the internal organs or a perforation). The crux of this algorithm is Runyon's Criteria for secondary bacterial peritonitis, which requires two of these three features: total protein >1 g/dL, glucose <50 mg/dL (2.8 mM), and lactate dehydrogenase above the upper limit of normal for serum.

Answer: A i.e., Spontaneous bacterial peritonitis

34. A young male comes to the OPD with history of jaundice since many years. He has noted that the jaundice may fluctuate but is often aggravated when he is fasting. There is no history of hospitalisation, no drug use, alcoholism or blood transfusion. Family history is not significant. Clinical examination is unremarkable except for mild scleral icterus. What is the likely diagnosis?

A. Dubin Johnson syndrome

B. Crigler Najjar syndrome type-I

C. Gilbert's syndrome

D. Rotor syndrome

Gilbert's syndrome (GS) is a mild liver disorder in which the liver does not properly process bilirubin. Many people never have symptoms. Occasionally a slight yellowish color of the skin or sclera may occur. Episodes of jaundice may be triggered by stress such as exercise, menstruation, or not eating.

Answer: C i.e., Gilbert's syndrome

35. **A right handed 70 years old man has a brain scan which reveals a lesion that has damaged his left angular and supramarginal gyrus. On examination, one would expect the following EXCEPT:**

A. Difficulty with left to right discrimination

B. Inappropriate affect

C. Finger agnosia

D. Inability to write

The angular gyrus is the part of the brain associated with complex language functions (i.e. reading, writing and interpretation of what is written). Lesion to this part of the brain shows symptoms of the Gerstmann syndrome: effects include finger agnosia, alexia (inability to read), acalculia (inability to use arithmetic operations), agraphia (inability to copy), and left-right confusion.

Answer: B i.e., Inappropriate affect

36. **A 34-week pregnant nurse comes in contact with a patient with chickenpox at her workplace. She has never had chickenpox in the past and is unvaccinated. The best option for her is:**

A, Varicella zoster immunoglobulin to be given within 7 days

B. Vaccinate for chicken pox

C. Start oral acyclovir

D. Wait and watch

Varicella (live attenuated vaccine) is not recommended in pregnancy. Varicella zoster immunoglobulin (VZIG) should be given to exposed non-immune patients as it reduces the morbidity.

Answer: A i.e., Varicella zoster immunoglobulin to be given within 7 days

37. **A 24 years old male presents with consumption of an unknown substance. His respiratory rate is 22/minute, pulse rate is 110/minute, BP is 150/94 mmHg and he has 2 episodes of seizures. There are tremors and hallucinations. The substance ingested most likely is:**

A. Amphetamines B Diazepam

C. Oxycodone D. Ethanol

Amphetamines increase the activity of the neurotransmitters dopamine and norepinephrine. Tachycardia and other arrhythmias are due to the sympathomimetic effects of amphetamines. Amphetamines cause tachycardia and hypertension and can cause significant cerebral blood flow which increases by 30%. Increased dopamine levels in the central nervous system (CNS) cause psychosis, euphoric effects, and other movement disorders. Amphetamine toxicity can also cause seizures due to neuronal death from the interaction between amphetamines and NMDA receptors.

Answer: A i.e., Amphetamines

38. **An 18 years old boy was brought to the emergency department after being bitten by a saw-scaled viper. The monitoring which is most crucial in this patient is:**

A. Single breath count

B. Neck flop

C. Whole blood clotting time

D. Creatine phosphokinase

Most of saw-scaled viper species have venom that contains factors that can cause a consumption coagulopathy and defibrination, which may persist for days to weeks. This may result in bleeding anywhere in the body, including the possibility of an intracranial hemorrhage. The latter classically occurs a few days following the bite.

Answer: C i.e., Whole blood clotting time

39. **A 35 years old man with history of alcoholism presents with ophthalmoplegia, ataxia and global confusion. The treatment of choice for this patient is:**

A. I.V. Glucose B. I.V. Thiamine

C. I.V. Mannitol D. I.V. Immunoglobulin

Classically, Wernicke encephalopathy is characterised by the triad – ophthalmoplegia, ataxia, and confusion. In patients suspected of WE, thiamine treatment should be started immediately. Blood should be immediately taken to test for thiamine, other vitamins and minerals levels. Following this an immediate intravenous or intramuscular dose of thiamine should be administered two or three times daily.

Answer: B i.e., I.V. Thiamine

40. Characteristic features of Horner's Syndrome are:

A. partial ptosis, enophthalmos, constricted pupil, decreased sweating

B. partial ptosis, exophthalmos, constricted pupil, decreased sweating

C. partial ptosis, enophthalmos, dilated pupil, decreased sweating

D. partial ptosis, enophthalmos, constricted pupil, increased sweating

Horner's syndrome, also known as oculosympathetic paresis, is a combination of symptoms that arises when sympathetic trunk is damaged. The signs and symptoms occur on the same side (ipsilateral) as it is a lesion of the sympathetic trunk. It is characterized by miosis (a constricted pupil), partial ptosis (a weak, droopy eyelid), apparent anhidrosis (decreased sweating), with apparent enophthalmos (inset eyeball)

Answer: A i.e., Partial ptosis, enophthalmos, constricted pupil, decreased sweating

41. A 40 years old woman presents with sudden onset palpitations. An ECG done reveals narrow-QRS complex tachycardia. The most likely diagnosis is:

A. Ventricular tachycardia

B. Pre-excited tachycardia

C. Paroxysmal supraventricular tachycardia with aberrancy

D. AV re-entry tachycardia

Findings on AV nodal re-entry tachycardia (AVNRT) on ECG include narrow complex tachycardia, a P wave that occurs after the QRS complex (a short RP interval) and tachycardia that quickly terminates with AV blocking manoeuvres (carotid massage or adenosine)

Answer: D i.e., AV re-entry tachycardia

42. A 21 years young man presents in emergency with high-grade fever with inflammation of knee and ankle joints which is fleeting in nature. There is history of occasional palpitations. There is no history of antecedent sore throat. On examination, splenomegaly is present. The ECG shows prolongation of PR interval. What is the most likely diagnosis in India?

A. Still disease B. Enteric fever

C. Rheumatic fever D. Reiter's syndrome

Rheumatic arthritis is an asymmetric, migratory / fleeting polyarthritis with predominant involvement of large joints of lower limbs and migrates to the upper limb. Classically the joints are red, tender, swollen and the child cannot tolerate any movement about the joint.

Answer: C i.e., Rheumatic fever

43. A 50 years gentleman with Type-2 Diabetes mellitus for 5 years presents in medical emergency with sudden onset of dyspnoea at rest, orthopnoea, and prostration. On examination, pulse is rapid and very weak in volume. His blood pressure is 100/70 mmHg. There are diffuse crepitations at lung bases. What is the most likely diagnosis of his conditions?

A. Mitral stenosis with bacterial endocarditis

B. Right heart failure

C. Left heart failure

D. Constrictive pericarditis

Common respiratory signs of left heart failure are increased rate of breathing (tachypnea) and increased work of breathing (nonspecific signs of respiratory distress). Rales or crackles, heard initially in the lung bases, and when severe, throughout the lung fields suggest the development of pulmonary edema (fluid in the). The person will have dyspnea (shortness of breath) on exertion and in severe cases, dyspnea at rest. Increasing breathlessness on lying flat, called orthopnea, occurs.

Answer: C i.e., Left heart failure

44. A 26 years old HIV infected male presents with odynophagia. Upper GI endoscopy demonstrates serpiginous ulcers in a normal surrounding mucosa in distal esophagus. The most likely diagnosis is:

A. Gastro esophageal reflux disease

B. Cytomegalovirus esophagitis

C. Candida esophagitis

D. Herpetic esophagitis

CMV classically causes serpiginous ulcers in the distal esophagus that may coalesce to form giant ulcers. Brushings alone are insufficient for diagnosis, and biopsies must be performed. Biopsies reveal intranuclear and intracytoplasmic inclusions with enlarged nuclei in large fibroblasts and endothelial cells.

Answer: B i.e., Cytomegalovirus esophagitis

45. Which of the following is the most important complication in a patient with coeliac disease, who was previously doing well on a gluten-free diet and is now not responding to gluten restriction?

A. Intestinal infection

B. Intestinal lymphoma

C. Resistant coeliac disease

D. Type II Diabetes mellitus

For a small number of people living with celiac disease, a gluten-free diet is not enough to stop the otherwise severe symptoms. These patients are classified as having refractory celiac disease (RCD), which usually affects between 2 and 5 percent of celiac disease patients. In one type of RCD called RCDII, the white blood cells found in the wall of the small intestine divide and multiply in excessive numbers. In approximately half of the RCDII patients, these cells, called lymphocytes, go on to develop into a particularly rare form of lymphoma. This rare and very aggressive form of white blood cell cancer is called enteropathy-associated T-cell lymphoma.

Answer: B i.e., Intestinal lymphoma

46. A middle aged diabetic male who has recurrent chest pain undergoes coronary artery angiogram. The following day, he develops haematuria, proteinuria and renal impairment. What is the most likely diagnosis?

A. Renal artery stenosis

B. Acute renal infraction

C. Atheroembolism

D. Haemolytic Uraemic syndrome

Cholesterol embolism occurs when cholesterol is released, usually from an atherosclerotic plaque, and travels as an embolus in the bloodstream to lodge (as an embolism) causing an obstruction in blood vessels further away. Most commonly this causes skin symptoms (usually livedo reticularis), gangrene of the extremities and sometimes kidney failure; problems with other organs may arise, depending on the site at which the cholesterol crystals enter the bloodstream. When the kidneys are involved, the disease is referred to as atheroembolic renal disease. it is a complication of medical procedures involving the blood vessels, such as vascular surgery or angiography.

Answer: C i.e., Atheroembolism

47. Which one of the following is a cause of early (0–4 weeks) infection in recipients of haematopoietic stem cell transplantation?

A. Cytomegalovirus

B. Pneumocystis jirovecii

C. Varicella zoster

D. Herpes simplex

HSV (herpes simplex virus) infection (especially of skin and mucous membranes) prior to the introduction of acyclovir was a major problem in the HSCT (hematopoietic stem cell transplantation) recipient. Occurring in the pre-engraftment period, HSV infection greatly exacerbated the severity of mucositis. Not only were ulcers observed in the oral cavity and anogenital areas, ulcerations of the esophagus, stomach and intestine were also observed. HSV pneumonia was also noted, with rare cases of cutaneous dissemination and encephalitis. The current standard of care is to test all candidates for HSCT for an antibody to HSV, with seropositive individuals then placed on antiviral prophylaxis, beginning prior to HSCT. Effective agents for HSV prophylaxis include acyclovir (intravenous or oral), valacyclovir or famciclovir.

Answer: D i.e., Herpes simplex

48. **A 24 years female presented with generalized weakness. Her thyroid function test is as follows. Serum T3 = Normal, T4 = Normal, TSH = 10mU/L. What is the most likely diagnosis?**

A. Primary hypothyroidism

B. Secondary hypothyroidism

C. Subclinical hypothyroidism

D. Non thyroidal illness

Subclinical hypothyroidism (SCH), also called mild thyroid failure, is diagnosed when peripheral thyroid hormone levels are within normal reference laboratory range but serum thyroid-stimulating hormone (TSH) levels are mildly elevated. This condition occurs in 3% to 8% of the general population. It is more common in women than men, and its prevalence increases with age. Of patients with SCH, 80% have a serum TSH of less than 10 mIU/L.

Answer: C i.e., Subclinical hypothyroidism

49. **A 32 years old HIV infected male presents with shortness of breath and moderate fever of two-week duration. On examination, cyanosis is present, with respiratory rate of 22/minute and some basal crackles in chest. The CT chest shows bilateral ground-glass pattern. The most likely etiologic diagnosis is:**

A. Streptococcus pneumoniae

B. Pneumocystis jirovecii

C. Mycobacterium tuberculosis

D. Staphylococcus sp.

The most common high-resolution CT finding of Pneumocystis jiroveci pneumonia is diffuse ground-glass opacity. The term ground-glass refers to parenchymal opacification, which does not obscure the underlying pulmonary architecture. This usually occurs in a bilateral, symmetrical, predominantly perihilar distribution and may be geographic or mosaic in appearance, with areas of normal lung adjacent to areas of affected lung.

Answer: B i.e., Pneumocystis jirovecii

50. **A 22 years old male is admitted with fever and altered consciousness for two days. Examination reveals nuchal rigidity and diffuse petechial rash on the trunk and lower extremities. The most likely etiologic agent is:**

A. Escherichia coli

B. Streptococcus pneumoniae

C. Neisseria meningitidis

D. Haemophilus infleunzae

The average incubation period of meningococcal meningitis is four days, but can range between two and 10 days. The most common symptoms are a stiff neck, high fever, sensitivity to light, confusion, headaches and vomiting. In addition, in infants bulging fontanelle and ragdoll appearance are commonly found. A less common but even more severe (often fatal) form of meningococcal disease is meningococcal septicaemia, which is characterized by a haemorrhagic rash and rapid circulatory collapse.

Answer: C i.e., Neisseria meningitidis

51. **A 36 years old chronic alcoholic, malnourished male is hospitalized with pneumonia. His condition worsens after aggressive treatment with intravenous dextrose and antibiotics. This phenomenon of 'Refeeding Syndrome' is accompanied by which one of the following biochemical alterations?**

A. Hypophosphatemia B. Hyponatremia

C. Hyperkalemia D. Hypermagnesemia

Hypophosphatemia is a potentially life-threatening complication of reinstating nutrition in a malnourished patient. Refeeding syndrome is a term that refers to various metabolic abnormalities that may complicate carbohydrate administration in subnourished patient populations.

Answer: A i.e., Hypophosphatemia

52. **A 31 years young man presents with fever, weight loss, pain with swelling of knee joint and low backache with stiffness. Three weeks earlier, he was treated for symptoms of urinary tract infection by local practitioner. The joint aspirate is leucocyte rich and contains multinucleated macrophages. His urine culture is sterile. What is the most probable diagnosis?**

A. Septic arthritis
B. Crystal arthritis
C. Reactive arthritis
D. Still disease

Reactive arthritis (ReA), formerly termed Reiter syndrome, is an autoimmune condition that develops in response to an infection. It has been associated with gastrointestinal (GI) infections with Shigella, Salmonella, Campylobacter, and other organisms, as well as with genitourinary (GU) infections (especially with Chlamydia trachomatis).

Answer: C i.e., Reactive arthritis

53. A 56 years old man presented with acute onset aphasia. Speech output was markedly reduced with preserved comprehension of spoken language. The area of brain involved is:

A. Posterior part of temporal lobe
B. Cerebellum
C. Midbrain
D. Inferior frontal gyrus

Expressive aphasia, also known as Broca's aphasia, is a type of aphasia characterized by partial loss of the ability to produce language (spoken, manual, or written), although comprehension generally remains intact. Broca's area is located in inferior frontal gyrus.

Answer: D i.e., Inferior frontal gyrus

54. A 30 years old male was being evaluated for paraparesis. On examination, there was severe muscle atrophy, with absent deep tendon reflexes and absent Babinski sign. The most likely possibility is:

A. Upper motor neuron disease
B. Lower motor neuron disease
C. Psychogenic cause
D. Cerebellar disease

In LMN (lower motor neuron) disease, the extensor plantar reflex is usually absent. Muscle paresis/paralysis, hypotonia/atonia, and hyporeflexia/areflexia are usually seen immediately following an insult. Muscle wasting, fasciculations and fibrillations are typically signs of end-stage muscle denervation and are seen over a longer time period. Another feature is the segmentation of symptoms – only muscles innervated by the damaged nerves will be symptomatic.

Answer: B i.e., Lower motor neuron disease

55. A 16 years old boy presented with fever and a diffuse maculopapular rash. Examination revealed generalised cervical lymphadenopathy and hepatosplenomegaly. After intake of Ampicillin (prescribed by a local practitioner), the rash worsened. The most likely diagnosis is:

A. Dengue fever
B. Measles
C. Drug-rash
D. Infectious mononucleosis

In adolescence and young adulthood, infectious mononucleosis presents with a characteristic triad: Fever – usually lasting 14 days; often mild; Sore throat – usually severe for 3–5 days, before resolving in the next 7–10 days and swollen glands – mobile; usually located around the back of the neck (posterior cervical lymph nodes) and sometimes throughout the body.

A small minority of people spontaneously present a rash, usually on the arms or trunk, which can be macular (morbilliform) or popular. Almost all people given amoxicillin or ampicillin eventually develop a generalized, itchy maculopapular rash, which however does not imply that the person will have adverse reactions to penicillin's again in the future.

Answer: D i.e., Infectious mononucleosis

56. Following the bite of a snake, a patient develops generalised myalgia's, rhabdomyolysis, and progressive flaccid paralysis. The most likely snake implicated is:

A. Cobra
B. Krait
C. Russel viper
D. Sea snake

The most important symptoms of sea snake bite are rhabdomyolysis (rapid breakdown of skeletal muscle tissue) and paralysis. Early symptoms include headache, a thick-feeling tongue, thirst, sweating, and vomiting. The venom is very slow acting and symptoms that happen from little as 30 minutes to several hours after the bite include generalized aching, stiffness, and tenderness of muscles all over the body. Passive stretching of the muscles is also painful, and trismus, which is similar to tetanus, is common. This is followed later on by symptoms typical of other elapid envenomations, a progressive flaccid paralysis, starting with ptosis and paralysis of voluntary muscles. Paralysis of muscles involved in swallowing and respiration can be fatal.

Answer: D i.e., Sea snake

57. **A 65 years old man, on Warfarin treatment, is started on antitubercular treatment. The pharmacologic effect of Warfarin is likely to:**

A. Increase

B. Decrease

C. Remain the same

D. Be unpredictable and variable

Rifampin has been reported to decrease the warfarin pharmacological effects in human subjects ingesting these agents simultaneously as rifampicin is an enzyme inducer (CYP2D6) enhancing the metabolism of warfarin. The concomitant administration of rifampin and warfarin resulted in the need for an unusually high maintenance dose of warfarin (20 mg per day) in order to produce a therapeutic effect.

Answer: B i.e., Decrease

58. **A chronic alcoholic develops a paroxysm of palpitations after alcohol binge. Which of the following Arrhythmia is most likely?**

A. Ventricular fibrillation

B. Ventricular premature complex

C. Atrial flutter

D. Atrial fibrillation

In 1978, Philip Ettinger described "Holiday heart syndrome" (HHS) for the first time, as the occurrence, in healthy people without heart disease known to cause arrhythmia, of an acute cardiac rhythm disturbance, most frequently atrial fibrillation, after binge drinking.

Answer: D i.e., Atrial fibrillation

59. **An elderly-man with history of Diabetes mellitus and Coronary Artery Disease comes for follow-up, with complaints of muscle pains. Which one of the following drugs could be the most likely cause?**

A. Aspirin
B. Glimepiride

C. Enalapril
D. Atorvastatin

Muscle aches are the commonest (10%) side effect of statins. Rise in CPK levels occur infrequently.

Answer: D i.e., Atorvastatin

60. **A 40 years old lady comes to outdoor clinic with complaints of sudden onset chest pain. The chest X-ray shows bilateral Pneumothorax. Examination reveals abnormalities of body habitus-including long arms, legs and finger (arachnodactyly), scoliosis, high arched palate, joint hypermobility, and a pansystolic murmur at cardiac apex. Which one of the following diseases is most likely?**

A. Takayasu's arteritis

B. Raynaud's syndrome

C. Marfan's syndrome

D. Rheumatic heart disease-Mitral regurgitation

Marfan syndrome (MFS) is a genetic disorder that affects the connective tissue. Those with the condition tend to be tall and thin, with long arms, legs, fingers & toes. They also typically have overly-flexible joints and scoliosis. The most serious complications involve the heart and aorta, with an increased risk of mitral valve prolapse and aortic aneurysm.

Answer: C i.e., Marfan's syndrome

61. **An 18 years old male has insulin dependent diabetes, with malabsorption syndrome and bilateral upper lobe bronchiectasis. A diagnostic work-up will include all EXCEPT:**

A. 24-hour fecal fat estimation

B. CT-chest

C. Lung biopsy

D. DNA sequencing study

Clinical presentation suggests the diagnosis of cystic fibrosis/ CF. Investigations done for CF include 24 hours fecal fat estimation (for malabsorption), CT scan chest (for bronchiectasis) and DNA sequencing study for CF.

Answer: C i.e., Lung biopsy

62. A 26 years old young lady attends medical emergency and is labelled as acute severe asthma by the emergency physician. Which one of the following is unlikely to be a part of the prescription?

A. Albuterol
B. Anti-leukotrienes
C. Aminophylline
D. Magnesium sulfate

Anti-leukotrienes (Montelukast) are used for maintenance therapy of asthma. They have no role in managing acute severe asthma.

Answer: B i.e., Anti-leukotrienes

63. Spontaneous oesophageal perforation after a bout of forceful vomiting or retching is characteristically seen in which one of the following conditions?

A. Menetrier's disease
B. Boerhaave's syndrome
C. Achalasia of the oesophagus
D. Barrett's oesophagus

Boerhaave syndrome is also known as spontaneous esophageal rupture or effort rupture of the esophagus. Although vomiting is thought to be the most common cause, other causes include those that can increase intra-esophageal pressure and cause a barogenic esophageal rupture.

Answer: B i.e., Boerhaave's syndrome

64. A 13 years old boy presents with hematuria, oliguria, edema and hypertension. He has history of sore throat two weeks prior to presentation. Laboratory investigations are remarkable for low C3 and increased titres of ASO and antiDNase. Which one of the following statements is NOT correct about management for this condition?

A. Renal biopsy is rarely required for making diagnosis
B. Antibiotic treatment is given for streptococcal infection
C. Treatment is largely supportive
D. Immunosuppressants are to be used for crescentic glomerulonephritis

Combination of glucocorticoids in pulsed doses, cytotoxic agents (azathioprine, cyclophosphamide), and intensive plasma exchange may be useful in crescentic GN.

Answer: D i.e., Immunosuppressants are to be used for crescentic glomerulonephritis

65. A 60 years old patient is admitted in emergency with seizure, aphasia and altered sensorium. He has history of fever and headache for the preceding 3 days. The CSF examination is unremarkable. What would be the probable diagnosis?

A. Multiple sclerosis
B. Tubercular meningitis
C. Pyogenic (bacterial) meningitis
D. Viral encephalitis

Sign & symptoms of encephalitis include headache, fever, fits, altered sensorium with or without neurological deficit, signs of increased intracranial tension, and meningeal signs. No organism is seen in CSF.

Answer: D i.e., Viral encephalitis

66. A 68-years old male presented in OPD with complaints of progressive small handwriting. On examination, he had resting tremor, bradykinesia, rigidity and postural instability. This patient is suffering most likely from:

A. Parkinson's disease
B. Vascular dementia
C. Alzheimer's disease
D. Fruntotemporal dementia

Features of Parkinson's disease include tremor (mainly at rest and described as pill rolling tremor in hands), bradykinesia, limb rigidity, gait and balance problems etc.

Answer: A i.e., Parkinson's disease

67. An elderly patient presents with abnormal gait. He has a wide base freezing gait with imbalance, comprising short strides, shuffling along the floor and difficulty with starts and turns. Heal-Shin test is normal. Which one of the following is most likely disorder?

A. Cerebellar ataxia

B. Sensory ataxia

C. Frontal gait disorder

D. Parkinson's disease

Frontal lobe gait apraxia: A broad-based (wide-based) gait with short stride, freezing, falls, and an inability to 'walk and talk', in the elderly, is most likely due to frontal lobe pathology. The commonest cause is cerebrovascular disease.

Answer: C i.e., Frontal gait disorder

68. A 35 years old man presents with history of low-grade fever and headache for last five weeks. Clinical examination is remarkable for signs of meningismus. He undergoes lumbar puncture (LP) and a day later reports worsening of headache. Which one of the following features is NOT consistent with diagnosis of "Post-LP" headache?

A. Post-LP headache usually begins within 48 hours

B. Post-LP headache worsens in sitting position

C. Post-LP headache is most severe upon waking up

D. Post-LP headache may improve with caffeine intake

Post-Lumbar puncture headache is defined as "bilateral headaches that develop within 7 days after an lumbar puncture and disappears within 14 days. The headache worsens within 15 min of resuming the upright position, disappears or improves within 30 min of resuming the recumbent position". This definition helps to avoid confusion with migraine or simple headache after lumbar puncture.

Answer: C i.e., Post-LP headache is most severe upon waking up

69. A young lady presents in outdoor clinic with complaints of menstrual irregularity, weight gain, hair loss, tiredness and weakness. What will be the investigation of choice?

A. FSH & LH level

B. Estrogen level

C. Free T3 and free T4 level

D. Free T4 and TSH level

Clinical findings suggest the diagnosis of hypothyroidism. Thyroid function tests include TSH, T_3 and T_4 levels estimation.

Answer: D i.e., Free T4 and TSH level

CHAPTER 12

SURGERY

RAPID REVISION NOTES

Commonest site

Condition	*Common site*
Keratoderma blenorrhagicum	**Sole of foot**
Tinea versicolor	**Trunk**
Inverse psoriasis	**Body folds**
Psoriasis	**Knee, elbow**
Erythema multiforme	**Extensor surfaces**
Hyperpigmentation in Addison disease	**Exposed areas and creases of palms**
Malignant melanoma in males	**Trunk**
Malignant melanoma in females	**Leg**
Kaposi sarcoma	**Legs**
Phlebolith	**Pelvis veins**
Dercum's disease	**Trunk**
Instrumental perforation of esophagus	**Crico-pharynx**
Dermoid cyst	**External angle of eye**
Implantation dermoid	**Hand & finger**
Keloid	**Sternum, face and neck**
Sebaceous cyst	**Scalp, face & scrotum**
Erysipelas	**Face & scrotum**

RISK FACTORS FOR BREAST Ca

- Risk factors for breast carcinoma:
  - o Ovarian malignancy
  - o Nulliparity (NOT multiparity)
  - o First pregnancy after 30 years
  - o Family history of breast carcinoma
  - o Fibroadenosis (particularly epitheliosis subtype)
  - o High fat diet
  - o Who avoids breast feeding
  - o BRCA1 & BRCA2
- Histological findings with increased risk of development of breast carcinoma: Atypical hyperplasia, florid hyperplasia

NIPPLE DISCHARGE

- Blood stained discharge from nipple is commonly due to: Intraductal papilloma (microdochectomy is done/ excising the involved duct)
- Black/ Green discharge from nipple indicates: Duct ectasia

INVESTIGATION FOR BREAST Ca

- Initial investigation for breast lump is: FNAC
- Preferred diagnostic method for breast lump: Core needle biopsy
- Best & definitive investigation is: Open excisional biopsy
- Triple assessment for carcinoma breast includes: Clinical examination, mammogram, FNAC

Sentinel node

- First node in the ipsilateral axilla to drain the tumor in the breast
- Sentinel node biopsy is done in carcinoma breast and malignant melanoma

MAMMOGRAPHY

- Screening mammography: Indicated in 50-70 years, mortality reduced by 30%, radiation due to mammography may cause carcinoma
- Features of malignant tumour on mammography: Spiculation (smooth in benign tumours) irregular mass, attenuated architecture of breast parenchyma (normal breast parenchyma in benign tumours), microcalcification/ less than 5 mm (microcalcifications / more than 5mm diameter, in benign tumours)
- Popcorn calcification in mammography suggests: Fibroadenoma

STAGING OF BREAST Ca

- T3N2a denotes: Tumour size more than 5 cm carcinoma, fixed ipsilateral axillary lymph node
- T2N1M0 denotes: Tumour size 2-5 cm, ipsilateral mobile axillary lymph node, no distant metastasis
- T3N3cM0 denotes: Tumour size more than 5 cm, metastasis to ipsilateral supraclavicular lymph nodes, no distant metastasis
- In breast cancer, chest wall involvement means involvement of: Ribs, intercostal muscle & serratus anterior muscle (NOT pectoralis major)

BREAST Ca (FEMALE)

- Commonest type of breast carcinoma: Infiltrative ductal carcinoma
- Multicentric & bilateral carcinoma of breast: Lobular (so biopsy of other breast is recommended)
- Type of mammary ductal carcinoma in situ (DCIS), most likely to result in a palpable abnormality in the breast: Comedo DCIS
- Features (in India): Incidence is 20/ 1,00,000; average age is 42 years; positive history is a risk factor; less commoner in muslims, less incidence with prolonged breast feeding, common in nulliparous
- Histologically, breast carcinoma with best prognosis is: Colloid (Mucinous)
- Familial carcinoma: Breast, colon, ovary, brain
- 'Peau D' orange appearance of the mammary skin is due to: Lymphatic permeation/ blockage of subdermal lymphatics
- Indicator of carcinoma breast: Recent retraction of nipple, cellular atypia
- Lymphatic spread of carcinoma breast commonly involves: Axillary nodes

BREAST Ca (MALE)

- Estrogen receptor positive
- Undescended testis is a risk factor
- History of gynaecomastia may be present

MANAGEMENT OF BREAST Ca

- Steps of Patey's mastectomy: Nipple & areola is removed, surrounding normal tissue around tumour is removed, pectoralis minor is removed (pectoralis major is NOT removed)
- Ideal management for an old lady with positive history for breast cancer, diffuse microcalcification on mammography & intraductal carcinoma in situ on biopsy: Simple mastectomy
- Carcinoma breast stage I & II is managed by: Modified radical mastectomy or lumpectomy, axillary clearance & radiotherapy
- Breast conservation surgery includes: Lumpectomy, radiotherapy, axillary lymph node dissection, sentinel lymph node biopsy

- Best chemotherapeutic regimen for breast carcinoma: Cyclophosphamide, methotrexate, 5-FU (nowadays some advocate use of anthracyclines like doxorubicin & taxanes like paclitaxel)

THYROID CARCINOMA

- Rarest: Anaplastic Ca
- Worst prognosis: Anaplastic Ca
- Best prognosis: Papillary Ca
- Associated with MEN II: Medullary Ca
- Developing in thyroglossal cyst: Papillary Ca
- Least malignant: Papillary Ca
- Developing in Hashimoto's thyroiditis: Papillary Ca
- MC type: Papillary Ca
- Associated with psammoma bodies: Papillary Ca

VASCULAR MALFORMATIONS

- Strawberry naevus: Resolve spontaneously (by intravascular thrombosis)
- Portwine stain/ Naevus flammeus: Persists
- Sturge Weber syndrome is associated with:
  - o Epilepsy
  - o Hemiplegia &
  - o Mental retardation

Vascular entities

Port- wine stain	Vascular malformation present at birth Doesn't regress
Strawberry angioma	Capillary haemangioma not present at birth Appears at 1-3 weeks slowly regresses
Salmon patch	Present at birth
Haemorrhage	
Primary haemorrhage	**Immediately post- Operative**
Secondary haemorrhage	**Within 7-14 days postoperative, due to infection**
Reactionary haemorrhage	**Within 24 hours of surgery, due to slippage of ligature or hypertension.**

ANEURYSM

- MC cause of abdominal aortic aneurysm: Atherosclerosis
- Cirsoid aneurysm commonly involves: Superficial temporal artery
- Pseudoaneurysm usually follows: Trauma
- IOC for peripheral aneurysm: USG
- MC cause of mycotic aneurysm: Staphylococcus

THROMBOANGITIS OBLITERANS/ BUERGER'S DISEASE

- TAO affects:
  - o Small & medium sized arteries
  - o Young
  - o Smokers
- Treatment of TAO:
  - o Lumbar sympathectomy
  - o Xanthinol nicotinate is used

Buerger's disease

- Thromboangiitis obliterans
- Inflammatory reaction in the arterial wall, and neighbouring veins and nerves
- More common in middle aged men
- Associated with smoking
- Segmental, small and medium sized arteries are affected
- Both distal extremities are affected

Arterial occlusion syndrome

- Leriche's Syndrome: Occlusion in the region of bifurcation of aorta and internal iliac arteries, leading to intermittent claudication
- Most common vessel to be involved in embolism is femoral

Stages seen in Raynaud's phenomenon

- Stage of local syncope /stage of blanching: Pallor

- Stage of local asphyxia/stage of dusky anoxia: Cyanosis
- Stage of recovery /stage of red engorgement: Redness

Signs/ symptoms of ischemia

- Pain
- Pulse - absent
- Pallor
- Paraesthesia
- Paralysis

Storage of blood

With CPD	3 Weeks
with CPDA-I	5 Weeks

Conditions indicating significant ischemia

- Ischemic ulceration
- Neuropathy
- Rest pain
- Gangrene
- Claudication is due to mild ischemia

Amputation level	***Stump length***
Arm	**8 inches**
Forearm	**8 inches**
Leg	**5.5 inches**
Thigh	**10-12 inches**
Amputation eponyms	***Description***
Lisfranc's	Disarticulation through tarso-metatarsal joint
Chopart's	Disarticulation through midrarsal joint
Syme's	Removal of foot anterior to medial malleolus
Burger's	Below knee
Gritti-stoke's	Supracondylar

Cranial haematomas with their causes

Type	***Causes***
Epidural haematoma	Rupture of middle meningeal artery
Subdural haematoma	Torn bridging veins (superior cerebral vein)
Subarachnoid haematoma	Aneurysm rupture
Intracerebral haemorrhage	Rupture of lenticulostriate arteries
Shape of Haematomas on CT- Scan	
Acute subdural haematoma	**Concavo-convex**
Extradural haematoma	**Biconvex**

DEEP VENOUS THROMBOSIS

- Clinical presentation:
  - o Unilateral leg swelling
  - o Local warmth
  - o Erythema &
  - o Pain
- Non-invasive test to diagnose DVT: Duplex venous USG
- Drug used for DVT prophylaxis: Heparin
- Treatment:
  - o Thrombolytic therapy
  - o Bandaging etc.
- Homans sign in DVT: Forced dorsiflexion of foot causes calf pain

Signs of DVT

- Homan's sign: Pain in the calf on dorsiflexion of the foot
- Moses's sign: Pain is caused by squeezing of the calf muscle from side to side

VARICOSE VEINS

- Gold standard method of diagnosing VV: Duplex imaging
- Sclerosant used in VV: Ethanolamine oleate
- Test to demonstrate sapheno-femoral incompetence: Brodie-Trendelenburg test
- MC complication of stripping: Ecchymosis
- Cocket & Dodds's operation: Subfascial ligation

ARTERIOVENOUS FISTULA/ AVF

- Physiological effects of AVF:
  - o Enhanced venous return &

- o Increased cardiac output
- o May cause overgrowth of limb later (if in young) etc.

- Nicoladoni/ Branham sign:
  - o Pressure on the artery proximal to fistula causes
  - o Swelling to reduce in size
  - o A thrill/ bruit to cease
  - o Fall in pulse rate &
  - o Pulse pressure returns to normal

Fistula & sinus

- Fistula: Communicating track between two epithelial surfaces. One connecting hollow viscus with surface is called external fistula. One connecting two hollow viscera
- Sinus: Blind track lined by granulomatous tissue, leading form the surface down to the tissues, which may contain cavity

Aneurysms

- True aneurysm: Contains all the three layers of arterial wall
- False aneurysm: Single layer of fibrous tissue as the wall of sac
- Mycotic aneurysm: Produced by the growth of microorganisms in the wall of the vessel
- Cirsoid aneurysm: Mass of dilated pulsating serpiginous vessels, found in congenital arteriovenous aneurysms
- Aneurismal varix: Artery and vein are communicating directly with a short wide channel
- Varicose aneurysm: Anastomosis between artery and vein is indirect through as intermediate sac

Remember

- Atherosclerotic aneurysms are the commonest.
- Cimino fistula – for renal dialysis temporary iatrogenic A –V fistula is made in the wrist or ankle
- Branham's sign:
  - o If a finger is pressed on the artery proximal to A-V fistula, there will be slowing of pulse rate and rise in the diastolic pressure

- Marjolin's ulcer:
  - o Squamous cell carcinoma, which arises in a chronic benign ulcer or scar
  - o Most commonly seen in long standing venous ulcer

TOTAL PARENTERAL NUTRITION

- TPN is used as a primary therapy in:
  - o Severe burns
  - o Short bowel syndrome etc.
- Complications of TPN:
  - o Air embolism
  - o Weight loss in 7 days etc.
- Metabolic changes in TPN:
  - o Essential fatty acid deficiency
  - o Electrolyte disorder etc.

Wallace's rule of nine

To estimate the total body surface area in burns patient

In adults	*In children*
Head – 9	Head –18
Chest front – 9	Chest front – 9
Abdomen front – 9	Abdomen front – 9
Chest back – 9	Chest back – 9
Lower back – 9	Lower back – 9
Each upper limb – 9	Each upper limb – 9
Each thigh – 9	Each lower limb – 13.5
Each leg – 9	Perineum –1
Perineum –1	

Infections in burns

- Most common nonbacterial opportunistic organism form burn wounds is candidiasis
- Most common bacterial infection in burn wounds is Pseudomonas

WOUNDS & TISSUE REPAIR

- Healing by primary/ 1st intention:
  - o Closed wounds

- o Edges approximated
- o E.g. clean skin incision closed with sutures
- Factors delaying wound healing:
  - o Vitamin C deficiency
  - o Presence of vitamin E (inhibitory role)
  - o Deficiency of trace metals (zinc, copper etc.)
  - o Absence of oxygen (reduced perfusion)
  - o Anemia
  - o Infection etc.

Healing

- Healing by primary intention: Clean, surgically closed wounds
- Healing by secondary intention: Unsutured, infected wounds healing by granulation tissue formation
- Healing by tertiary intention: Delayed closure for infected surgical wounds, in which skin was kept open in initial operation

Classification of wounds

Clean	Viscus not opened
Clean contaminated	Viscus opened without spillage
Contaminated	Viscus opened with spillage
Dirty	Infected wounds, like abscesses

KELOID

- Appears after few days of surgery
- May be familial
- Rarely subsides
- Recurrence is common
- May turn malignant
- MC site is: Sternum
- Treatment of keloid:
  - o Intralesional steroid
  - o Excision & repair

SUTURES

- Absorbable sutures:
  - o Catgut
  - o Dexona (polyglycolic acid) etc.
- Non absorbable sutures:
  - o Prolene
  - o Silk etc.

Absorbable sutures	*Nonabsorbable*
Catgut	Polyester
Vicry1	Polyamide
Homopolymer of glycolide	Polypropylene
Homopolymer of polydioxanone	Polyethylene skin cotton

SKIN GRAFTS

- Partial thickness skin grafts/ Thiersch graft: Consist of epidermis & variable thickness of dermis
- Full thickness/ Wolfes graft: Consists of epidermis & all of the dermis
- Composite grafts: Consist of skin & some underlying tissue (fat, cartilage etc.)

Skin grafts

- Partial thickness graft
  - o Thin graft/ thiersch graft: Through the tips of papillae
  - o Thick graft /split skin grafts: All of epidermis and variable part of dermis
- Whole thickness skin graft/ Wolfe's graft: Includes entire epidermis and dermis

Partial thickness graft	*Full thickness graft*
Includes whole of dermis	Includes whole of epidermis and part of epidermis, and dermis
Wound contraction is more	Wound contraction is minimal
Skin on the donor site can regenerate on its own	Skin on the donor site cannot regenerate and hence Needs to be closed
Used for resurfacing large areas	Used for resurfacing small areas, as they match color and texture
Donor sites include upper	Donor site includes post-thighs, buttocks auricular and upper eyelids

Skin graft

- Skin graft can be stored in refrigerator for 2 weeks at 4 degrees centigrade

Skin graft survive in recipient bed by

- Imbibition: Absorption of nutrients into the graft which serves to feed the graft for the first 24 hours to 48 hours
- Inoculation: Process whereby donor and recipient capillaries become aligned
- Revascularization: Differentiation of connecting vessels into the arterioles and venules

Graft type	*Characteristic*
Autograft	Received from self
Allograft	Received from same species
Isograft	Received from different individual who is genetically identical
Xenograft	Received from different species.

SEBACEOUS CYST

- Retention cyst
- May lead to Cock's peculiar tumour

BASAL CELL CARCINOMA

- MC site of BCC: Face
- MC type of BCC: Nodulo-ulcerative type
- Mode of spread: Direct
- Excision procedure done: Moh's micrographic excision

Rodent ulcer/ Basal Cell Carcinoma

- 90 percent of basal cell carcinomas are seen in the face
- Majority occur above the line-connecting angle of mouth with lobule of the ear
- Commonest site is around the inner canthus of eye (Tear cancer)
- Typical rolled edge
- Spreads by local spread
- Geographical or 'field fire' basal cell carcinoma has irregular raised edge around the flat white scar
- Regional lymph node metastasis is characteristic
- Superficial radiotherapy is the treatment of choice

MELANOMA

- Mode of spread of MM: Lymphatic channels or hematogenous
- Cutaneous melanoma arises from: Epidermal melanocytes
- MC site involved in lentigo maligna (least common): Face
- MC type of MM: Superficial spreading
- Most malignant type of MM: Nodular melanoma

Melanomas

- Lymphatic spread is the commonest route of spread
- Radioresistant
- Best treated by surgery and local regional and perfusion with high doses cytotoxic agents

Melanoma

Most common type	**Superficial spreading**
Least common type	**Lentigo maligna melanoma**
Least malignant	**Lentigo maligna / Hutchinson's freckle**
Most malignant	**Nodular variety**
Most common site in males	**Lower back**
Most common site in females	**Legs**

RHABDOMYOSARCOMA

- MC soft tissue tumour in a child: Rhabdomyosarcoma
- MC type of RMS: Embryonal RMS
- Mode of spread of embryonal RMS: Lymphatic
- Prognosis depends upon: Grade of tumour

SALIVARY GLANDS

- MC benign parotid gland tumour: Pleomorphic adenoma
- Treatment of pleomorphic adenoma: Superficial parotidectomy (Patey's operation)

- Warthin's tumour (2nd MC benign parotid tumour) consists of: Epithelial & lymphoid elements (adeno-lymphoma)
- Treatment of Warthin's tumour: Superficial parotidectomy
- Adenoid cystic Ca/ cylindroma/ treacherous tumour invades: Perineural space & lymphatics
- Muco-epidermoid Ca arises from: Mucin secreting cells & epidermal cells
- MC benign salivary gland tumour: Pleomorphic adenoma
- Most of the minor salivary gland tumours are: Malignant
- Calculi are MC in: Submandibular duct

Salivary gland	*Histological type*
Parotid	**Serous**
Submandibular	**Mixed**
Sublingual	**Mucous**

Pleomorphic adenoma

- Commonest benign tumour of salivary glands
- Radioresistant
- Patey's operation/ superficial parotidectomy is done

Warthin's tumour

- Benign tumour
- Only involves parotid and usually lower portion
- Shows hot spot on Tc 99m pertechnetate scan
- Superficial parotidectomy is done
- Haemangioma is the most common benign tumour of parotid in children

Indications of radiotherapy in parotid tumors

- Recurrent disease
- Residual disease left at surgery
- High grade lesion
- Those who refuse surgery
- Unfit for surgery
- Unresectable local lesion

Triad of Mikulicz's disease

- Enlargement of salivary glands
- Narrow palpebral fissure
- Parchment like dryness of mouth

BREAST

- Peau'd orange is due to: Lymphatic permeation
- Risk factors for breast Ca:
    - o Positive family history
    - o Nullipara
    - o Fatty food intake
    - o Mammary dysplasia/ atypical hyperplasia/ sclerosing adenosis
- Management of stage I & II of breast Ca: Lumpectomy/ breast conservative therapy + axillary clearance + radiotherapy
- Mondor's disease is: Thrombophlebitis of breast (superficial veins)
- Cystosarcoma phyllodes:
    - o Serocystic disease of Brodie
    - o Benign breast tumour

Carcinoma breast

- Carcinoma breast is more common on: Left side
- Most common site: Upper outer quadrant
- Most common histological variant: Ductal carcinoma
- Histological variant with good prognosis even in presence of axillary lymph node metastasis: Medullary carcinoma

Lymphoedema grading

Grade	*Characteristic*
0	Subclinical
1	Pits on pressure, disappears on elevation /rest
2	Non-pitting; does not disappear on elevation and rest
3	Irreversible skin changes like fibrosis and papillae

CYSTIC HYGROMA

- Fluid filled lesions of lymphatic origin (lymphangioma)
- Brilliantly translucent
- Cough impulse is positive
- Associated with:
  - o Turners syndrome
  - o Trisomies etc.
- Treatment of choice: Excision

Cystic hygroma

- Cystic swelling containing clear lymph
- It is caused due to sequestration of apportion of a jugular sac from the lymphatic system, which fails to join and regular lymphatic system
- Commonest site is posterior triangle of neck
- Manifests in early infancy
- Brilliantly translucent
- Excision is the treatment of choice

BRANCHIAL CYST & RANULA

Branchial cyst

- MC site: Upper part of neck
- Wall is made of: Lymphoid tissue

Ranula

- Retention cyst of sublingual glands

CHEMODECTOMA

- Non chromaffin paraganglioma
- Origin from Schwann cells
- Rarely metastasizes
- Good prognosis
- Surgical excision is the treatment of choice

THYROGLOSSAL CYST

- MC site:
  - o Beneath the hyoid
  - o Occupies the midline usually (except in the region of thyroid cartilage)
- Swelling moves upwards on protrusion of the tongue as well as on swallowing (attachment with foramen caecum)
- Painless

Tongue carcinoma

- Most common site is Anterior 2/3rd
- Near the lateral margin

Thyroglossal cyst

- Cystic swelling developing from the remnant of thyroglossal tract
- Subhyoid position is the commonest
- Moves with deglutition
- Excision is treatment

Thyroglossal fistula

- Never congenital
- Caused by the external opening of an infected thyroglossal cyst

Sternomastoid tumour/ Congenital torticollis

- Caused by the infarction of the central portion of one of the sternomastoid muscle at the time of birth

De QUERVAIN'S THYROIDITIS

- Due to viral infection
- Increased ESR
- Self-limiting

SOLITARY THYROID NODULE

- MC in female
- Investigation of choice is: FNAC
- Hemi-thyroidectomy is done for solitary nodule

The thyroid moves with deglutition due to its attachment with the larynx and trachea by

- Ligament of berry
- Posterior lamina of the pretracheal fascia
- Levator glandulae thyroideae

MEN SYNDROME

- MEN-I:
    - o Parathyroid neoplasm
    - o Pancreas neoplasm &
    - o Pituitary (anterior) adenoma
- MEN-IIA:
    - o Medullary Ca (thyroid)
    - o Phaeochromocytomas &
    - o Parathyroid hyperplasia
- MEN-IIB:
    - o Medullary Ca (thyroid)
    - o Phaeochromocytomas &
    - o Mucosal neuromas (with distinctive marfanoid habitus)

THYROID-MEDULLARY Ca/ MTC

- 80% cases are sporadic
- 20% are familial (MEN-IIa or MEN-IIb)
- MTC is the first abnormality expressed in MEN-IIa/ IIb
- Stroma of MTC shows material with staining properties of amyloid
- MTC can be diagnosed by demonstrating calcitonin within the MTC cells (on immuno-histochemical studies)
- Total thyroidectomy is the TOC

THYROID PAPILLARY Ca

- MC thyroid tumour
- Encapsulated
- Psammoma bodies are seen
- Multifocal
- Least malignant
- Follicular type is a variety of papillary Ca

MISCELLANEOUS (THYROID)

Thyroid lymphoma

- Rapidly growing
- Diffuse large type is variant

Thyroidectomy

- Neck swelling immediately following thyroid surgery is due to: Tension hematoma (so open immediately)

Thyroid surgeries

- Superior thyroid artery: Ligated close to superior pole to avoid external laryngeal nerve
- Inferior thyroid artery: Ligated away from pole to avoid recurrent laryngeal nerve

ESOPHAGUS

- MC cause of esophagitis: Reflux esophagitis
- Young women with koilonychias, iron deficiency anemia & dysphagia: Plummer-Vinson syndrome/ Brown Kelly Syndrome/ Sideropenic dysphagia
- Schatzki's ring:
    - o Circular submucosal ring in the distal esophagus
    - o Usually at squamocolumnar junction:
- Barium study of a lady with non-progressive dysphagia (for solids) shows: Dilated esophagus with narrowing of lower part of esophagus
- Diffuse esophageal spasm, on barium swallow: Cork screw appearance
- Dysphagia lusoria: Secondary to vascular anomalies (double aortic arch, right aortic arch etc.)
- Zenker's diverticulum:
    - o Presents with intermittent dysphagia, regurgitation, gurgling sounds etc.
    - o Managed by: Excision of pouch/ cricopharyngeal myotomy
- Sliding hernia:
    - o Dislocation of cardia of stomach into posterior mediastinum

- o Complicated cases require surgery
- Mallory Weiss syndrome:
  - o Common in alcoholics
  - o MC site is cardia of stomach (NOT esophagus)
- Boerhaave's syndrome:
  - o Forceful vomiting may produce perforation of the esophagus
  - o Presents with acute chest pain

Zenker's diverticulum

- Most common complication of esophageal atresia
- Seen in elderly
- Characteristic site is within inferior pharyngeal constrictor, between the oblique fibres and horizontal fibres, at Killian's triangle
- Lung abscess due to aspiration is the most common complication

Plummer – Vinson syndrome/ Brown-kelly-Paterson syndrome/ Sideropenic dysphagia

- Esophageal web with iron deficiency anemia
- Permalignant- Pre-cricoid carcinoma
- Palmar and solar keratosis is seen in esophageal cancer

Sclerosing agents for endoscopic sclerotherapy

- Polidocanol / polydochy
- N-buty1- cyanoacrylate (glue injection)
- Absolute alcohol, phenol
- Ethanolamine maleate /oleate
- Sodium teradecy1 sulphate
- Stomach is the conduit of choice after oesophagectomy

ACHALASIA CARDIA

- Dysphagia is the presenting symptom
- Increased difficulty in swallowing both solids & liquids
- Failure of relaxation of lower esophageal sphincter
- Increased pressure
- X-ray shows bird beak appearance

BARRETTS ESOPHAGUS

- Metaplasia is seen at lower end of esophagus
- Squamous to columnar epithelial metaplasia is seen
- As a result of prolonged GERD
- MC type is intestinal metaplasia
- May lead to development of
  - o AdenoCa
  - o Barret ulcer
  - o Stricture etc.

Vomiting

Features	*Condition*
Vomiting since birth; often bile stained	**Duodenal atresia**
Non-bile stained vomitus with peak incidence at 3-6 weeks after birth	**Congenital hypertrophic pyloric stenosis**
Effortless, blood stained vomiting or small amounts soon after birth	**Hiatus hernia**
Continuous pouring out of saliva	**Esophageal atresia**

CONGENITAL/ INFANTILE HYPERTROPHIC PYLORIC STENOSIS

- Presents about 4 weeks after birth
- Weight loss
- Hypochloremic alkalosis
- Fluid of choice: Isotonic normal saline

Congenital/ Infantile Hypertrophic pyloric stenosis

- Shows hypochloremic alkalosis
- Congenital pyloric stenosis is best diagnosed by USG
- Hypertrophied pyloric muscle mass > 4 mm or pyloric length >14 mm

ESOPHAGEAL Ca

- Predisposing factors:
  - o Smoking
  - o Chronic achalasia

- o Tylosis
- o Barret's esophagus etc.
- MC type: Squamous cell Ca
- MC site: Lower end of esophagus
- MC site of adenoCa: Lower end
- MC site of squamous cell Ca: Middle 1/3rd
- Chemotherapeutic agents used: Cisplatin, bleomycin & 5-FU

GASTRIC Ca

- MC site: Antrum
- Predisposing factors:
  - o H. Pylori (causes gastritis, gastric atrophy),
  - o Blood group A etc.
- MC feature: Weight loss
- Early gastric Ca:
  - o Primary lesion limited to mucosa & submucosa
  - o Excellent prognosis
- Sister Mary Joseph's nodule: Metastatic involvement of para-umbilical nodes from intrapelvic/ intraabdominal malignancies (stomach)
- Gastric lymphoma:
  - o Vast majority of gastric lymphoid tumours are non-Hodgkin's lymphoma of B cell origin
  - o Surgery is indicated in bleeding, perforation etc.
- Gastro-intestinal stromal tumours/ GIST: MC in stomach

GI ULCERS

- MC site of duodenal ulcer: Duodenal cap
- Curling's ulcer: GI ulcers in severe burns
- Site of bleeding in duodenal ulcer: Gastroduodenal artery
- Treatment of perforated peptic ulcer:
  - o Exploratory laparotomy
  - o Nasogastric suction
  - o Acid suppression
  - o Antibiotics etc.
- Management of duodenal ulcer:
  - o Highly selective vagotomy (least chances of diarrhea/ dumping syndrome)
  - o Truncal vagotomy & antrectomy (lowest chances of recurrence)
- Cause of early dumping syndrome: Due to rapid emptying of hyperosmolar gastric contents into the small intestine

Dumping syndrome

Early dumping syndrome	*Late dumping syndrome*
Immediately after meals	Second hour after meals
Relief by lying down	Relief by exercise
Symptoms of epigastric fullness, tachycardia, colic	Symptoms of tremor, sweating, light headedness, fainting, prostration

Site of duodenal ulcer perforation & effect

- Posterior duodenal: Intense hemorrhage due to rupture ulcer perforation of gastro-duodenal artery
- Anterior duodenal: Pneumoperitoneum and peritonitis ulcer perforation

Vagotomy

- Truncal vagotomy/ vagectomy: Both the trunk of vagus nerves are resected
- Selective vagotomy: Removal of all gastric fibres of the vagus nerves, leaving the hepatic and celiac branches
- Highly selective vagotomy: Denervation of acid secreting part of stomach, keeping supply to the alkali secreting part of the stomach and other abdominal viscera intact

Typhoid

- Typhoid ulcers are placed longitudinally along the ileum
- Perforation of typhoid ulcer usually occurs in the 3rd week
- Most common complication of typhoid: Paralytic ileus
- Most common presentation: Intestinal bleeding
- Most common site involved: Ileum

Remember

- Tubercular ulcer is placed transversely along the ileum
- Acute mesenteric lymphadenitis is the disease with symptoms and signs most similar to those of acute appendicitis

- Strawberry lesion of recto-sigmoid is due to infection by spirochete vincenti and bacillus fusiformis. Carcinoid tumor is most frequently found in distal third of appendix
- Most common position of appendix: Retrocecal
- Bleeding is the earliest complication of rectal carcinoma followed by alteration of bowel movements
- Treatment of duodenal atresia is duodeno-jejunostomy or duodeno-duodenostomy
- Red currant jelly stool is seen in intussusception
- Most serious complication of end colostomies is parastomal hernia
- Bishop koop's operation is done in meconium ileus

Type of edge	*Ulcer*
Undermined edge	**Tuberculous ulcer**
Punched out edge	**Gummatous ulcer, deep trophic ulcer**
Sloping edge	**Healing traumatic ulcer**
Raised beaded edge	**Rodent ulcer**
Rolled out edge	**Squamous cell carcinoma**
Ulcer with eponyms	
Bazin's ulcer	Small multiple in ankle region Associated with: Erythrocyanosis frigida; seen exclusively in young women. Low grade ischemia of ankle, due to abnormally small or absent perforating arteries arising from the posterior tibial or peroneal arteries
Footballer's ulcer	Non-healing ulcer over shin Due to direct trauma by football
Phagedenic ulcer	Tropical ulcers seen in malnourished, poorly immunized with history of trauma or insect bite. Infection is caused by Vincent's organisms
Hunner's ulcer	Interstitial cystitis. Bladder capacity is reduced to 30-50 ml

APPENDIX

- Acute appendicitis: Left sided appendicitis is diverticulosis
- Enlarged lymphoid follicles associated with:
  - o Viral infections
  - o Inspissated barium etc.
- Pelvic & post-ileal appendicitis presents as: Diarrhea
- USG is helpful in diagnosis
- USG & CT are confirmatory
- Mucocele of appendix: Retention cyst/ benign tumour
- Appendicular carcinoid: MC malignant tumour of appendix

Blind loop syndrome

- Stagnation of small intestinal contents by strictures, stenosis, blind- pouch syndrome, or diverticula
- The bacterial flora in the stagnant area is increased in number
- Leading to anemia, hypoproteinemia, steatorrhea
- In distal small intestine, the abnormal bacterial flora compete for vitamin B12, leading to deficiency
- In proximal small intestine, they deconjugate bile salts, leading to steatorrhea
- Also leads to hypoproteinemia and avitaminosis

PERITONEAL CAVITY

- MC causative organism of acute bacterial peritonitis: E. Coli (2nd MC is klebsiella)
- Peritoneal mesotheliomas are associated with: Asbestos exposure
- MC malignant neoplasm of retroperitoneum: Lymphoma & retroperitoneal sarcoma
- Idiopathic retroperitoneal fibrosis is also known as: Ormond's disease
- Appendices epiploicae is also known as: Peritoneal mice
- MC site of intraperitoneal abscess: Pelvic
- Pneumococcal peritonitis is associated with: Nephritic syndrome

Tumour & their common appearance

Site	*Clinical type*
Vagina	Cauliflower growth
Glottis	Papillary variety
Penis	Flat/ infiltrating ulcer and papilliferous growth
Rectum	Ulcerating growth
Colon left sided	Stenosing growth
Colon right sided	Cauliflower type growth
Stomach	Ulcerating growth
Tongue	Fungating and ulcerating growth

NON NEOPLASTIC POLYPS

- Hyperplastic polyp
- Hamartomatous polyp
- Inflammatory polyp

Remember

- Villous adenoma has the highest malignant potential

Polyposis coli

Not premalignant	*Premalignant*
Juvenile polyposis Peutz-jegher's Syndrome	Tubular adenoma Villous adenoma **Familial adenomatous** **polyposis coli-** 100 percent Malignancy risk, autosomal dominant Gardner's syndrome **Turcot's syndrome – 100** Percent progression to malignancy

MECKEL'S DIVERTICULUM

- True congenital diverticulum
- Vestigial remnant of omphalomesenteric duct/ vitelline duct
- 2 feet from ileocaecal valve
- 2 types of ectopic tissue are common:
  - o Gastric &
  - o Pancreatic
- Torsion may lead to obstruction, ischemia & necrosis
- IOC to diagnose Meckel's diverticula: Technetium-99m pertechnetate (99mTc)
- It can be a leading point of intussusception

Meckel's diverticulum

- Meckel's diverticulum is a true diverticulum situated on antimesenteric border
- Present in 2 percent population 2 inches long
- 2 feet proximal to ileo-colic valve
- Most common complication of Meckel's diverticulum is intestinal obstruction followed by bleeding and diverticulitis

Remember

- Meckel's diverticulum: Result of partial obliteration of vitelline duct
- Persistent vitelline fistula: Result of failure of closure of vitelline duct

Classic quartet of intestinal obstruction

- Pain
- Abdominal distention
- Vomiting
- Constipation

INTUSSUSCEPTION

- Outer tube is known as: Intussuscipiens
- Inner tube is known as: Intussuscipiens
- Sign de dance: Emptiness in Iliac fossa
- MC type: Ileo-colic

COLORECTAL Ca

- MC site: Rectum
- MC site in colon: Sigmoid colon
- MC type: AdenoCa
- Presentation of right sided tumour: Anemia
- Left sided tumour presents as: Obstruction/ pain

- Risk factors:
  - o Increased dietary fats & oil
  - o Elevated serum cholesterol
  - o Ulcerative colitis & Crohn's disease
  - o Familial adenomatous polyps
- MC site of metastasis: Liver (33% patient may have metastasis)
- Treatment of choice: Surgery

Remember

- Aspirin/ NSAID are protective against colorectal Ca

Carcinoma colon

Carcinoma colon left	*Carcinoma colon right*
Obstructive syndromes	Anemia is more common predominate

Duke's classification of colon carcinoma

Stage A	Growth is limited to the bowel
Stage B	Spread into adjoining structures, without lymphatic metastasis
Stage C	Lymphatic metastases

Duke's classification of rectal carcinoma

Stage A	Growth limited to rectal wall
Stage B	Beyond rectal wall, but no involvement of lymph nodes.
Stage C	Growth beyond rectal wall, with involvement of regional lymph nodes.

Tumour markers

Tumour marker	*Associated tumours*
HCG	Trophoblastic tumours, nonseminomatous testicular tumours
Calcitonin	Medullary carcinoma of thyroid
Alpha fetoprotein	Liver cell cancer, nonseminomatous germ cell tumours of Testis
CEA	Carcinoma colon, pancreas, lung, stomach, breast.
Acid phosphatase	Prostate cancer
PSA	Prostate cancer
Neuron specific Enolase	Small cell lung cancer, Neuroblastoma
Immunoglobulins	Multiple myeloma
CA 125	Ovarian cancer, pancreatic cancer
Ca 19-9	Colon cancer, pancreatic cancer
Ca 15-3	Breast cancer
5-HIA	Carcinoid tumors
S. alkaline phosphatase	Osteosarcoma
Homovanillic acid, VMA	Neuroblastoma, pheochromocytoma
Ca 50 / Ca 242	Colorectal, pancreatic, gastric.
NSE	Neuroendocrine tumours Small cell lung carcinomas, Medullary thyroid carcinomas

Remember

- Characteristic of AML- Auer rods
- Philadelphia chromosome – CML
- Kaposi's sarcoma is the most common neoplasm in patients with AIDS
- Commonest malignancy in women in developing countries is cervical cancer
- Commonest malignancy in women in developed countries is breast cancer
- Commonest cancer in elderly is prostate cancer
- Burkitt's lymphoma – most rapidly progressive tumour
- Most common inherited malignancy is retinoblastoma

Intestinal lesions & common sites

Condition	*Common site*
Amoebiasis	**Sigmoid colon**
Rupture in blast injury	**Pelvic colon**
Ischemic colitis	**Splenic flexure**
Volvulus in small intestine	**Lower ileum**
Volvulus neonatorum	**Midgut (whole small intestine plus caecum)**
Intussusception in infant	**Last 50 cm of ileum**
Pneumatosis cystoides	**Small intestine**
Perforation in typhoid	**Small intestine near ileocecal junction**

Diverticulosis	**Sigmoid colon**
Hirschsprung's disease	**Upper limit is recto-sigmoid junction**
Ulcerative colitis	**Starts at rectum**
Crohn's disease	**Starts at or near ileocecal valve**
Typhoid ulcer	**Small intestine (ileum)**
Carcinoma colon	**Sigmoid colon & recto-sigmoid junction**
Carcinoma small intestine	**Jejunum**
ZES/ gastrinoma	**Pancreas**
Familial polyposis & Gardner's syndrome	**Colon**
Polypi in Peutz Jeghers syndrome	**Jejunum**
Non-hodgkin lymphoma	**Stomach**
Lipoma	**Caecum**

MISCELLANEOUS (GIT)

- Acute gastric dilatation:
  - o Patient is dehydrated &
  - o Has electrolyte disturbances (vomits oftenly)
  - o Neglect can cause sudden massive vomit & aspiration (lungs)
  - o Surgery is NOT advised (do nasogastric suction)
- Phytobezoars: Made of vegetable matter
- Short bowel syndrome:
  - o Diarrhea/ steatorrhea
  - o Gastric hypersecretion of acid

Short bowel syndrome

- Massive bowel resection.
- Minimum amount of small bowel required to prevent short bowel syndrome is 100 cm
- Absorption of fat, water, electrolytes, and vitamin B12 is affected
- Associated with hypergastrinemia

Causes

- Massive intestinal resection
- Regional enteritis with multiple bowel reactions
- A jejuno- ileal bypass for morbid obesity

Grading of piles

First degree	Contained within the anal canal
Second degree	Extruded on defecation, but return at the end or act
Third degree	Prolapse on defecation and then need to be manually reduced
Fourth degree	Prolapse on defecation and then cannot be reduced

Treatment of piles

First degree	Sclerosants
Second degree	Sclerosants, rubber banding
Third degree	Sclerosants, rubber banding
Fourth degree	Rubber banding, haemorrhoidectomy

Goodsall's rule

- Anal fistulae with an external opening in relation to anterior half of anus tends to have a straight path, whereas those related to posterior half, usually have curving tracks and may be of the horseshoe variety

HERNIA

- Spigelian hernia: Interparietal hernia (sub-umbilical/ level of arcuate line)
- Littre's hernia: Hernia of Meckel's diverticulum
- Morgagni's hernia: Hernia between costal & sternal parts of diaphragm
- Hernia en glissade/ sliding hernia:
  - o Content on left side are sigmoid colon & mesentery
  - o Right side content is caecum
- Femoral hernia:
  - o MC in Female
  - o MC on Right side
  - o MC strangulates

Hernia

- Hernia through foramen of Moragnite: Herniation through the retrosternal defect between sternal and costal attachment of diaphragm

- Hernia through foramen of Bochdalek: Herniation posterolaterally through pleuro-parietal opening
- Spigelian: Interparietal and subumbilical herniation, lateral to rectus muscle at the level of arcuate line
- Richter's hernia:
  Herniation of circumference of intestine
- Littre's hernia: Herniation of Meckel's diverticulum
- Maydl's hernia: Hernia en W

Remember

- Landmark for differentiating femoral hernia from inguinal hernia is the pubic tubercle
  - o Neck of the sac of inguinal hernia is above and medial to it, while that of femoral hernia is below and lateral to it
- Landmark for differentiating direct form indirect inguinal hernia is inferior epigastric vessels
  - o Neck of direct is medial to it, while that of indirect is lateral to it

Hernia surgeries

- Herniotomy: Neck of the sac is transfixed and ligated and then the hernial sac is excised, no repair is done
- Herniorrhaphy: Herniotomy with repair of posterior wall of the inguinal canal
- Hernioplasty: Herniorrhaphy with reinforced repair of the posterior wall of the inguinal canal by filling the gap between the conjoined tendon and inguinal ligament

PANCREAS

- MC site of heterotopic pancreatic tissue: Stomach
- Annular pancreas:
  - o 2nd part of duodenum is surrounded by a ring of pancreatic tissue
  - o Managed by duodeno-duodenostomy

ACUTE PANCREATITIS

- MC cause: Gallstones
- Investigation which can cause acute pancreatitis: ERCP
- Grey turner sign: Blue-red-purple or green-brown discoloration due to catabolism of hemoglobin
- Diagnosis: Fecal fat estimation
- CT scan is the diagnostic modality
- Best prognosis: Gall stone pancreatitis
- Recurrent pancreatitis occurs in: Methylmalonic acidemia
- Conditions with raised serum amylase:
  - o Pancreatitis
  - o Renal failure
  - o Ruptured ectopic pregnancy etc.

PANCREATIC PSEUDOCYST

- MC cause in children: Trauma
- MC cause in adults: Pancreatitis
- MC presentation: Upper abdominal pain
- MC complication: Infection

PANCREATIC Ca

- Most consistent risk factor: Cigarette smoking
- MC site: Pancreatic head (70%)
- MC symptom: Weight loss & pain

Trousseau's sign of malignancy / Trousseau's syndrome

- Some malignancies, especially adenocarcinomas of the pancreas and lung, are associated with hypercoagulability
- In patients with malignancy–associated hypercoagulable states, the blood may spontaneously form clots in the portal vessels, the deep veins of the extremities, or the superficial veins anywhere on the body
- When recurrent clots form in different superficial veins around the body, this is described as migratory thrombophlebitis
- Armand Trousseau first described this finding in himself; he was subsequently found to have pancreatic cancer

Mesna –Sodium 2 – mercapto ethane sulphate

- Protective agent in cancer chemotherapy (Cyclophosphamide) to prevent hemorrhagic cystitis
- Acrolein is thought to be responsible for its action

GASTRINOMA/ ZES

- MC site: Duodenum
- Non beta cell tumour
- Neuro-endocrine tumour/ NET secreting: Gastrin
- Most important investigation: Secretin injection test
- DOC for ZES: Proton pump inhibitors
- Hepatic metastasis occurs (33%)

PANCREATIC TUMOURS (ENDOCRINE)

Insulinoma

- MC endocrine tumours of pancreas (from beta cells)
- Usually single
- Whipple's triad is seen
- Distributed equally throughout pancreas
- Total capsule removal is ensured to prevent tumour recurrence

Somatostatinoma

- Endocrine tumours that secrete excessive amount of somatostatin
- Characterized by
  - o DM
  - o Gallbladder disease
  - o Diarrhea &
  - o Steatorrhea

VIPoma:

- VIP is secreted
- Characterized by:
  - o Large volume watery diarrhea
  - o Dehydration &
  - o Hypokalemia

Pancreatic duct

Duct of Wirsung	Major pancreatic duct
Duct of Santorini	Minor pancreatic duct

Pancreatitis

- Most commonly elevated and tested enzyme: Serum amylase
- Low serum amylase is seen in: Serum protein loss in congestive heart failure
- Single best enzyme for pancreatitis: Serum lipase
- Pancreases the only source of: Serum trypsinogen
- Drugs inducing pancreatitis: L - asparaginase, thiazides, steroids
- Organism causing pancreatitis: Mumps
- Best prognosis: Gall stone pancreatitis

Pancreatitis

- Grey Turner's sign: In hemorrhagic pancreatitis, bluish discoloration in the flank is seen
- Cullen's sing–In hemorrhagic pancreatitis, bluish discoloration in the peri-umbilical area is seen
- Most common site of pseudopancreatic cyst is body and tail pancreas
- Pseudocyst >5 cm in diameter is an indication of drainage
- Pseudocyst <5 cm and <6 weeks duration should be observed only

Pancreatic tumours

Gastrinoma/ Zollinger-Ellison syndrome	Arises from G-cells, Secretes gastrin, Malignant tumour
Insulinoma	Most common, Arises from beta cells, Hypoglycemia
Glucagonoma	Arises from alpha cells. Cause diabetes, anemia, thrombosis, skin rashes
Somatostatin-Oma	Arises from delta cells. Causes diabetes, gallstone, steatorrhea, hypochlorhydria, malignant
VIPoma	Verner-Morrison syndrome, D1tumour, diarrhea with hypokalemia, hypochlorhydria (pancreatic cholera)

Whipple's criteria for diagnosis of hypoglycemia

- Symptoms of hypoglycemia
- Serum glucose < 2.8 moles/L
- Prompt relief of symptoms after glucose administration

SPLEEN

- MC cyst of spleen: Pseudocyst
- MC symptom of pseudocyst of spleen:
  - o Left upper quadrant pain
  - o Radiating to shoulder
- Splenunculi:
  - o Single/ multiple accessory spleen
  - o Near the hilum of the spleen commonly

SPLENIC TRAUMA

- Characteristic sign of splenic rupture: Kehr's sign (referred pain) in left shoulder
- Kehr' sign may also be seen in:
  - o Diaphragmatic lesions
  - o Hemoperitoneum etc.
- X-ray features of splenic injury:
  - o Obliteration of splenic shadow
  - o Obliteration of psoas shadow
  - o Elevation of left diaphragm

SPLENECTOMY

- Done in:
  - o Hereditary spherocytosis
  - o Portal hypertension
  - o Hypersplenism etc.
- Splenectomy is not done in:
  - o Hereditary hemolytic anemia
  - o Porphyria etc.
- Splenectomy increases risk for:
  - o Pneumococcal infections
  - o H. Influenzae infections etc.

OVERWHELMING POST-SPLENCETOMY INFECTIONS/ OPSI

- Caused by Streptococcus pneumoniae mostly
- Left lower lobe atelectasis is MC complication

OPSI/ Opportunistic Post Splenectomy Infection

- Streptococcus pneumoniae
- N. meningitides
- H. influenza
- Babesia microti

Blood disorders treatable by splenectomy

- Hereditary spherocytosis
- Hereditary elliptocytosis
- Thalassemia major
- Acquired hemolytic anemia
- ITP
- Idiopathic myelofibrosis
- Opitz's disease

Kehr's sign

- Splenic rupture
- Peritoneal hemorrhage irritates diaphragm, causes referred pain to the left shoulder
- Balance sign: Rupture spleen shows non-shifting dullness in the left flank

Hypersplenism

- Splenomegaly
- Anemia, leucopenia, and thrombocytopenia
- Compensatory bone marrow –hyperplasia
- Improvement after splenectomy
- Banti's syndrome
- Congestive splenomegaly with hypersplenism associated with cirrhosis and portal hypertension

LIVER

Couinaud's segments:

- Based on hepatic vein & portal vein division

- Segment I is caudate lobe
- Segment I has independent vascular supply
- Segment IV is quadrate lobe

PORTAL VEIN

- Formed behind neck of pancreas
- By union of splenic vein & superior mesenteric vein
- Portal hypertension: More than 10 mm Hg
- Sites of porto-systemic anastomosis:
    - o Rectum & anal canal (hemorrhoids)
    - o Lower end of esophagus (varices) etc.

Portal circulation

Normal portal pressure	6-12cm of Hg 10-15 mm of water
Portal hypertension	> 40 mm of Hg

Portosystemic venous shunts

- Anastomoses between veins of falciform ligament and superior and inferior epigastric veins- caput medusae
- Anastomoses between gastric vein and esophageal veins- esophageal varices
- Anastomoses between superior hemorrhoidal vein and middle and inferior rectal veins- hemorrhoids
- Anastomoses between veins of retropeitoneal structures and the body wall (veins of Retzius)

LIVER ABSCESS

Amoebic !iver abscess

- MC site: Right lobe (postero-superior surface)
- Anchovy sauce pus (chocolate coloured pus due to RBC lysis)
- Complications of amoebic liver abscess:
    - o Pleuro-pulmonary involvement
    - o Rupture into pleural space etc.

Pyogenic liver abscess

- Usually single & large
- MC route of infection: Infection through bile duct (hematogenous route is 2nd MC route)

HYDATID DISEASE

- ELISA is sensitive
- No role of blood culture
- Crumbled egg appearance
- PAIR technique is used for management:
    - o **P**ercutaneous **A**spiration
    - o **I**njection of scolicidal agent
    - o **R**easpiration of cyst contents
- Most effective drug: Albendazole

HEPATIC NEOPLASMS

Hepatocellular Ca

- Predisposing factors:
    - o HBV
    - o HCV
    - o Alcoholic liver disease etc.
- Commonest marker for HCC: Alpha Fetoprotein
- Other markers:
    - o Neurotensin
    - o PIVKA 2
- Imaging modality for screening HCC: USG
- Percutaneous biopsy (USG/ CT guided) can be diagnostic

Fibrolamellar Ca

- Not associated with cirrhosis
- Slow growing
- Good prognosis, if treated

LIVER TRANSPLANTATION

Indications

- Biliary atresia (children's)
- Primary sclerosing cholangitis (adults)
- Fulminant hepatitis (adults) etc.

Child –pugh Grading

Features	*1 point*	*2 points*	*3 points*
Encephalopathy	-	Grade1/2	Grade 3,4
Ascites	Absent	Sight	Moderate
Serum bilirubin	1-2 mg	2-3 mg	> 3 mg
Serum albumin	> 3.5 mg	2.8- 3.5 mg	<2.8 mg
Prothrombin time (seconds prolonged)	1-4	4-6	>6

Most common indication for liver transplantation

- Adults: Chronic liver failure
- In children: Biliary atresia is the most common indication

Metabolic diseases, which can be cured by liver transplantation

- Wilson's disease
- Alpha 1 antitrypsin deficiency
- Oxalosis

Hogarth pringle maneuver

- Hepatic artery is compressed between fingers and thumb in lesser omentum through foramen, to stop bleeding from injured cystic artery, when it cannot be controlled by packing, suction and ligation of bleeding artery

Gall stones

	Cholesterol	*Pigmented*	*Mixed*
Number	Single	Multiple	Multiple
Frequency	6-8%	12%	80%
Shape	-	Coral/ mulberry	Faceted, laminated
Formed in	Stasis bladder	-	In infection

CHOLELITHIASIS

- Pigment stones:
  - o Chronic hemolysis
  - o Alcoholic cirrhosis
  - o Chronic biliary tract infection etc.
- Complications of gallstones:
  - o Acute & chronic cholecystitis
  - o Carcinoma of gall bladder
  - o Acute pancreatitis
  - o Gallstone ileus (acute intestinal obstruction) etc.
- CBD stone:
  - o MC cause of obstructive jaundice
  - o On USG, bile duct diameter of more than 6 mm is suggestive of CBD stone
  - o Meniscus sign (cholangiography)

Gall bladder

Condition	*Description*
Pyocele/ empyema	Sterile pus in inflamed obstructed gall bladder
Mucocele	Obstruction of neck of sterile gall bladder by single stone
Limey bile	Due to gradual obstruction of common bile duct
White bile	Not white, opalescent secretion by bile duct with distal obstruction contains mucus, cholesterol and traces or none of bile salts

MISCELLANEOUS (GALL BLADDER)

Gallstone ileus

- MC site of obstruction is: Ileum
- Management: Enterotomy & removal of stone

Acalculous cholecystitis

- Associated with:
  - o DM
  - o Total parenteral nutrition
  - o Major surgeries etc.
- Investigation of choice for acalculous cholecystitis: USG

Hemobilia

- Causes:
  - o Trauma

- o Gallstones etc.
- Triad of hemobilia:
  - o Abdominal pain
  - o Obstructive jaundice &
  - o Melena

Charcot's triad is seen in cholangitis and bile duct stones

- Pain
- Jaundice
- Fever

Hemobilia –triad

- Biliary colic
- Jaundice
- Melaena

Emphysematous cholecystitis

- Associated with presence of gas in the gallbladder
- Seen in diabetics, due to infection with gas forming bacilli
- Ultrasound shows gas in the gallbladder
- Needs to be operated immediately

Structures in free border of lesser peritoneum from anterior to posterior

- Common bile duct
- Hepatic artery
- Portal vein

Saint's triad

- Gallstones
- Diverticulosis coli
- Hiatus hernia

Calot's triangle

- Cystic artery superiorly
- Cystic duct inferiorly
- Common hepatic duct medially
- Contents: Lymph node of Lund

Remember

- Blood supply to the liver is derived 80 percent from portal vein and 20 percent from hepatic artery
- CAROLI's disease - Congenital dilatation of intrahepatic biliary tree
- Caterpillar turn or Moynihan's hump- tortuous right hepatic artery
- Most common route of infection of liver is along the bile ducts followed by via the hepatic artery
- Commonest cause of liver abscess is pyogenic 80 percent
- Honeycomb liver is found in actinomycosis
- In Budd-Chiari syndrome, obstruction occurs at hepatic vein
- Haemangioma is the commonest benign tumour of the liver
- Commonest primary lesion causing metastasis to liver is colon carcinoma, pancreas, and breast
- Gold standard for liver imaging is triple phase spiral CT scan
- Up to 80 percent of liver resection may be tolerated
- Acute cholecystitis - Most commonly caused by E. coli

Renal stones

	Oxalate	*Phosphate*	*Urate*	*Cystine*
Urine	Acid	Alkaline	Acid	Acid
Shape	Mul-berry	Staghorn	Faceted	Hexa-gonal crystals
Number	Single	Single	Many	Many
Hemat-uria	Early	Late	-	-

RENAL CALCULI

- MC stones: Calcium stones (75-85%)
- Radiolucent stones: Uric acid
- Stones MC in men: Calcium
- Renal calculi overlies spine in lateral view

- Dietl's crisis:
  - o Renal colic
  - o Swelling in loin &
  - o Disappearance of swelling with micturition
- Pain in ureteric calculi is due to ureteric peristalsis
- Stones MC in females: Struvite stones
- Stones MC in UTI with urease producing bacteria (proteus spp.): Struvite stones
- Stone which grows in alkaline urine: Struvite stones
- Stone which grows in infected urine: Struvite stone
- Stone hard to break in ESWL: Cysteine stone

Indications of percutaneous nephrolithotomy

- Stones bigger than 3 cm
- Staghorn calculus
- Hard stones
- Anatomic abnormality like scoliosis or obesity
- Stones unresponsive to ESWL
- Coexisting obstructive uropathy

Contraindications to ESWL

- Pregnant women
- Abdominal aortic aneurysm
- Uncorrectable coagulation disorders
- Hard stones
- Stones in poorly draining hydronephrotic kidney

Management of ureteric stones

Upper third	ESWL
Middle third	ESWL/Ureteroscopic removal
Lower third	Ureteroscopic extraction

Triple phosphate stones

- Consists of calcium- ammonium – magnesium phosphate
- Usually formed as a result of inflammation
- Form Staghorn calculus

Three glass urine test

Observation	*Diagnosis*
1st glass is hazy, 2nd is clear	**Urethritis**
If the 1st glass contains thread	**Prostatitis**
If 1st glass is clear, 2nd is cloudy	**Diverticulitis**
If the 2nd glass is cloudier	**Cystitis**

RENAL CELL CA

- Associated with:
  - o Von Hippel Lindau syndrome
  - o Tuberous sclerosis &
  - o Polycystic kidney disease
- MC type of RCC: Clear cell Ca (60%)
- Causes expansile osteolytic lesions
- Paraneoplastic syndromes are seen:
  - o Hypercalcemia
  - o Erythrocytosis
  - o Cushing's syndrome etc.
- MC site of metastasis:
  - o Lung
  - o Followed by soft tissue
- Standard management of stage I or II, few cases of stage III: Radical nephrectomy

URINARY BLADDER Ca

- MC type: Transitional cell Ca
- Pure squamous Ca may be seen in:
  - o Schistosomiasis
  - o Stones
  - o Smoking etc.
- MC symptom: Painless hematuria
- Vaccine used in initial stages (trial): BCG (intravesical)

Chemical	*Associated cancer*
Benzene	Leukemia's
Vinyl chloride	Angiosarcoma of liver
Beta- naphthylamine	Urinary bladder carcinoma
Azo dyes	Hepatoma
Aflatoxin	Hepatoma

Tumors associated with absolute erythrocytosis

- Hypernephroma (renal cell carcinoma)
- Cerebellar hemangioblastoma
- Hepatoma
- Adrenal adenoma
- Pheochromocytoma
- Meningioma
- Uterine fibromyoma

MISCELLANEOUS (EXCRETROY SYSTEM)

- Secondary vesical calculus: Stone formed in urinary bladder after infection
- Tear drop bladder: Pelvic hematoma
- Kiss cancer: Benign tumour of urinary bladder
- Schistosomiasis: Calcification & small contracted urinary bladder
- Terms associated with Tuberculous (urinary system) infection:
  - o Cobble stone appearance
  - o Thimble bladder (long standing cases)
  - o Golf hole ureter

Renal TB

- Sterile pyuria is a consistent feature
- Most sensitive technique for early detection: IVU

Thimble bladder

- Seen in late stages of tuberculosis
- Fibrosis leads to reduced capacity

TB urinary system

- Sterile pyuria is seen in tuberculosis
- Golf hole ureteric orifice is seen in late stages of tuberculosis of urinary system as the ureter is pulled upward

Remember

- Duplication of renal pelvis is the commonest congenital abnormality of the upper tract
- Commonest cause of lower urinary tract infection in boys is posterior urethral valve
- Meatal ulcer with scabbing is the most common cause of acute retention in boys

Urine examination

Feature	*Condition*
Hematospermia (blood in semen)	**Tuberculous prostatitis, chronic seminal vesiculitis**
Drop of blood at the beginning or end of micturition	**BPH**
Uniform, intermittent & painless hematuria	**Lesions of kidney**
Painless, profuse, paroxysmal hematuria for long period	**Vesical neoplasm**
Few drops of blood stained urine or blood stained debris at the end of micturition	**Cystitis**
Few drops of bright red blood at the end of micturition	**Vesical calculus**
Few drops of hematuria at the beginning	**Ulcer**

URETHRA

- MC cause of urethral stricture: Trauma
- Part of urethra injured in pelvic fracture: Membranous urethra
- Mechanism of urethral injury: Fall astride a projecting object (History of blow to perineum)
- Triad of ruptured bulbar urethra (Avoid catheterization):
  - o Retention of urine
  - o Perineal hematoma &
  - o Bleeding from external urinary meatus

POSTERIOR URETHRAL VALVE

- Usually found distal to the verumontanum
- Occurs in males
- MC cause of urinary obstruction in male infant
- Diagnosis is done by: VCUG & endoscopy

TESTICULAR CA

- Bilateral in 10% of cases
- Abdominal cryptorchid testes are at higher risk as compared to inguinal cryptorchid testes
- Testicular feminization syndrome increases the risk of testicular germ cell tumour
- MC Ca of testes in young: Seminoma
- MC Ca in elderly: Lymphoma
- MC Ca in infants: Yolk sac tumour

Highly radiosensitive tumors	*Highly radioresistant*
Seminoma	Hepatoma
Ewing's tumor	Melanoma
Lymphoma	Osteosarcoma
Wilm's tumor	Pancreatic cancer
Multiple myeloma	
Dysgerminoma	

Remember

- Most radiocurable tumor is Hodgkin's disease

Locations of ectopic testis

- Superficial inguinal pounch (commonest)
- In front of the pubis
- Superficial perineal pouch
- Near the Saphenous opening

Undescended testis	*Ectopic testis*
The testis is arrested in its	Testis deviates from its normal path of descent normal path of descent
Usually undeveloped	Fully developed
Scrotum is not well developed	Scrotum is well developed
Spermatogenesis is poor	Spermatogenesis is perfect
May be associated with indirect inguinal hernia	Never associated with indirect inguinal hernia

Seminoma

- Radiosensitive
- Corresponds to dysgerminoma of ovary &
- Treatment of choice is: Surgery

MISCELLANEOUS (GENITOURINARY SYSTEM)

Hypospadias

- Hooded prepuce
- Meatal stenosis
- Bifid scrotum
- Best time of surgery: 6-10 months of age

Paraphimosis

- Complication: Gangrene (due to hampering of venous & lymphatic return from glans)
- May require circumcision (if manipulation fails)

Peyronie's disease

- Hard plaques of fibrosis can be felt in the tunica
- Usually idiopathic
- May be associated with:
    - o Trauma
    - o Dupuytren's contracture
- Histologically similar to keloid or Dupuytren's contracture
- Self limiting

Incomplete descent of testes

- Complication: Malignant change (even if the testes have been brought down surgically)
- Best time to operate: 9-15 months of age

Spermatocele

- Diverticulum of epididymis, which:
    - o Contains fluid (with spermatozoa) resembling barley fluid &
    - o Can be transilluminated

Varicocele

- MC on: Left side
- Negative tranillumination test
- MC cause of male infertility, which is surgically treated

Testicular torsion

- Urine analysis is negative
- Elevation will not decrease the pain (negative Phen's sign)
- Roche's sign
- In torsion of testis, the epididymis cannot be distinguished from the body of the testis, whereas in epididymitis, the body of the testis can be felt in the enlarged crescent of the epididymis
- Operation should not be delayed for more than 4 hours from the time of onset of symptoms

PROSTATE GLAND

- Carcinoma arises from: Peripheral zone
- BPH arises from: Periurethral zone
- MC complication of TURP: Retrograde ejaculation
- Irrigation fluid used in TURP: 1.5% glycine
- Drowsiness & altered sensorium after TURP may point toward: Hyponatremia

PROSTATIC Ca

- McNeal's zone refers to Ca zone,
- Earliest marker/ screening test: PSA
- MC nodes to be affected in lymphatic spread: Obturator
- Metastasis to vertebrae is via: Batson's vertebral venous plexus
- Gleason's staging is used
- Most sensitive test for screening of prostate Ca: Digital rectal examination & PSA

SURGICAL PROCEDURES

- Delorme's procedure: Prolapse rectum
- Anderson Hynes pyeloplasty: Hydronephrosis

MC ABOUT CARCINOMA

- MC esophageal Ca: Squamous cell Ca
- MC site of adenoCa: Lower end
- MC site of squamous cell Ca: Middle third
- MC site of pancreatic tumour: Pancreatic head
- MC symptom of pancreatic Ca: Pain & weight loss
- MC type of rectal Ca: AdenoCa
- MC type of anal Ca: Epidermoid Ca

Indication for operative treatment of penetrating thoracic injuries

- Caked haemothorax
- Large air leaks with inadequate ventilation or persistent collapse of lung
- Drainage of more than 1500 ml of blood when chest tube is first inserted
- Continuous hemorrhage of more than 200 ml per hour for > 3 consecutive hours
- Esophageal perforation
- Pericardial tamponade

Timings of operation

Cleft lip operation	Done at 3-6 months
Cleft palate operation	Done between 6 months to 1.5 years

Remember

- Suture removal after cleft lip operation is done on fifth day.

Conditions related to dental tissue

Epulis	A swelling situated on the gum arising from the alveolar margin
Dental cyst	Associated with chronically infected Pulpless tooth. Always associated with a normally erupted tooth
Dentigerous cyst	Associated with non-erupted permanent tooth. Cyst contains molar tooth
Adamantinoma	True neoplasm of odontogenic epithelium Epithelial tumour arising from ameloblasts

Coagulation system

Vitamin K dependent factors are 2, 7, 9, 10, proteins C and S	
Extrinsic system of coagulation	Factor 7
Common system of coagulation	Factors 1, 2, 5, 10
Intrinsic system of coagulation	Factors 8, 9, 11, 12
PT	Detects deficiency of common and extrinsic system of coagulation. Elevated in deficiency of factors 1, 2, 5, 7, 10 Also elevated in liver disease and early vitamin K Deficiency
PTT (aPTT/ PPTk)	Detects deficiency of intrinsic and common system of coagulation. Elevated in deficiency of factors 1, 2, 5, 8, 9, 10, 11, 12. Also elevated in liver disease and late vitamin K deficiency, Von Willebrand's disease, lupus anticoagulants
Clot solubility in urea	Detects factor 13

Frey's syndrome

- Damage to the auriculotemporal nerve and greater auricular nerve
- On healing there is cross joining, go that when the patient eats, there is sweating in the parotid region

Crocodile tears

- Following facial nerve paralysis, due to inaccurate regrowth of fibers
- So on eating, there is lacrimation

Beck' s triad of cardiac tamponade

- Muffled heart sounds
- Distended neck veins
- Hypotension

Biological fractionation of radiotherapy is explained by

- Repair of sublethal damage
- Repopulation between fractions
- Redistribution of cells in the cell cycle
- Reoxygenation of tumor
- Inherent radiosensitivity
- Recruitment of cells into the proliferating fraction

Remember

- Most radiosensitive portion of cell cycle G2-M phase
- Thimble chamber - Used for detection and measurement of radiation

Penetrating power

- Neutron >Gamma >X-ray>Beta > Alpha (Helium)

Ionizing power and damaging power

- Alpha (Helium) >Beta >X-ray > Gamma

Translocations

Cancer	*Translocation*
CML	**t (9, 22)**
Burkitt's lymphoma	**t (8, 14)**
Ewing's tumour	**t (11, 22)**
Acute promyelocytic leukemia	**t (15, 17)**

Tumor suppressor genes

Rb	Retinoblastoma and osteogenic sarcoma
p53	Many tumors and Li Fraumeni syndrome
Wt 1	Wilms' tumors and aniridia
Nf1	Neurofibromatosis

p53

- p53 is the guardian of genome
- p53 mutation is the most common genetic alteration seen in human cancer
- It is the causative in Li- Fraumeni familial cancer syndrome

Ann Arbor staging for Hodgkin's disease

- Stage I: Involvement of single lymph node region
- Stage II: Involvement of 2 or more lymph node regions on same side of diaphragm
- Stage III Involvement of lymph node region on both sides of diaphragm
- Stage IV Disseminated involvement of one or more extra lymphatic organs with or without

Half lives

Tc-99m	**6 hours**
I-131	**8 days**
I-125	**60 days**
Co-60	**5.2 years**
Ra 226	**1699 years**

Terms

- Pott's puffy tumour is seen in chronic frontal osteomyelitis, it is subperiosteal swelling with edema of scalp
- Dercum's disease/Adiposis dolorosa: Variant of lipoma in which there are tender lipomatosis on the trunk
- Tietze disease: Painful and non-suppurative swelling of 2nd and 3rd costal cartilage
- Fournier's gangrene: Idiopathic gangrene of scrotum, mostly by hemolytic streptococci

Proctalgia fugax

- Intermittent
- Levator muscle spasm
- Painful spasm of anal sphincter which awakens the patient at night

Felon

- Infection of the distal pulp space, usually secondary to a puncture wound
- Late osteomyelitis may develop

Remember

- Enlargement of Krause's nodes (located at jugular foramen) leads to jugular foramen syndrome (compression of 9th, 10th , 11th cranial nerve)
- PSA over 4 ng/ml is abnormal
- Superior vena cava syndrome is most commonly caused by lung cancer
- TURP syndrome is seen due to glycine absorption
- Thymoma is the most common mediastinal tumour
- Most common malignant tumor of the mediastinum is Seminoma
- Honeymoon pyelitis: Acute pyelitis occurring in females soon after marriage
- Seminoma is the most common testicular tumour
- Thrombosis of splenic veins leading to thrombophlebitis splenomegaly
- Hypospadias - Commonest type Glandular
- Champagne urine: Fistula into urinary tract by diverticulosis gives rise to pneumaturia
- Intussusception is the most common cause of intestinal obstruction in children under 2 years of age

Raspberry tumour

- A small part of vitello-intestinal duct remains patent near the umbilicus
- Giving to rise to a mucus-discharging sinus, with its epithelium everted

Common site of metastasis

Tumour	*Metastasis to*
Prostate	Pelvic bones, lumbar vertebrae
Breast	Lumbar vertebrae
Kidney (Wilms tumour)	Lungs (along veins)
Choriocarcinoma	Lungs
Teratoma	Lungs
Lung	Adrenal
Rectum	Liver
GIT	Liver
Seminoma	Aortic lymph nodes

CLINICAL QUESTIONS

1. **A young female presented with a 3×3 cm mass in the right breast, which was freely mobile. Most likely diagnosis:**

   A. Carcinoma breast

   B. Fibroadenoma

   C. Mastitis

   D. Cystosarcoma phyllodes

   Clinical presentation is suggestive of fibroadenoma.

   A fibroadenoma is a very common benign (not cancer) breast condition. Fibroadenomas often develop during puberty so are mostly found in young women.

   Answer: B i.e., Fibroadenoma

2. **A 60 years old smoker male presented with cough, breathlessness and dysphagia. A lump was palpated in the neck. Most likely condition:**

   A. Squamous cell carcinoma of the lung

   B. Adenocarcinoma of the lung

   C. Mixed cell carcinoma of the lung

   D. Large cell carcinoma of the lung

   Clinical presentation is suggestive of squamous cell carcinoma of the lung

   Squamous-cell carcinoma (SCC) of the lung is a histologic type of non-small-cell lung carcinoma (NSCLC). It is the second most prevalent type of lung cancer.

   Answer: A i.e., Squamous cell carcinoma of the lung

3. **A young female was washing clothes in the winter season. She noticed color changes in her hand ranging from white to red. Such a patient would be benefitted by giving:**

   A. Beta adrenergic blockers

   B. ACE inhibitors

   C. Calcium channel blockers

   D. Alpha adrenergic blockers

   Clinical presentation is suggestive of Raynaud's phenomenon.

   Raynaud's phenomenon (RP) is a disorder resulting in vasospasm, a particular series of discolorations of the fingers and/or the toes after exposure to cold.

   Answer: C i.e., Calcium channel blockers

4. **A 12 years old boy came with absence of testis in left scrotal sac. On clinical examination, the testis was found to be in superior inguinal pouch on the left side. This is known as:**

   A. Undescended testis B. Ectopic testis

   C. Retractile testis D. Testicular atrophy

   Clinical presentation is suggestive of ectopic testis.

   Ectopic testis refers to the testis entering a location other than the scrotum after passing the inguinal canal.

   Answer: B i.e., Ectopic testis

5. **A lactating mother presented with pain and swelling in the right lower quadrant of right breast. She was also having fever. Local temperature was raised. USG demonstrated fluid collection. Best management is:**

   A. Antibiotics only B. USG guided aspiration

   C. Incision and drainage D. Excision biopsy

   Clinical presentation is suggestive of breast abscess.

   Breast abscess is a common condition in lactating females. It is painful accumulation of pus that develops from untreated infection.

   Answer: C i.e., Incision and drainage

6. **A 28-year old chronic smoker male is having pain in the legs on walking hardly for 200 meters and then he has to sit down. Previously, he could easily walk around 400 steps, before the pain starts. Most probable cause:**

   A. Prolapsed inter-vertebral disc

   B. Deep venous thrombosis

   C. Buerger's disease

   D. Malingering

   Clinical presentation is suggestive of Buerger's disease.

   Buerger's disease is characterized by narrowing or blockage (occlusion) of the intermediate and/or small sized arteries and veins of the extremities.

   Answer: C i.e., Buerger's disease

7. **Emergency tracheostomy was done in a patient but after the procedure, he developed subcutaneous emphysema. Most likely cause for this:**

A. Blockage of the tube

B. Application of sutures tightly, around the tracheostomy tube

C. Puncture of posterior wall of trachea

D. Wrong level of tracheostomy

One of the rare complications of tracheostomy is retropharyngeal emphysema. A combination of vigorous cough and tight peristomal sutures of the tracheostomy promotes this.

Answer: B i.e., Application of sutures tightly, around the tracheostomy tube

8. **A female patient sustained burn injuries and was brought to the Emergency department. On examination, she was found to have burns involving posterior aspect of neck, whole of back and the gluteal region. Preferred way of management:**

A. Dressing of the wounds only

B. Intravenous antibiotics only

C. Resuscitation followed by skin grafting

D. Wait and watch

A skin graft is a patch of skin that is removed by surgery from one area of the body and transplanted, or attached, to another area.

Answer: C i.e., Resuscitation followed by skin grafting

9. **A patient presented with features if bronchospasm. On evaluation, a tumour was found in ileum. There was increased level of 5-Hydroxy Indole Acetic Acid in urine. Most likely diagnosis:**

A. Carcinoma ileum B. Carcinoid syndrome

C. Carcinoma bronchus D. Bronchial asthma

Clinical presentation is suggestive of carcinoid syndrome.

Carcinoid syndrome is a paraneoplastic syndrome comprising the signs and symptoms that occur secondary to carcinoid tumors. Carcinoid tumors are of neuroendocrine origin and derived from primitive stem cells in the gut wall, especially the appendix.

Answer: B i.e., Carcinoid syndrome

10. **A 48 years old male presented with episodes of palpitations, sweating and headache. On examination, a small left sided supra-renal mass was demonstrated. Next step in confirming the diagnosis:**

A. Urinary VMA level estimation

B. Serum 5-HIAA level estimation

C. Secretin test

D. Short ACTH test

Clinical presentation is suggestive of pheochromocytoma.

A pheochromocytoma is a rare, catecholamine-secreting tumor derived from chromaffin cells.

Answer: A i.e., Urinary VMA level estimation

11. **A chronic alcoholic male has features of chronic liver disease. Now he presented with hematemesis of sudden onset. What could be the most likely cause?**

A. Peptic ulcer disease

B. Mallory-Weiss syndrome

C. Boerhaave's syndrome

D. Esophageal variceal bleed

Clinical presentation is suggestive of esophageal variceal bleed.

Esophageal varices are dilated submucosal distal esophageal veins connecting the portal and systemic circulations.

Answer: D i.e., Esophageal variceal bleed

12. **What should be the immediate management of cystic duct stump leakage after laparoscopic cholecystectomy?**

A. Exploratory laparotomy

B. Antibiotics only

C. ERCP with stent

D. Wait and watch

Cystic duct stump leaks occur in 0.12% of cholecystectomies.

Initial management is typically endoscopic and includes sphincterotomy or biliary stenting.

Answer: C i.e., ERCP with stent

13. **In a 50 years old grocery store cashier, with 9 months history of leg edema, increasing over the course of a workday, associated with moderate to severe lower leg bursting pain, the most appropriate investigation would be:**

A. Doppler USG

B. Brodie- trendelenburg test

C. Ascending and descending phlebography

D. Venous reflux plethysmography

Clinical presentation is suggestive of deep venous thrombosis

Deep vein thrombosis (DVT) is a type of venous thrombosis involving the formation of a blood clot in a deep vein, most commonly in the legs or pelvis.

Doppler ultrasonography is USG technique that employs the Doppler effect to perform imaging of the movement of tissues and body fluids (usually blood), and their relative velocity to the probe.

Duplex ultrasonography sometimes refers to Doppler ultrasonography or spectral Doppler ultrasonography.

Doppler ultrasonography consists of two components: brightness mode (B-mode) showing anatomy of the organs, and Doppler mode (showing blood flow) superimposed on the B-mode.

Answer: A i.e., Doppler USG

14. **An intern was doing saphenous cannulation for a burn patient. After the procedure the patient developed pain along the medial border of the corresponding foot. Which nerve has been accidentally ligated?**

A. Sural nerve

B. Deep peroneal nerve

C. Saphenous nerve

D. Genicular nerve

Clinical presentation is suggestive of injury to saphenous nerve neuralgia.

Saphenous nerve neuralgia is a painful disorder of the saphenous nerve due to damage and/or loss of function in saphenous nerve.

Answer: C i.e., Saphenous nerve

15. **Kalavati, a 40 years old female presented with a progressively increasing lump in the parotid region. On oral examination, the tonsil was pushed medially. Biopsy showed it to be pleomorphic adenoma. Most appropriate management:**

A. Superficial parotidectomy

B. Lumpectomy

C. Conservative total parotidectomy

D. Enucleation

Pleomorphic adenoma, the most common salivary gland tumor, is also known as benign mixed tumors (BMT›s), because of its dual origin from epithelial and myoepithelial elements. It is the commonest of all salivary gland tumors constituting up to two-thirds of all salivary gland tumors.

Answer: C i.e., Conservative total parotidectomy

16. **Cystic spaces lined by double layer of neoplastic epithelial cells resting on dense lymphoid tissue is a feature of:**

A. Dermoid cyst

B. Warthin's tumour

C. Pleomorphic adenoma

D. Hashimoto's thyroiditis

Presentation is suggestive of Warthin's tumour

Warthin tumor is a relatively frequent and benign neoplasm of the major salivary glands. It is histologically characterized by a dense lymphoid stroma and a double layer of oncocytic epithelium with a papillary and cystic architectural pattern. Its etiology remains uncertain.

Answer: B i.e., Warthin's tumour

17. **The tumour which may occur in the residual breast or overlying skin following wide local excision and radiotherapy for breast carcinoma is:**

A. Leiomyosarcoma

B. Squamous cell carcinoma

C. Basal cell carcinoma

D. Angiosarcoma

Clinical presentation is suggestive of angiomyosarcoma.

Angiosarcoma (AS) is a rare and highly aggressive malignant tumor, originating from lymphatic or vascular endothelial-cell. Many times, it's a complication of previous radiation treatment to the breast. It can happen 8-10 years after getting radiation treatment to the breast.

Answer: D i.e., Angiosarcoma

18. A 25 years old woman presents with a firm and mobile lump in the breast. Most likely diagnosis:

A. Fibroadenoma

B. Carcinoma breast

C. Paget's disease of nipple

D. Cystosarcoma

Clinical presentation is suggestive of fibroadenoma/ breast mouse.

A fibroadenoma is a painless, unilateral, benign (non-cancerous) breast tumor that is a solid, not fluid-filled, lump.

Answer: A i.e., Fibroadenoma

19. A 45 years old female has undergone mastectomy for Ca breast. After mastectomy, patient is NOT able to extend, adduct and internally rotate the arm. Nerve supply to which of the following muscle has been damaged:

A. Pectoralis major B. Teres minor

C. Latissimus dorsi D. Long-head of triceps

Clinical presentation is suggestive of paralysis of Latissimus dorsi.

Latissimus Dorsi is one of four muscles responsible for the thoracobrachial motion. It is large, flat and triangular in shape.

The thoracodorsal nerve, a branch of the posterior cord of the brachial plexus (C6 to C8 with C7 predominant) provides innervation to the latissimus dorsi.

Answer: C i.e., Latissimus dorsi

20. Ca breast was operated and followed by radiotherapy in a 50 years old woman. Now she suddenly developed blue nodule on same side of surgery. Most likely diagnosis:

A. Angiosarcoma B. Recurrence

C. Hemangioma D. Cellulitis

Clinical presentation is suggestive of angiosarcoma.

Angiosarcoma (AS) is a rare and highly aggressive malignant tumor, originating from lymphatic or vascular endothelial-cell. Many times, it is a complication of previous radiation treatment to the breast. It can happen 8-10 years after getting radiation treatment to the breast.

Answer: A i.e., Angiosarcoma

21. A 55 years old lady comes with blood-stained discharge from the nipple and a positive family history of breast Ca. Next best step:

A. Ductoscopy

B. Nipple discharge cytology

C. Sono-mammogram

D. MRI

Clinical presentation is suggestive of possibility of carcinoma breast.

MRI is useful in screening females with high-risk group.

Answer: D i.e., MRI

22. A lady noticed mass in her left breast with greenish discharge. Histopathology revealed duct ectasia. Management is:

A. Simple mastectomy B. Microdochectomy

C. Lobectomy D. Hadfield operation

Duct ectasia, also known as mammary duct ectasia, is a benign (non-cancerous) breast condition that occurs when a milk duct in the breast widens and its walls thicken.

Answer: D i.e., Hadfield operation

23. A 26 years old female complains of discharge of blood from a single duct in her breast. Most appropriate treatment is:

A. Radical excision B. Microdochectomy

C. Radical mastectomy D. Biopsy to rule out Ca

Clinical presentation is suggestive of duct papilloma.

Intraductal papillomas are benign (non-cancerous), wart-like tumors that grow within the milk ducts of the breast. They are made up of gland tissue along with fibrous tissue and blood vessels (called fibrovascular tissue).

Answer: B i.e., Microdochectomy

24. A 22 years old female came with a mass in her left breast since past 6 months. There are no associated symptoms. Examination shows a freely mobile mass not attached to the overlying skin or underlying tissue. Most likely diagnosis:

A. Fibroadenoma

B. Cysto-sarcoma phyllodes

C. Scirrhous Ca

D. Fibroadenosis

Clinical presentation is suggestive of fibroadenoma.

A fibroadenoma is a very common benign (not cancer) breast condition. Fibroadenomas often develop during puberty so are mostly found in young women

Answer: A i.e., Fibroadenoma

25. A 50 years old female presented with lump in the left breast, which has developed suddenly in weeks. Peri-menstrual symptoms were present. There is no associated family history. On examination, the lump is well circumscribed, fluctuant, 1.5 cm oval in shape. Most likely diagnosis:

A. Breast cyst B. Galactocele

C. Fibroadenoma D. Breast Ca

Clinical presentation is suggestive of breast cyst

A firm, round lump in breast tissue could be a fluid-filled cyst. Typically, not cancerous, ***breast cysts*** *often need no treatment.*

Answer: A i.e., Breast cyst

26. A 68 years old female underwent right radical mastectomy 10 years back. Now she presents with multiple subcutaneous nodules in the right upper limb. Most likely diagnosis:

A. Lymphangiosarcoma

B. Multiple lipomas

C. Varicose veins

D. Metastasis

Clinical presentation is suggestive of lymphangiosarcoma.

Lymphangiosarcoma is characterized by skin changes in the form of purple colored raised cutaneous lesions progressing to ulceration in a lymphedematous arm within a median of ten years following mastectomy.

Answer: A i.e., Lymphangiosarcoma

27. A 50 years post-menopausal lady was on adjuvant hormonal treatment with Tamoxifen for 3 years for Ca breast. She came to OPD with history of passing blood clots per vaginum. She is probably suffering from:

A. Ca vulva B. Ca vagina

C. Ca endometrium D. Uterine fibroid

Clinical presentation is suggestive of carcinoma endometrium.

Endometrial cancer begins in the lining (endometrium) of the uterus.

Answer: C i.e., Ca endometrium

28. Cystic, compressible and translucent swelling in the posterior triangle of neck is most probably:

A. Cystic hygroma B. Branchial cyst

C. Thyroglossal cyst D. Dermoid cyst

Clinical presentation is suggestive of cystic hygroma.

Cystic hygromas are the cystic variety of lymphangioma, common locations being cervico-facial regions and axilla.

Answer: A i.e., Cystic hygroma

29. A central midline neck swelling is noted in a 5 years old girl, posted for tonsillectomy. The swelling is painless, mobile, and cystic, just below the hyoid bone and measure 2×1.1×1 cm. Ultrasound shows a thick- walled cystic lesion. Management is:

A. Surgical removal

B. Antibiotics

C. Percutaneous aspiration

D. Chest X-ray

Clinical presentation is suggestive of thyroglossal cyst.

A thyroglossal cyst is a fibrous cyst that forms from a persistent thyroglossal duct. Thyroglossal cysts can be defined as an irregular neck mass or a lump.

Answer: A i.e., Surgical removal

30. A 65 years old male with history of weight loss and dysphagia. He can take liquid only. He is a chronic smoker. Most likely diagnosis:

A. Achalasia cardia

B. Barrett's esophagus

C. Carcinoma esophagus

D. Corrosive injury

Clinical presentation is suggestive of carcinoma esophagus.

Answer: C i.e., Carcinoma esophagus

31. An elderly male presents with history of dysphagia, regurgitation, foul breath and cough. Bilateral lung crepitations are noted on examination. Most likely diagnosis:

A. Schatzki's ring

B. Zenker's diverticulum

C. Diffuse esophageal spasm

D. Plummer-Vinson syndrome

Clinical presentation is suggestive of Zenker's diverticulum.

Zenker's diverticulum (ZD) results from posterior herniation of esophageal mucosa into Killian›s triangle, an area of least resistance.

Answer: B i.e., Zenker's diverticulum

32. A 50 years old male presented with occasional dysphagia for solids, regurgitation of food and foul-smelling breath. Most likely diagnosis:

A. Achalasia cardia B. Zenker's diverticulum

C. Carcinoma esophagus D. Diabetic gastroparesis

Clinical presentation is suggestive of Zenker's diverticulum.

A Zenker's diverticulum, also pharyngeal pouch, is a diverticulum of the mucosa of the human pharynx, just above the cricopharyngeal muscle

Answer: B i.e., Zenker's diverticulum

33. A 44 years old patient presented with dysphagia to both liquids and solids and regurgitation for 3 months. The dysphagia was non-progressive. Most likely diagnosis:

A. Carcinoma of esophagus

B. Lower esophageal mucosal rings

C. Achalasia cardia

D. Reflux esophagitis with esophageal stricture

Clinical presentation is suggestive of achalasia cardia.

Achalasia cardia is a rare oesophageal motility disorder caused by autoimmune neurodegeneration of the oesophageal myenteric plexus.

Answer: C i.e., Achalasia cardia

34. An old man presenting to the emergency following a bout of prolonged vomiting with excessive hematemesis following alcohol ingestion is likely to suffer from:

A. Mallory-Weiss syndrome

B. Esophageal varices

C. Gastric carcinoma

D. Bleeding disorder

Clinical presentation is suggestive of Malory Weiss syndrome.

Mallory-Weiss syndrome is characterized by upper gastrointestinal bleeding secondary to longitudinal mucosal lacerations.

Answer: A i.e., Mallory-Weiss syndrome

35. A male executive, 50 years of age is seen in casualty with hypotension and hematemesis. There is previous history of alcohol intake of 100 mL daily. The blood loss is around 2 litres. Most likely diagnosis:

A. Gastritis B. Duodenal ulcer

C. Mallory-Weiss tear D. Esophageal varices

Clinical presentation is suggestive of duodenal ulcer.

A duodenal ulcer is a peptic ulcer that develops in the first part of the small intestine (duodenum).

Answer: B i.e., Duodenal ulcer

36. **A 4 weeks old infant presents with refractory non-bilious vomiting, abdominal distension, poor feeding and lethargy. Most likely diagnosis:**

A. Jejunal atresia

B. Congenital hypertrophic pyloric stenosis

C. Necrotizing enterocolitis

D. Tracheo-esophageal fistula

Clinical presentation is suggestive of congenital hypertrophic pyloric stenosis.

Infantile hypertrophic pyloric stenosis (IHPS) is a disorder of young infants caused by hypertrophy of the pylorus, which can progress to near-complete obstruction of the gastric outlet, leading to forceful vomiting.

Answer: B i.e., Congenital hypertrophic pyloric stenosis

37. **Make the diagnosis of a 26 days old infant presenting with recurrent non-bilious vomiting with constipation and loss of weight:**

A. Esophageal atresia B. Choledochal cyst

C. Ileal atresia D. Pyloric stenosis

Clinical presentation is suggestive of pyloric stenosis.

Pyloric stenosis is a narrowing of the opening from the stomach to the first part of the small intestine (the pylorus).

Answer: D i.e., Pyloric stenosis

38. **A 60 years old male had a sudden fall in the toilet. His BP was 90/ 50 mm Hg and pulse rate of 100/ minute. His relatives said that he is a known case of hypertension and Coronary Artery Disease and is regularly taking aspirin, atenolol and sorbitrate. Most likely diagnosis:**

A. Gastric ulcer with bleeding

B. Acute myocardial infarction with cardiogenic shock

C. Acute cerebrovascular accident

D. Pulmonary embolism

Clinical presentation is suggestive of gastric ulcer with bleeding,

Gastric ulcers are a break in the mucosa of the stomach lining that penetrates through the muscularis mucosa and extends more than 5 mm in diameter.

Answer: A i.e., Gastric ulcer with bleeding

39. **A twenty-eight years old male presents with symptoms of epigastric pain radiating to back those wakes him up at night and is relieved by taking food. He gives history of similar pain in the past which was diagnosed as perforated duodenal ulcer and treated with omental patch surgery on two occasions. Proton pump inhibitors and analgesics have controlled pain before surgery and after surgery. Likely diagnosis on this occasion:**

A. Duodenal ulcer B. Gastric ulcer

C. Atrophic gastritis D. Chronic pancreatitis

Clinical presentation is suggestive of duodenal ulcer.

Duodenal ulcers occur when there is a disruption to the surface of the mucosa of the duodenum. These ulcers are part of peptic ulcer disease

Answer: A i.e., Duodenal ulcer

40. **A female in her twenties presents with complaints of pain abdomen, abdominal distension and vomiting. On examination, she was found to have alopecia and a crepitus in the abdomen. Most likely diagnosis:**

A. Trichobezoar

B. Carcinoma pyloric region

C. Peptic ulcer disease

D. Ascites

Clinical presentation is suggestive of trichobezoar.

Trichobezoar consists of a compact mass of hair occupying the gastric cavity to a various extent.

Answer: A i.e., Trichobezoar

CHAPTER 13

OBSTETRICS

RAPID REVISION NOTES

Physiological changes during pregnancy

Structure/ organ	*Changes*
Skin	Chloasma or pregnancy mask appears on face, striae gravidarum
Breast	Ductal development (estrogen), alveolar development (progesterone), Montgomery tubercles are hypertrophied sebaceous glands
Ovary	Persistent corpus luteum reaches maximum size at 8th week, colloid degeneration at 12th week
Isthmus of uterus	Portion between anatomical and histological internal os; forms lower uterine segment; unfolding of isthmus begins from 12th week; failure of sphincteric action of internal os leads to mid-term abortion
Uterus	Dextro-rotation
Cervix	Levo-rotation

EMBRYOLOGY

- Oogonia are derived from: Yolk sac
- MC site of fertilization: Ampulla
- Zygote reaches uterine cavity at: 16 celled stage
- Placental circulation is established on: 17th day of fertilization
- Vessels in umbilical cord: 2 arteries, 1 vein
- Nitabuch's layer: Zone of fibrinoid degeneration; where trophoblasts & decidua meet (in placenta)

AMNIOTIC FLUID

- Amount at 12 weeks: 50 ml
- Amount at term: 600-800 ml
- It is replaced every: 3 hours
- Green coloured amniotic fluid indicates: Fetal distress
- Causes of oligohydramnios:
  - o Renal agenesis
  - o Multicystic dysplastic kidneys etc.
- Polyhydramnios is seen in:
  - o Esophageal atresia
  - o Duodenal atresia etc.

Amniotic fluid colour & conditions

- Straw: Normal
- Golden colour: Rh incompatibility

- Greenish yellow (saffron): Post-maturity
- Dark coloured: Concealed accidental hemorrhage
- Dark brown (tobacco juice): Intrauterine death
- Meconium stained (green): Fetal distress
- Thick with flakes (pea-soup): Chronic fetal distress
- Purulent: Chorioamnionitis

Polyhydramnios

- Liquor amnii exceeds 2000 ml. OR
- AFI > 20 cm / > 90th percentile for the gestational age

Oligohydramnios

- Liquor amnii is less than 100ml. OR
- AFI < 5 cm/ < 10th percentile for gestational age

CHORIONIC VILLOUS SAMPLING/ CVS

- CVS is preferably done at: 10-12 weeks (transabdominally 10 weeks to term)
- CVS if done before 10 weeks results in: Oromandibular limb defects

Procedure & Preferred time

- Chorionic villous sampling: 10-12 weeks
- Placental villi sampling: > 12 weeks
- Amniocentesis: 14-16 weeks
- Cordocentesis: After 18 weeks

HCG

- HCG is secreted by: Syncytiotrophoblasts
- Structurally HCG has: 2 subunits
- It is a glycoprotein

Shape of uterus

Period	*Shape*
Non-pregnant	Pyriform
12 weeks	Globular
28 weeks	Oval
36 weeks	Spherical

SIGNS OF PREGNANCY

- Congestion of pelvis causing bluish/ purplish hue of vagina/ cervix: Chadwick sign
- Cyanosis & softening of cervix: Goodell's sign
- Compressibility of isthmus on bimanual examination: Hegar's sign
- Softening of cervix with lateral implantation: Piskacek's sign
- Pulsations in lateral vaginal fornix: Osiander's sign
- Rhythmic contractions of uterus: Palmer's sign

DIAGNOSING PREGNANCY

- Earliest detection of pregnancy by USG is by demonstrating: Gestation sac
- Pregnancy is confirmed by:
  - Fetal heart rate
  - Fetal movements
  - Fetal sac on USG

Weight gain

- 1 kg in first trimester
- 5 kg each in second and third trimester

ANTENATAL VISIT

- Minimum number of antenatal visit: 4
- Ideal number of antenatal visits: 12-14

MATERNAL PELVIS

- MC type: Gynaecoid
- Platypelloid/ flat pelvis: Transverse diameter is more than AP diameter
- Least common type of pelvis: Platypelloid
- Deep transverse arrest/ persistent occipito posterior position is common in: Android pelvis
- AP diameter more than transverse diameter: Anthropoid pelvis

- Face to pubis delivery is common in: Anthropoid pelvis
- Shortest diameter of pelvic inlet: Obstetric conjugate

Pelvis

- Naegele's pelvis: Ala on one side is absent
- Robert's pelvis: Ala on both sides is absent

FETAL SKULL

- Shortest diameter of fetal skull: Bimastoid (7.5 cm)
- Largest diameter of fetal skull: Mentovertical (14 cm)

Diameter

- Bimastoid: 7.5 cm
- Bitemporal: 8 cm
- Submento –bregmatic: 9.5 cm
- Biparietal: 9.5 cm
- Suboccipto-bregmatic: 9.5 cm
- Suboccipto-frontal: 10 cm
- Occipito-frontal: 11.5 cm
- Sub-mento-vertical: 11.5 cm
- Mentovertical: 14 cm

ENGAGING DIAMETER & PRESENTATION

- Presentation is defined as: Fetal part which lie over the inlet
- Presentation in Sub-mento-vertical diameter: Face
- Presentation in Sub-mento-bregmatic diameter: Face
- Presentation in Sub-occipito-bregmatic & Sub-occipito-frontal diameter: Vertex (MC type of vertex presentation: Left Occipito-Anterior)

PLACENTA

- Placenta succenturiata: One or more small lobes of placenta, size of a cotyledon, may be placed at varying distances, from the main placental margin
- Placenta extrachorialis Circumvallate placenta-The fetal surface of placenta shows a central zone surrounded by a thickened white ring, which is composed of double fold of amnion
- Placenta marginata: A thin fibrous ring is present at the margin of the chorionic plate where fetal vessels appear to terminate
- Placenta membranacea: Unduly large and thin placenta
- Battledore placenta: Cord is attached to the martin of placenta
- Velamentous placenta: Cord is attached to membranes
- Placenta accrete: Placenta is directly anchored to the myometrium, partially or completely without intervening decidua
- Placenta increta: Varying degree of penetration of the villi into the muscle bundles
- Placenta percreta: Penetration of the villi up to the serosal surface

BISHOP SCORING

- Used for labour
- Total score of 13
- 6-13 is favourable
- 5 or less is unfavourable
- Includes:
    - Dilatation of cervix
    - Effacement of cervix
    - Consistency of cervix
    - Position of cervix
    - Station of head
- Partogram is:
    - Graphical representation of stages of labour
    - Assessment of labour
- Cervicograph is: Graph showing relationship between cervical dilatation & labour

Manning's score

- Non-stress test
- Breathing movement – At least 1 in 30 minutes for 30 seconds duration
- At least 3 fetal movements in 30 minutes

- Fetal tone: At least 1 in 30 min
- Adequacy of amniotic fluid
- Maximum score – 10
    - o 10-8 is Normal
    - o 6 is Equivocal
    - o 4 or less is Abnormal

STAGES OF LABOR

- 1st stage: Onset of labor to dilatation of cervix
    - o 6-20 hours in primigravida
    - o 2-10 hours in multigravida
- 2nd stage: From full dilatation of cervix to complete birth of baby
- 3rd stage: Birth of infant to delivery of placenta

Prolonged latent phase of labor

- Latent phase exceeds:
    - o 20 hours in primigravida and
    - o 14 hours in multigravida

Prolonged labour

- Combined duration of first and second stage is more than 18 hours
- Labour is considered to be prolonged when:
    - o Cervical dilatation rate is less than 1 cm/hr
    - o Descent is less than 1 cm/hr for a period of more than 4hrs

Precipitate labour

- Combined duration of the first and second stage is less than 2 hours

Premature rupture of membranes

- Spontaneous rupture of membranes:
    - o Any time beyond 28th week of pregnancy
    - o But before the onset of labour

LOCHIA

- L. rubra: Reddish (1-4 days)
- L. serosa: Yellowish (5-9 days)
- L. alba: Pale white (10-15 days)

Puerperium

Condition	*Time of appearance*
Post-partum pituitary necrosis	**4th to 20th day**
Mastitis parenchymatosa	**10-20 days**
Thrombophlebitis	**15-20 days**
Deep phlebothrombosis	**7th to 10th day**
Superficial phlebothrombosis	**4th to 5th day**
Post-puerperal infection, fever	**2nd or 3rd day**

PUERPERIUM

- Puerperium lasts for: 6 weeks after delivery
- Uterus becomes a pelvic organ after: 2 weeks of delivery
- Involution of uterus is complete by: 6 weeks
- MC cause of puerperal infection: Streptococcus
- MC route of spread of puerperal infection: Direct spread

ABORTION

- Definition: Expulsion of fetus less than 500 gms/ before 20 weeks
- Causes of 1st trimester abortion:
    - o Chromosomal aberrations
    - o Embryonic defect etc.
- MC cause of 1st trimester abortion: Trisomy
    - o MC is trisomy 16 amongst all trisomies
- Management of cervical incompetence:
    - o Shirodkar's procedure
    - o McDonald's procedure etc.
- Female with recurrent abortion & raised APTT is suggestive of: Antiphospholipid antibody syndrome

Inevitable abortion

- It's a clinical type of abortion where the changes have progressed from where continuation of pregnancy is impossible
- Increased vaginal bleeding

- Dilated internal os, through which products of conception are felt

Incomplete abortion

- Entire products of conception are not expelled but a part of it is left inside the uterine cavity
- Persistence of vaginal bleeding
- Patulous cervical os

Threatened abortion

- Process of abortion has started but has not reached stage, form where recovery is impossible
- External os is closed
- Slight vaginal bleeding
- USG indicates a healthy fetus
- Fetal cardiac movements are present SS

Complete abortion

- Products of conception are expelled en masse
- Vaginal bleeding is absent /trace, following expulsion
- Cervical os is closed

Missed abortion/ Silent miscarriage

- When the fetus is dead and retained inside the uterus for a vaginal discharge
- Absent fetal heart sounds
- Cervix firm
- Empty gestational sac

ECTOPIC PREGNANCY/ EP

- Ectopic pregnancy is associated with:
    - o Tubal disease (MC cause)
    - o Endometriosis
    - o PID
    - o Progestasert etc.
- MC presentation of EP is: Pain
- Expelled products in EP have origin from: Decidua vera
- MC type of EP which ruptures is: Isthmic
- Medical management of EP:
    - o Methotrexate
    - o Actinomycin-D etc.
- Surgery for unruptured tubal pregnancy: Salpingostomy
- Clinical presentation of EP:
    - o A young girl with 8 weeks amenorrhea & presenting with shock
    - o A young girl with 6 weeks amenorrhea with abdominal mass & empty uterus on USG
    - o A young girl with 6 weeks amenorrhea with abdominal pain & fluid in pouch of douglas, aspiration of which reveals a dark coloured fluid which doesn't clot

HYDATID MOLE

- Investigation of choice to diagnose H. mole: USG
- H. mole is associated with:
    - o PIH
    - o Thyrotoxicosis
    - o Hyperemesis
- Treatment of choice: Suction – evacuation
- Histological feature of H. mole: Hydropic degeneration
- Molar pregnancy is usually diagnosed in: 1st trimester

Hydatidiform mole/ vesicular mole

- Incomplete H. mole: Focal affection of the chorionic villi
- Complete H. mole: Have only placental parts, as sperm fertilizes an empty ovum
- Complete H. moles have 46 XX karyotype (molar chromosomes derived entirely from the father)
- MC presentation: Vaginal bleeding
- White currant in red currant juice: Blood may be mixed with fluid from the ruptured cysts
- USG findings: Snow storm appearance and bunch of grapes appearance
- High HCG titre
- Routine follow-up must be done for at least 1 year (by regularly checking beta-HCG levels, and chest X-rays)

Risk factors for development of choriocarcinoma

- Risk of development of choriocarcinoma: 2-10%
- Initial HCG level in urine > 1 lac IU/hour
- Histologically proven infiltrative mole
- Previous history of molar pregnancy
- Age > 35 years
- Parity >3

Development of fetus

Time	*Remark*
12th week	Sex of the fetus can be determined; maternal IgG crosses placenta
16th week	Lanugo hair appears
20th week	Sebaceous gland appears, meconium appears
24th week	Surfactant appears in lungs

TWIN PREGNANCY

- MC type on conjoined twins: Thoracophagus
- MC cause of mortality in twins is: Prematurity

Indications of medical management in ectopic pregnancy

- Hemodynamically stable patient
- Unruptured pregnancy
- Gestational sac size <3.5 cm in diameter
- HCG < 2500 IU/ml

Maneuvers in breech

Maneuver	*Indication*
Marshall burns technique, Mauriceau-Smellie-viet technique	Delivery of after-coming head in breech presentation
Lovset's maneuver	Delivery of extended arms in breech

COMPLICATED PREGNANCY

- Procedures for delivery of head in breech presentation:
  - o Burn Marshall technique
  - o Maureciau-Smeille-Veit method etc.
- Management of shoulder dystocia:
  - o Apply suprapubic pressure
  - o McRoberts procedure (legs in flexion) etc.

RETRACTION RING

- Eponym: Bandl's ring
- Cause: Obstructed labor
- Tenderness: Present
- Palpation: Fetal parts not felt; Ring felt; Round ligaments felt
- FHS usually absent
- Vaginal Examination: Ring is not felt
- Location: Always at junction of upper and lower segment; Progressively moves upward
- Management: To relieve obstruction

Constriction ring

- Eponym: Schroeder's ring
- Cause: Undue irritability of uterus
- Location: Usually at the junction of Upper and lower segment; May occur at other places; Position doesn't alter
- Tenderness: Absent
- Palpation: Fetal parts felt; Ring not felt; Round ligament not felt
- Fetal Heart Sounds present
- Vaginal Examination: Ring is felt
- Management: To relax ring after delivery of body

Rh INCOMAPTIBILITY

- Also known as: Immune hydrops/ IH
- Earliest sign of IH on USG: Skin edema
- Feto-maternal transfusion is detected by: Kleihauer-Betke test
- Prognosis depends upon: S. bilirubin
- Management is:
  - o Immediate cord ligation
  - o Anti-D to mother (with 72 hours)

HEART DISEASES/ HD & PREGNANCY

- MC HD associated with pregnancy: Mitral stenosis/ MS
- HD carrying worst prognosis in pregnancy: Eisenmenger complex
- HD showing highest mortality: Eisenmenger complex
- Pathological murmur heard in pregnancy: Diastolic murmur
- Conditions in which pregnancy is to be terminated:
  - o Primary pulmonary HTN
  - o Eisenmenger syndrome etc.

HIV & PREGNANCY

- Incidence of perinatal transmission of HIV can be reduced by:
  - o LSCS
  - o Antiretroviral prophylaxis (zidovudine)
  - o Avoid breast feeding
  - o Intrapartum nevirapine etc.

DIABETES & PREGNANCY

Effects of pregnancy on diabetes

- More insulin is required
- Progression & worsening of diabetic nephropathy

Effects of diabetes on mother

- Chorioamnionitis
- Endometritis
- Postpartum bleeding
- Increased risk of death in patients with diabetic Cardiomyopathy.

WHO criteria for diagnosis of gestational diabetes mellitus

- Fasting:
  - o Normal values: Less than 105
  - o Impaired glucose tolerance: 105-139
  - o Diabetes: More than 140
- 2 hours post glucose administration:
  - o Normal values: Less than 160
  - o Impaired glucose tolerance: 160-199
  - o Diabetes: More than 200

HYPERTENSION IN PREGNANCY

- Earliest sign is: Raised BP
- Can be predicted by: Rolling over test
- Eclampsia is defined as:
  - o HTN
  - o Proteinuria &
  - o Convulsions
  - o Edema
- MC eclampsia is: Antepartum
- Cause of convulsion in eclampsia is: Cerebral anoxia
- Earliest sign of PIH: Rapid gain in weight
- Sudden loss of vision in PIH is due to: Retinal detachment
- Treatment for eclampsia: Magnesium sulphate
- Toxicity of $MgSO_4$ is monitored by:
  - o Urinary output
  - o Respiratory rate
  - o Knee jerk
- DOC in severe pre-eclampsia: Labetalol
- Complications of pre-eclampsia:
  - o Cerebral hemorrhage
  - o Pulmonary hemorrhage etc.
- Drugs absolutely C/I in pregnancy: ACE inhibitors

Diagnostic Criteria of PIH

- Hypertension:
  - o An absolute rise of blood pressure of at least 140/90 mm Hg, OR
  - o A rise in systolic blood pressure of atleast 30 mm Hg, over the previously known blood pressure

  - A rise of 20 mm Hg MAP over the previous reading, OR
  - When the MAP is 105 mm Hg, of more
  - The rise of blood pressure should be evident at least on two occasions, at least 4 hours apart
- Edema:
  - Pitting edema over the ankles, after 12 hours of bed rest, Or
  - Rapid gain of weight of more than 1 pound/ week, or more than 5 pound a month
- Proteinuria:
  - Protein in 24 hours urine, of more than 0.3 gm OR
  - More than 1 gm per litre
  - In 2 or more midstream specimens
  - Obtained 6 hours apart
  - In the absence of UTI

HELLP syndrome

- **H**emolysis
- **E**levated **L**iver enzymes
- **L**ow **P**latelet count
- A complication of PIH

Pritchard's Regime

- Magnesium sulphate- 4 gm IV and 10 gm deep IM, 5 gm in alternate buttocks 4 hourly
- Repeat injection only after ensuring
  - Urine output is more than 30 ml/ hour
  - Respiration rate is > 12/ minute
  - Knee jerk is present
- Therapeutic level of serum magnesium is 4-7 mEq/l

PLACENTA PRAEVIA

- Type I (lateral):
  - Major part of placenta is attached to the upper segment and
  - Only lower margin encroaches onto the lower segment
  - But not upto the os
  - Up to 5 cm above the os
- Type II (marginal):
  - Placenta reaches the internal os
  - But does not cover it
- Type III (Incomplete central):
  - Placenta completely covers the internal os when close
  - But does not entirely do so when fully dilated.
- Type IV (central):
  - Placenta completely covers the internal os even after it is fully dilated
- Mild placenta praevia: Type I and II anterior
- Major degree: Type II posterior, Type III and IV
- Dangerous placenta praevia:
  - Type II posterior
  - As it prevents engagement of the head, preventing the compression of the separated placenta to stop bleeding.

Placenta praevia

- Painless, causeless, recurrent bleeding
- Fetal heart sounds usually present
- Placenta is present in lower segment, so malpresentation is common
- Bleeding is always revealed
- Uterus is soft and relaxed

ABRUPTIO PLACENTAE

- Painful, due to pre-eclampsia or trauma, continuous bleeding
- Fetal heart sounds usually absent
- Placenta is present in upper segment
- No Malpresentation
- Bleeding may be revealed, concealed or mixed
- Uterus is tense, tender, and rigid

POST PARTUM HEMORRHAGE

- MC cause of PPH: Atonic uterus (grand multipara, prolonged labor etc.)
- PPH is said to occur if: Blood loss is more than 500 cc
- Drugs used for PPH:
  - o Misoprostol
  - o Ergometrine etc.

UTERINE INVERSION

- Cause of uterine inversion: Mismanaged 3rd stage of labor
- Complications of 3rd stage of labor:
  - o Hemorrhage (MC)
  - o Neurogenic shock etc.

IDIOPATHIC CHOLESTASIS OF PREGNANCY/ ICP

- ICP occurs in: Last/ 3rd trimester
- MC symptom: Generalized pruritus
- ICP shows raised serum levels of:
  - o Alkaline phosphatase
  - o ALT & AST etc.
- Treatment of ICP: Urso-deoxy-cholic acid/ ursodiol

FETAL HEART RATE/ FHR

- Early deceleration in FHR shows: Head compression
- Late deceleration in FHR is indicative of:
  - o Placental insufficiency
  - o Fetal distress
- Variable deceleration: Cord compression

Amniotic fluid indicators of fetal maturity

- Creatinine > 2mg/ 100 ml
- Orange colored cells > 50% when stained with 0.1 percent Nile blue sulphate
- Osmolarity of 250 mosmol/litre
- L:S ratio of >2
- Identification of phosphatidyl glycerol
- Optical density difference (at 650 m) greater than 0.15

BIOPHYSICAL PROFILE/ BPP

- BPP predicts:
  - o +/– of fetal asphyxia
  - o Risk of fetal death in antenatal period
- Parameters in BPP: 5 components
  - o Includes FBM, FBM i.e.
  - o Breathing & body movements of fetus

DRUGS IN PREGNANCY

Indicated

- Propylthiouracil
- INH

C/I

- Streptomycin
- Primaquine
- Valproate (causes NTD)
- Methotrexate
- Yellow fever vaccine

MATERNAL SERUM ALPHA-FETO-PROTEIN

Raised in

- Wrong gestational age
- Anterior abdominal wall defects
- Open neural defects
- Multiple pregnancy
- Renal anomalies
- IUFD

Lowered in

- Trisomies

Triple test

- Used in detection of Down's syndrome

- Low MSAFP
- High HCG
- Low Estriol

INFECTIONS

Organisms crossing placenta

- Syphilis
- Parvovirus
- Hepatitis B and C
- Toxoplasma
- Rubella
- HIV
- CMV

TORCH

- Toxoplasmosis
- Others (syphilis, tuberculosis)
- Rubella
- Cytomegalovirus
- Herpes

Toxoplasmosis transplacental transmission

- First trimester:
    - o Low incidence of transplacental infection
    - o But disease is more severe
- Third trimester:
    - o High incidence of transmission
    - o But severity is less

VERSION

External version

- Conversion is done by External manipulation only
- Done for Breech presentation and Transverse lie

Internal version

- Done in Transverse lie in case of second baby of twins
- Conversion is done by one hand introduced into the uterus and the other on the abdomen

FORCEPS APPLICATION

Indications

- Delay in the second stage of labor
- Low birth weight baby
- Postmaturity
- Maternal distress
- Appearance of fetal distress
- Cord prolapse
- After coming head of breech
- Pre-eclampsia
- Post-caesarean pregnancy

Conditions to be fulfilled

- Membranes must have ruptured
- Head must be engaged; station must be > +2
- No obstruction should be present
- Suitable presentation and position
- Cervix must be fully dilated and effaced
- Live baby
- Uterus should be actively contracting and relaxing

Advantages of forceps over ventouse

- Useful in suspected pelvic contraction
- Quicker, hence more useful in fetal distress
- Safer in premature babies
- Can be used in face presentation and after coming head of breech
- Incidence of hemorrhages in fetus is less

VENTOUSE

Indications

- As an alternative to forceps operation
- Deep transverse arrest with adequate pelvis
- Delay in descent of head of the second baby of twins

- Delay in first stage due to uterine inertia or primary cervical dystocia

Contraindications

- Prematurity
- Head not engaged
- Fetal distress
- Pelvic contraction
- Transverse lie
- After coming head of breech
- Partially dilated cervix
- Congenital anomalies
- Dead fetus

Complications

- Cephalohematoma
- Subaponeurotic or subgaleal haemorrhage
- Chignon
- Retinal hemorrhage

Advantages of ventouse over forceps

- It can be applied through incompletely dilated cervix (atleast 6 cm)
- Not space occupying
- Can be used in unrotated and malrotated Occipito-posterior position
- Lesser traction force required
- Can be applied at higher station

CAESAREAN SECTION

Indications of classical caesarean section

- Previous classical cesarean section
- Neglected shoulder with anhydramnios
- Structural abnormality making approach to lower segment difficult
- Constriction ring due to neglected labor
- Fibroids in lower segment
- Anterior placenta accreta and praevia
- Postmortem caesarean section
- Very preterm fetus, where lower segment is poorly formed

Contraindications of caesarean section

- Dead fetus
- Baby so premature that it can't survive ex-utero
- Presence of blood-coagulation disorders

Indication of caesarean section

Absolute indications	*Relative*
Central placenta previa	Cephalopelvic disproportion
Severe degree of contracted pelvis	Previous uterine scar
Cervical or broad ligament fibroid	Fetal distress during first stage of labour
Advanced carcinoma cervix	Abnormal uterine contraction In severe degree of placenta previa In lesser degree Of placenta previa when bleeding continues despite low rupture of membranes Abruptio placentae Malpresentation –transverse lie brow, mentoposterior Position. Bad obstetric history Hypertensive disorders- acute fulminating pre-eclampsia not responding to treatment Uncontrolled eclampsia Failed surgical induction Elderly primigravidae Medical gynaecological disorders-chronic hypertension or chronic nephritis Uncontrolled diabetes Uncorrected heart disease Pelvic tumours Vaginal atresia

Naegele's formula

- If the periods are regular
- Add 9 months and 7 days to the first days to the first day of the last menstrual cycle
- If the cycle length is more than 28 days, then extra days are to be added, if less, then they should be subtracted

Intrauterine fetal death

- Blair Hartley's sign: Attitude of hyperextension or hyperflexion of fetal body. Seen after 3-4 weeks
- Robert's sign: Gas translucencies are seen in fetal heart and great vessels. Seen after 12 hours
- Halo sign of Deuel: Radiolucent halo around fetal cranium, due to edema of pericranial fat. Seen after 2 days
- Helix sign: Presence of gas in umbilical cord

Terms

- Superfecundation: Fertilization of two ova released in same menstrual cycles, by separate acts of coitus, within a short period of time
- Superfetation: Fertilization of two ova related in different menstrual cycles

Physiological causes of hyperprolactinemia

- Early morning/sleep
- High protein meal
- Stress, physical or psychological
- Late follicular phase of menstrual cycle
- Pregnancy, suckling
- Prolonged breast manipulation
- Coitus
- Exercise

Changes in fetal circulation at birth

Structure	*Functional closure*	*Anatomical closure*
Foramen ovale	At birth	1 year
Ductus arteriosus	At birth, after establishment of pulmonary circulation	1-3 month
Umbilical vein	A little later than arteries	-
Umbilical arteries	At birth	2-3 month

CLINICAL QUESTIONS

1. **A 25 years old lady with a 24 months baby has heavy irregular bleeding during menstruation. The baby is on breast feed. Which of the following contraceptive agent is advised to such a patient?**

   A. Depot formulation   B. Cu-T 380A

   C. Progestasert   D. Mala-N

   Here we need to prescribe an agent, which serves 3 purposes: Contraception, relief in menorrhagia without affecting lactation.

   Depot formulation/ Injectable progestins include DMPA (like depot medroxy-progesterone acetate) and NET-EN (norethisterone enanthate).

   Advantages: It can be used safely during lactation.

   Menstrual symptoms e.g., menorrhagia and dysmenorrhoea are reduced.

   Answer: A i.e., Depot formulation

2. **A primigravida pregnant lady was in labor with a fetus in right occipito-posterior presentation. Uterine contractions are good. Next step in management of such a patient:**

   A. Cesarean section

   B. Wait and watch for normal vaginal delivery

   C. Start oxytocin drip

   D. Forceps delivery

   In otherwise uncomplicated cases of occipito-posterior position, the labor is allowed to proceed in a manner similar to normal labor.

   Favorable factor includes good uterine contractions and favorable pelvis (gynecoid).

   Occipito-posterior position per se is not an indication of cesarean section.

   Answer: B i.e., Wait and watch for normal vaginal delivery

3. **On 7th day of a normal vaginal delivery, a lady was brought to the emergency department at midnight with the complaints of loss of appetite, depression, difficulty in sleeping and occasional crying. General examination and pelvic examination were normal. What could be the most likely diagnosis?**

   A. Puerperal blues   B. Postpartum depression

   C. Postpartum psychosis   D. Postpartum insomnia

   Puerperal blues/ Baby blues is observed 4-5 days after delivery and presents as depression, anxiety, tearfulness, insomnia, helplessness and negative feelings toward the infant.

   Answer: A i.e., Postpartum blues

4. **A 25 years old lady complains of right sided lower abdominal pain and mild bleeding per vaginum for one day after a period of amenorrhoea of 6 weeks. Her general condition is satisfactory and the vitals were stable. There is tenderness in the right iliac fossa. HCG level was 1400 IU/ ml. Transvaginal ultrasound scan does not reveal any adnexal mass or any intrauterine pregnancy but the uterus was bulky and trilaminar endometrium was seen. There was no fluid in the pouch of Douglas. What is the next best step in management?**

   A. Perform a laparoscopic examination

   B. Repeat beta-HCG after 48 hours

   C. Repeat USG after a week

   D. Give progesterone

   Clinical history is indicative of an ectopic pregnancy since there is no intrauterine pregnancy.

   A trilaminar appearance of endometrium has 94% specificity but 40% sensitivity to diagnose ectopic pregnancy.

   Transvaginal sonography provides visualization of a well-formed intrauterine gestational sac as early as 4-5 weeks from the last menstrual period. The lowest level of serum beta-HCG at which a gestational sac is consistently visible using TVS (discriminatory zone) is 1,500 IU/ L. The corresponding value of serum beta-HCG for transabdominal sonography is 6,000 IU/ L.

   (1) When the beta-HCG value is greater than 1,500 IU/ L and there is an empty uterine cavity, ectopic pregnancy is more likely.

   (2) Failure to double the value of beta-HCG by 48 hours along with an empty uterus is very much suggestive of ectopic pregnancy.

   So, in the given MCQ, we would repeat the beta-HCG values after 48 hours to see whether it doubles or not. If it fails to double, then it's an indicator of ectopic pregnancy (as per criteria number 2).

   Answer: B i.e., Repeat beta-HCG after 48 hours

5. **A primigravida with full term pregnancy and in labor presented with sign and symptoms of dehydration. Her heart rate was 105 beats/ minute and a BP of 130/ 90 mm of Hg. Per abdominal examination showed a fundal height of 32 weeks and the fetus was having right occipito transverse position. Fetal heart sounds were feeble and mild uterine contractions were felt. Per vaginal examination revealed a fully dilated cervix, head is at the level of ischial spine, caput was present and moulding was also present. Pelvis was found to be inadequate. What will be the most appropriate management of such a case?**

A. Injection oxytocin

B. Lower segment cesarean section

C. Ventouse delivery

D. Forceps application

Clinical history suggests the diagnosis of deep transverse arrest.

The head is deep into the cavity; the sagittal suture is placed in the transverse bispinous diameter and there is no progress in descent of the head even after half to one hour following full dilatation of cervix.

When vaginal delivery is not found to be safe as in case of big baby or inadequate pelvis, perform cesarean section.

Operative vaginal delivery (Ventouse or forceps) for DTA should only be performed by a skilled obstetrician. Otherwise, cesarean delivery is always preferred.

Answer: B i.e., Lower segment cesarean section

6. **A pregnant lady with 32 weeks pregnancy develops hypertension and edema. Urine examination shows presence of protein. Treating doctor suspected it to be a case of preeclampsia. Which of the following theory defines it?**

A. Incomplete invasion of extra-villous cytotrophoblast into uterine artery

B. Incomplete invasion of extra-villous cytotrophoblast into radial artery

C. Incomplete invasion of extra-villous cytotrophoblast into basal artery

D. Incomplete invasion of extra-villous cytotrophoblast into spiral artery

Normally placenta has villi and intervillous spaces. The villi are lined by trophoblast and into the villi, open fetal blood capillaries.

In the intervillous space, spiral arterioles carrying maternal blood open.

The endovascular trophoblast replaces the lining of these maternal spiral arteries, making them low resistance, low pressure and high flow vessels.

In PIH, this trophoblastic invasion is incomplete, so maternal blood vessels have high resistance and high pressure causing PIH.

Answer: D i.e., Incomplete invasion of extra-villous cytotrophoblast into spiral artery

7. **A lady with 22 weeks of pregnancy presented with lower abdominal pain and severe vaginal bleeding. A clinical diagnosis of unruptured ectopic pregnancy was made. Most likely site of implantation is:**

A. Fallopian tube B. Ovary

C. Abdomen D. Cervix

Abdominal pregnancy can continue up to term.

Isthmic ectopic pregnancy rupture usually occurs at 6-8 weeks, the ampullary one at 8-12 weeks and the interstitial one at about 4 months.

Answer: C i.e., Abdomen

8. **Blood test reports of a 24 weeks pregnant lady revealed AST & ALT >70 IU/ L, bilirubin >1.2 mg/ dL and platelet counts 90,000/ mm^3. Most likely diagnosis:**

A. Obstructive jaundice

B. Viral hepatitis

C. HELLP syndrome

D. Dengue hemorrhagic fever

HELLP syndrome is an acronym for Hemolysis, Elevated Liver enzymes and Low Platelets (below 100,000/ mm^3). This is a rare complication of preeclampsia (10-15%).

Parenchymal necrosis of liver causes elevation in hepatic enzymes and bilirubin.

Answer: C i.e., HELLP syndrome

9. A lady with pre-eclampsia presented to the Emergency department with absent patellar reflexes and bilateral plantar reflexes. She was having a respiratory rate of 11 breaths/ minute and decreased urinary output. On auscultation, lung fields were clear. Her random blood sugar value was 210 mg/ dl. Most likely diagnosis:

A. Magnesium sulphate toxicity

B. Eclampsia

C. HELLP syndrome

D. Diabetes mellitus

Magnesium toxicity and serum magnesium levels: (a) Loss of deep tendon reflexes at more than 7 mEq/ L; (b) Respiratory depression at more 10 mEq/ L and (c) Cardiac arrest at magnesium levels of more than 25 mEq/L.

Answer: A i.e., Magnesium sulphate toxicity

10. A 26 years old primipara with normal BMI attended the antenatal clinic. She is having amenorrhoea of 35 weeks and a single live fetus in breech presentation. USG demonstrated complete breech presentation and adequate liquor volume. There was no other abnormality on USG scan. Her pregnancy is otherwise uncomplicated. What should be done next?

A. Perform an elective cesarean section at 39 weeks of pregnancy

B. Perform an external cephalic version at 36 weeks of pregnancy

C. Perform normal vaginal delivery at term

D. Induction of labor, if not delivered till 40 weeks

Everything is normal so ECV can be attempted. Successful version is likely in cases of complete breech, non-engaged breech, adequate liquor, sacro-anterior posterior position (fetal back anteriorly) and non-obese patient.

Answer: B i.e., Perform an external cephalic version at 36 weeks of pregnancy

11. A 24 years old primigravida had post-partum hemorrhage, hypotension, shock and disseminated intravascular coagulation following normal vaginal delivery of a full-term healthy infant. Uterus is well contracted and hard. Fetus is normal. Most likely diagnosis:

A. Amniotic fluid embolism

B. Ruptured uterus

C. Vaginal laceration

D. Uterine atony

Features of shock and DIC goes in favour of the diagnosis of amniotic fluid embolism.

Liquor amnii is forced into the maternal circulation either through a rent in the membranes or placenta. Thromboplastin rich liquor amnii containing the debris, blocks the pulmonary arteries and triggers the complex coagulation mechanism leading to DIC.

Amniotic fluid embolism is one important cause of extracardiac shock in obstetrics.

Answer: A i.e., Amniotic fluid embolism

12. A known case of cervical incompetence with previous abortion presented at 12 weeks of pregnancy. Doctor planned her for cerclage operation. Which of the following is an absolute contraindication for cervical cerclage operation:

A. Previous abortion

B. Bag of water projecting into vagina

C. Rupture of membranes

D. Previous history of ectopic pregnancy

Contraindications of cerclage operation: (1) Intrauterine infection. (ii) Ruptured membranes. (iii) Presence of vaginal bleeding. (iv) Severe uterine irritability. (v) Cervical dilatation greater than 4 cm. (vi) Fetal death or defect.

Answer: C i.e., Rupture of membranes

CHAPTER 14

GYNECOLOGY

RAPID REVISION NOTES

Development of structures

	Female	*Male*
Mesonephros	Epoophoron, paroophoron	Efferent ducts, head of epididymis, paradidymis, aberrant ductules
Mesonephric duct	Gartner's duct, urethra	Vas deferens, ejaculatory duct, prostatic urethra
Mullerian duct	Fallopian tubes, uterus, upper 2/3rd of vagina	Appendix of testes, prostate
Genital swelling	Labia majora	Scrotum
Urethral folds	Labia minora	Penile urethra

EMBRYOLOGY

- Genital ridge forms: Ovary
- Genital tubercle forms: Clitoris
- Genital folds forms: Labia minora
- Labia swelling forms: Labia majora

Development of vagina

- Upper 4/5th, above the hymen is developed from: Mucus membrane from endoderm of the canalized sinovaginal bulbs
- Musculature: from the mesoderm of two fused Mullerian ducts
- Lower 1/5th, below the Hymen is developed from: Endoderm of the urogenital sinus.

Rokitansky–kuster–Hauser syndrome

- Congenital hypoplasia/ absence of vagina in combination with an abnormal or absent uterus
- Second most common cause of primary amenorrhoea
- Gonadal dysgenesis is the most common cause of primary amenorrhoea

ANATOMY

Fallopian tube

- Lined by: Ciliated columnar epithelium
- Length: 10 cms

Female urethra

- Length: 4 cm/ 40 mm (diameter: 6 mm)
- Lining: Transitional epithelium

Fallopian tube has four parts

- Interstitial (narrowest part)
- Isthmus

- Ampullary (fertilization taken place here)
- Infundibulum

Female genital tract

- Uterus measures 8cm and weighs 50-80gm
- Female urethra measures 4cm
- Gland of Cloquet or Rosenmuller–uppermost deep femoral gland

Uterine position

Anteversion	Long axis of the uterus is bent forward on the long axis of vagina, making an angle of 90 degree
Anteflexion	Long axis of the body of uterus is bent forward at the level of internal os with the long axis of the cervix, ma king an angle of 120 degrees

PHYSIOLOGY

- Best predictor of ovulation: Pre-ovulatory rise in progesterone
- In normal menstrual cycle, progesterone is secreted by: Corpus luteum
- Inhibin is secreted by: Graafian follicle
- LH precedes ovulation by: 24 hours (Ovulation coincides with LH surge)
- Ovulatory period: Corresponds to 14 days before next menstruation
- FSH stimulates: Growth of granulosa cells (measure of ovarian reserve)
- LH stimulates: Follicle rupture & ovulation

Common sites in vagina

Lesion/ procedure	*Site*
Spontaneous tear	Upper part of posterior wall
Coital tear	Anterior wall
Implantation cyst	Posterior vaginal wall
Gartner duct cyst	Upper part of anterior wall
Secondary's	Suburethral
Carcinoma	Upper third of posterior vaginal wall
Biopsy for carcinoma	Posterior fornix
Biopsy for hormonal changes	Upper part of lateral walls

VAGINA

- It lacks mucus secreting glands
- Clue cells in vagina, fishy odour, positive Whiff test signifies: Infection with Hemophilus vaginalis (bacterial vaginosis)
- Senile vaginitis is due to: Estrogen deficiency
- Protective bacterium in normal vagina: Lactobacillus

Doderlein's bacillus

- It appears on vagina after birth, then disappears by 10-14 days; to reappear at puberty and then disappears at menopause
- It converts glycogen present in vaginal mucosa into lactic acid, to maintain acidic vaginal pH which protects against infection by pathogenic organisms

VAGINAL DISCHARGE

- Foamy, frothy discharge & motile trophozoites (flagellate protozoa with motility): Trichomonas vaginalis
- Pruritus, vulvovaginitis, cottage-cheese discharge: Candidiasis
- pH less than 5, clue cells, amine odour: Bacterial vaginosis
- Urethral discharge, gram negative diplococci in PMN's: N. Gonorrhea
- Culture negative specimen with inclusion bodies: Chlamydiae trachomatis
- Urease positive organism without cell wall: Ureaplasma urealyticum

CHANCROID

- Presents as:
  - o Genital ulcer (painful)
  - o Inguinal adenitis

- Culture appearance: School of fish appearance
- DOC: Ceftriaxone

CANDIDIASIS

- Presentation:
    - o Profuse curdy
    - o White discharge (cottage cheese appearance)
    - o Intense itching

TRICHOMONIASIS

- Caused by: Trichomonas vaginalis (flagellate parasite)
- Clinical presentation:
    - o Profuse
    - o Thin
    - o Greeny discharge (malodourous)
- Appearance of vagina: Strawberry vagina/ Colpitis macularis appearance
- DOC: Metronidazole

BACTERIAL VAGINOSIS

- Caused by: Multi-bacterial (Hemophilus vaginalis, Gardnerella vaginalis etc.)
- Clinical presentation:
    - o Milky
    - o Homogenous &
    - o Adherent discharge
- Vaginal pH: Alkaline (greater than 4.5)
- Histological feature: Clue cells
- DOC: Metronidazole

LYMPHOGRANULOMA VENERUM/ LGV

- Clinical presentation:
    - o Esthiomene (Chronic ulcerated state of vulva & clitoris)
    - o Genital elephantiasis
- The 'groove sign' characteristic of LGV (if both the inguinal and the femoral nodes are involved)
- DOC: Doxycycline

GENITAL TB

- MC site of primary infection: Lungs (50%)
- MC site of affection in genital TB: Fallopian tubes

Fern test

- Cervical mucus shows characteristic fern pattern on microscopic examination, during the estrogenic phase of cycle
- It is due to sodium chloride in mucus
- It disappears after 21 days

ENDOMETRIOSIS

- MC in: Nullipara
- MC accepted etiological theory: Sampson's theory of retrograde menstruation
- MC presentation: Pelvic pain
- Associated feature: Chocolate cysts
- Treatment:
    - o Progesterone
    - o Clomiphene (in fertile women)
    - o GnRH analogues
- Surgical procedures: Ovarian cystectomy/ oophorectomy/ wedge resection

Failure rates of contraceptive agents

Method	*Failure rates (per 100 woman years)*
Douching	40
Spermicidal agents	30
Coitus interruptus	25
Rhythma method	25
Condoms	10-14
Dutch cap	4-6
IUCD	2-6
Mini pills	2-3
Norplant	1.1
Combined oral pills	0.1

CONTRACEPTION

- Contraceptive for post partum: Lactational amenorrhea
- Ideal contraceptive for newly married couple: OCP
- Ideal contraceptive for couple staying away & meeting occasionally: Barrier contraception
- OCP of choice in lactating females is: Mini pill

Missed oral pills

Problem	*Solution*
One pill missed	Two pills next day (one in the morning, one in the evening)
Three pills forgotten	Use additional method for that cycle

OCP

- Protects against:
    - o Uterine Ca
    - o Ovarian Ca
    - o RA
    - o Endometriosis etc.

OCP	*Progestin*	*Oestrogen*
Mala N	Norgestrel 30 μg	Ethinyl estradiol 30 μg
Ovral L	Levonorgestrel μg	Ethinyl estradiol 30 μg
Mala D	D-Norgestrel 30 μg	Ethinyl estradiol 30 μg
Femilon	Desonorgestrel μg	Ethinyl estradiol 20 μg

Contraindications to use of OCP

Absolute	*Relative*
Thromboembolism	Hypertension
Active liver disease	Diabetes
Liver adenoma	Epilepsy
Gall bladder disease	Smokers over 35
Cholestatic jaundice	Age over 45
During pregnancy	Obesity
Surgery within 1 month	Lactation
General/ breast carcinoma	Past liver disease
Focal migraine	Recent history of depression Adolescence Sickle cell disease Hyperlipidemia

OC pills

Tumors associated	*Provides protection*
Cervical cancer	Ovarian tumors
Hepatic adenoma	Uterine tumors
Pituitary adenoma	Benign breast disease

Oral pills

Following child birth, start	After 6 weeks (preferably at the conclusion of first menstruation)
After procured abortion, start pills	From 5th day
Protection starts from	2nd course
After discontinuation of oral pills, ovulation returns after	3 months (in 98%)

Centchroman /Saheli

- Nonhormonal OCP
- Dose 30 mg twice weekly for 3 months then once a week
- Weak estrogenic and potent antiestrogenic effect
- Suppresses endometrial proliferation
- Interferes endometrial with nidation of embryo
- Can be used in DUB and emergency contraception

Half lives

Cu-T 200/ Cu-T 200B/ Multiload Cu 250	**3 years**
Cu T- 380 A	**10 years**
Nova T	**5 years**
Progestasert	**1 years**
LNG- IUS	**5 years**

Timing for IUCD insertion

- Postmenstrual day 4/5
- Postabortal after MTP

Indications of MTP

- S- Social
- H-Humanitarian
- E- Eugenic fetal anomalies
- L- Life saving
- F- Failure of contraception

Indications of therapeutic termination of pregnancy

- Primary pulmonary hypertension
- Eisenmenger's syndrome
- Pulmonary veno-occlusive disease

Failure rates of sterilization procedures

Method	*Failure rates (per 100 woman years)*
Hysteroscopic sterilization	**15**
Laparoscopic sterilization	**0.6**
Minilap	**0.4**

STERILIZATION

- Criteria for sterilization:
  - o Age of female > 22 years
  - o Male < 60 years
  - o Couple should have at least 2 children
- MC site for laparoscopic sterilization (female): Isthmus
- Portion ligated in Pomeroy's method (female sterilization): Isthmo-ampullary portion

PROLAPSE

- Cystocele is: Prolapse of upper 2/3rd of anterior vaginal wall
- Complications: Decubitus ulcers (due to venous congestion) etc.
- Management of prolapsed in women < 40 years with complete family; wanting to retain menstrual function: Fothergill's repair
- Management in young women:
  - o Sling operation
  - o Perineal exercises
- Management in 2nd trimester: Spontaneous resolution
- Management in 1st trimester: Pessary

Degree of retroversion

- First degree: Fundus is vertical and pointing towards the sacral promontory
- Second degree: Fundus lies in the sacral hollow but not below the internal os
- Third degree: Fundus lies below the level of internal os

Degrees of uterine prolapse

- First degree: Uterus descends from the normal position
- Second degree: External os protrudes outside the vaginal introitus but the uterine body still remains inside the vagina
- Third degree procidentia/ complete prolapsed: Uterine body descends to lie outside the introitus

Indications of pessary treatment

- Early pregnancy, up to 18 weeks
- Patients unfit for surgery
- Puerperium
- Patients unwilling of surgery
- Patients waiting to complete family

Menstrual cycle

Feature	*Seen in*
Regeneration of endometrium	**48 hours after cessation of menses**
Saw tooth appearance seen in	**Late secretory phase**
Corkscrew appearance is seen in	**Late secretory phase**
Telescoped glands are seen in	**Late proliferative phase**
Spear shaped/ Assegai shaped cells are seen in	**Secretory phase**

MENSTRUATION

- Amount of blood loss in menstruation: 20-80 ml (Average 50 ml)
- Premature menopause: When menstruation ceases before 40 years of age
- MC cause of post menopausal bleeding in India:
  - o Indiscriminate use of Hormonal Replacement Therapy
  - o Ca endometrium
- MC cause of secondary amenorrhea in India: Endometrial TB

- Primary amenorrhea: Failure of menses in a girl by 16 years of age

DYSFUNCTIONAL UTERINE BLEEDING/ DUB

- Associated with: Metropathia hemorrhagica
- Commonly endometrium in DUB is: Hyperplastic (irregular shedding, irregular ripening)
- Hormonal status:
  - o Increased estrogen
  - o Deficient progesterone

Metropathia hemorrhagica/ Schroeder's disease

- Cystic glandular hyperplasia
- Swiss cheese appearance of endometrium on microscopy

Terms

- Menorrhagia (Hypermenorrhoea): Excess and /or prolonged bleeding
- Epimenorrhoea (polymenorrhoea): <21 days
- Oligomenorrhoea: >35 days
- Hypomenorrhoea: Scant bleeding
- Metrorrhagia: Irregular, Acyclic bleeding

Mittelschmerz

- Lower abdominal pain cyclically 2 weeks before menstruation (in mid menstrual period)

MULLERIAN AGENESIS/ 46XX

- Normal ovarian functions (cyclic ovulation), Absence/ hypoplasia of vagina

CLINICAL PRESENTATIONS

- Girl with cystic swelling at the junction of lower 1/3rd & upper 2/3rd of anterior vaginal wall (10 O'clock): Gartner cyst
- 16-year old girl with primary amenorrhea, feminized breast, has no pubic hairs. USG shows no uterus & ovaries & blind vagina: Testicular feminization syndrome
- An 11-year old girl has primary amenorrhea with absent breast & malformed uterus: Turner syndrome
- A girl with primary amenorrhea has normal ovaries, absent internal genitalia but normal external genitalia: Mullerian agenesis

Swellings

- Cystic swelling at junction of lower1/3rd and upper 2/3rd of vaginal wall should be Gartner's duct
- Cystic swelling at the junction of posterior 1/3rd and anterior 2/3rd of labium majus should be Bartholin's cyst

Follicular ovarian cyst

- Arises due to failure of rupture of follicle
- Usually unilateral
- Spontaneously disappear within 2 months

Remember

- Corpus luteal cyst appears due to failure of regression of corpus luteum in14 days. It can cause delayed mense
- LH surge precedes ovulation by 24-36 hours
- Subnuclear vacuole seen on day 16 is the first sign of ovulation

CERVICAL Ca

- Arises from: Squamo-columnar junction
- Earliest symptom: Post-coital bleeding
- MC site: Ectocervix
- MC agent: Human Papilloma Virus 16
- Other type of HPV which are associated with cervical Ca: HPV 18, 31, 45, 51, 52 & 53
- Predisposing factors: HPV, HSV & HIV infections
- Lymph nodes affected: Obturator, hypogastric & external iliac
- Time taken for conversion of CIN to invasive Ca: 10 years
- MC type: Squamous cell Ca
- Best method for diagnosing: Cervical biopsy

- 100% cure rates are seen in: CIS
- MC cause of death: Renal failure
- Best method of screening: Pap smear
- Management of stage II (disease extends beyond cervix, but not to the pelvic wall/ lower third of vagina):
    - o Extended hysterectomy
    - o Chemotherapy &
    - o Intracavitary brachytherapy
- Stage III is: Disease extends to the pelvic wall or lower third of the vagina or causes hydronephrosis
- Management of stage IIIB:
    - o Radiotherapy &
    - o Chemotherapy

Pap smears is used to diagnose

- HPV
- Herpes infection
- Trichomoniasis
- Cervical cancer
- It is taken from posterior part of vaginal wall
- For hormonal cytological evaluation it is taken from lateral part of vaginal wall

Histological findings

Call Exner bodies	Granulosa cell tumor
Reinke's crystal	Hilus cell tumor
Signet ring	Krukenberg tumor
Schiller-Duval bodies	Endodermal sinus tumor
Psammoma bodies	Serous cystadenocarcinoma

Remember

- Meig's syndrome – Fibroma
- Pseudo-Meig's syndrome - Brenner tumor
- Clue cells – diagnostic of bacterial vaginosis
- Strawberry appearance of vagina is seen in Trichomoniasis
- Endometrial biopsy is done between 21st – 23rd days of menstrual cycle; If cycle is irregular then, it is done within 24 hours period
- Fibroid is the most common pelvic tumour
- Mucinous cystadenoma- is the largest benign ovarian tumour
- Commonest site of endometriosis is ovary
- Premature ovarian failure, when before 40 years

FIBROID

- Red degeneration of fibroid:
    - o Seen in 2nd half of pregnancy or puerperium
    - o Due to thrombosis of large veins of the tumour
    - o Infection has no role (this process is an aseptic one)
- Management is conservative (analgesics & sedatives)
- Fibroids are associated with:
    - o Follicular ovarian cysts
    - o Endometriosis
    - o Endometrial hyperplasia
    - o Endometrial Ca
- MC type of fibroid: Intramural/ interstitial
- MC type of degeneration: Hyaline (starts from the centre)
- MC to undergo malignant change: Intramural
- MC to undergo calcareous degeneration: Subserous
- Most fibroid starts as: Interstitial fibroids

ENDOMETRIAL CARCINOMA

- MC type: Adenocarcinoma (upto 80%)
- Most malignant type: Clear cell Ca
- Predisposing factors:
    - o Family history
    - o Obesity
    - o DM
    - o Tamoxifen therapy
    - o PCOD
- Adjuvant radiotherapy is given in cases of:
    - o Deep myometrial involvement

- o Ca In Situ/ CIS
- o Lymph node involvement etc.
- MC cause of endometrial Ca: Unopposed estrogen
- Treatment of atypical endometrial hyperplasia: Hysterectomy (panhysterectomy in elderly)

Age incidence of tumours

Tumour	*Age group*
Pseudo-mucinous cystadenoma	**30-60 years**
Dermoid	**20-30 & 40-50 years**
Dysgerminoma	**Childhood**
Fibroma	**30-40 years**
Secondary ovarian carcinoma	**35-50 years**
Adenocarcinoma uterus	**50-55 years**
Carcinoma cervix	**45-50 years**
Sarcoma uterus	**40-50 years**

OVARIAN TUMOURS

- Meig's syndrome:
  - o Ascites
  - o Hydrothorax (right side) &
  - o Benign tumour of ovary (fibroma)
- Malignant ovarian tumour is included in: Pseudomeig syndrome
- Masculinizing ovarian tumours:
  - o Hilus cell tumour
  - o Sertoli cell tumour
  - o Leydig cell tumour
- Feminizing cell tumour:
  - o Theca cell tumour
  - o Granulosa cell tumour
- MC ovarian tumour (in < 20 years): Dysgerminoma
- Most radiosensitive ovarian tumour: Dysgerminoma

HISTOLOGICAL FEATURES & OVARIAN TUMOURS

- Rokitansky bodies: Teratoma
- Schiller Duval bodies: Endodermal sinus tumour
- Reinke's crystal: Hilus cell tumour
- Call Exner bodies: Granulosa cell tumour

Ovarian tumours

Cut section of teratoma shows	Peculiar trabeculated appearance
Brenner tumour is	Always yellow
Commonest complication of operations on ovarian tumours	Post-operative bleeding
Most common complication of ovarian cyst	Torsion
Tumour producing features resembling metropathia hemorrhagica (Schroeder's disease)	Granulose cell tumour
Dermoid cyst usually co-exst with	Pseudo-mucinous cystadenoma
Secondary's from ovarian tumour earliest goes to	Peritoneum
Commonest primary for krukenberg tumour	Stomach carcinoma (70%)
Commonest malignancy	Serous papillomatous, cystadenocarcinoma
Krukenberg tumours	Atypical secondary's, due to retrograde lymphatic spread, signet ring cells on histology, freely mobile, always bilateral, no adhesions
Reinke crystal are seen in	Hilus cell tumour, leydig/ interstitial cell tumour
Meig's syndrome occurs with	Fibroma
Unilateral malignant tumours	Arrhenoblastoma, Brenner tumour, theca cell tumour, malignant melanoma
Largest, commonest and torsion is a common complication of	Pseudo-mucinous cystadenoma

OVARIAN TUMOURS & MARKERS

- Placental alkaline phosphatase: Dysgerminoma

- LDH: Dysgerminoma
- Inhibin: Granulosa cell tumour
- CA 125: Ovarian tumours

DRUGS IN GYNAECOLOGY

Clomiphene

- Antiestrogenic effect
- Chances of pregnancy are increased (3 fold)
- Risk of ectopic pregnancy is increased (6-10 fold)
- Used in the treatment of:
  - o PCOS (Stein Levinthal syndrome) &
  - o Infertility in males with oligospermia

Normal sperm values

- Volume: > 2ml
- Sperm: > 20 million / ml
- Motility: > 50 percent
- Morphology: > 30 percent normal forms

Terms

- Infertility is inability of a couple to achieve conception after 1 year of unprotected sex
- Oligospermia / Oligozoospermia: Count is less than 20 million spermatozoa per ml
- Polyzoospermia: When the count is more than 350 million per ml
- Azoospermia: No spermatozoa in the semen
- Asthenospermia: Means reduction in the vitality of spermatozoa
- Necrospermia/ Necrozoospermia: Condition in which the spermatozoa are dead or motionless
- Teratospermia/ teratozoospermia: Presence of high number of malformed spermatozoa in the semen

Semen

- Normal pH 7.5
- Seminal vesicle contributes to the bulk of volume
- Also contributes fructose, which is source of energy
- Prostate alkalinizes semen, contributes clotting enzyme and fibrinolysin

Clomiphene

Indicated in	*Contraindicated in*
Anovulatory infertility	Ovarian cyst
Polycystic ovarian disease associated with infertility	Chronic liver disease
In in vitro fertilization, GIFT technique and ART	Scotoma

Tamoxifen

- Non steroidal antiestrogenic

Danazol

- Androgen derivative
- Gonadotropin inhibitor
- Used in:
  - o Endometriosis
  - o Cyclic & non-cyclic mastalgia
  - o Primary menorrhagia
  - o Precocious puberty etc.

Other drugs

- Antitubercular C/I in pregnancy:
  - o Streptomycin
  - o Pyrazinamide

Precocious & delayed

- Precocious menstruation: If menstruation starts before the child reaches the age of 10
- Precocious puberty: Appearance of appropriate secondary characters before the age of 8 years in girls
- Delayed puberty: Breast tissue and/ or pubic hair have not appeared by 13-14 years or menarche has not occurred by 16 years.

Timing of test in infertility

Procedure	*Time of menstrual cycle*
Fern test	Before 21 days (negative after that)
Vaginal cytology and endometrial cytology	21-28 days
Cervical mucus (profuse and spinnbarkeit)	Ovulation time
Air insufflation & hysterosalpingogram	5th – 14th day
Biopsy in TB endometritis	Pre- menstrual phase

CONDITIONS & PRESENTATIONS

Teratoma

- 25 years old female
- Abdominal pain & adnexal mass
- USG shows:
    - o Heterogeneous
    - o Well circumscribed mass with
    - o Solid & cystic components and
    - o Dense calcification

Turner syndrome

- 16 years female with amenorrhea
- Webbed neck
- Low hair line &
- Widely spaced nipples
- USG showing streaky gonads (ovaries)

Turner's syndrome

- 45 X
- Gonads are streaky
- Sex chromatin study is negative
- Hypergonadotropic hypogonadism
- Presents with primary amenorrhoea with delayed appearance of secondary sexual characteristics

McCune-Albright syndrome

- Sexual precocity
- Multiple cystic bone lesions
- Endocrinopathies
- Café-au-lait spots on the skin

Klinefelter's syndrome

- Sex chromatin is positive
- Karyotype is XXY or XXXY
- Small and underdeveloped male genitalia
- Eunuchoid appearance
- Gynecomastia
- Azoospermia

Androgen insensitivity syndrome/ testicular feminization

- X-linked recessive inheritance
- Testicular feminization syndrome is the most common from of male intersex
- Primary amenorrheoea phenotypically and psychologically females with adequate breast development
- Absence of axillary and pubic hair. Normal external genitalia
- Short and blind vagina
- Testes are placed in labia, inguinal canal or abdomen
- Sex chromatin is negative
- Karyotype is 46,XY
- Normal testosterone level

Endometrial Ca

- 60 years female
- Hypertensive & DM with
- Vaginal bleeding

Sheehan syndrome

- 24 year female
- 2 weeks after delivery with
- Inability to breast feed her baby
- Weakness & fatiguability with
- Low ACTH, LH, FSH

Condyloma acuminata (HPV)

- 28 years female with
- Soft, pinkish, cauliflower like lesions
- H/O multiple partners
- Responding to Imiquimod

Toxic shock syndrome

- Female with fever
- Hypotension
- Skin rash
- Headache &
- Diarrhea and altered mental status
- H/O using vaginal tampon

Adenomyosis

- 35 years female with
- Dysmenorrhea
- Menorrhagia
- Chronic pelvic pain
- Symmetrically enlarged uterus
- Smooth & tender on palpation

Endometriosis

- 36 years female
- Dysmenorrhea
- Dyspareunia with
- Fixed retroverted uterus &
- Nodularity of uterosacral ligaments

Premenstrual syndrome

- 20 years female with irritability
- Breast tenderness
- Headache & bloating before menstrual cycles

Ovarian Ca

- 60 years female with
- Abdominal & pelvic swelling
- Increased CA 125 level

Bacterial vaginosis

- 28 years female, with
- Profuse watery
- Dirty grey discharge
- Positive Whiff test

Herpes simplex II/ herpes genitalis

- 24 years female with
- Paraesthesia
- Burning pain in perineal area &
- Vesicles showing Cowdry inclusions
- Painful inguinal lympho-adenopathy

Trichomonas vaginalis

- 28 years female with
- Foul smelling
- Frothy
- Light green coloured vaginal discharge
- Strawberry cervix &
- Vaginal erythema

PCOD

- 21 years obese female with
- Irregular menses
- Acne
- Insulin resistance &
- Raised LH:FSH ratio

Diagnostic criteria of PCOS

Major

- Chronic anovulation
- Hyperandrogenism
- Clinical signs of hyperandrogenism
- Exclusion of other etiologies

Minor

- Insulin resistance
- Perimenarchal onest of Hirsutism and obesity
- Elevated LH to FSH ratio

- Intermittent anovulation associated with hyperandrogenism

Ultrasound criteria

- Increased ovarian area/ volume
- 10-15 microcytes organized in a peripheral rosary pattern
- Increased echogenicity of ovarian stroma

Stein- Leventhal syndrome

- Increased androgens
- Increased estrogens
- Increased LH
- Increased GNRH
- Decreased FSH
- Hirsutism and Amenorrhoea
- Decreased ovarian follicular maturation
- HAIR-AN syndrome – hyperandrogenism, insulin resistance, acanthosis nigricans
- LH: FSH ratio is > than 3:1
- Treatment:
    - o Clomiphene
    - o Surgical resection

Incontinence

- Stress incontinence: Leakage of urine coincides with stress. No prior urge to void. Small amount. Patient aware Micturition is normal
- Urge incontinence: Unable to control escape of urine once there is urge to void. Large amount. Patient aware Urgency and frequency
- Detrusor instability: Incompetence may occur abruptly without a full bladder. Large amount. Patient no aware Frequency and nocturia

Triple swab test for fistulas

- Uppermost swab: Placed in vaginal vault
- Second in middle part
- Third: Placed in the lower part, just above introitus
- Methylene blue dye is instilled in the bladder

Results

- Ureterovaginal fistula: Uppermost swab soaked with urine but unstained with dye, lower two swabs remain dry
- Vesicovaginal fistula: Upper and lower swabs remain dry but the middle swab stained with dye
- Urethrovaginal fistula: Upper two swabs remain dry but the lower swab stained with Dye

Fistula	*Symptoms*
Ureterovaginal	Urge present. Can pass urine normally
Vesicovaginal	Urge absent
Urethrovaginal	Urge present. Cannot pass urine normally

Remember

- Vesicovaginal fistula is the commonest genitourinary fistula
- Most commonly caused by obstructed labour in developing countries and following operative injury in developed countries

Mode of action of contraceptives

Mode of contraception	*Action*
IUCD	Anti-implantation effect on blastocyst and foreign body reaction in endometrium
Injectable contraceptive	Suppression of ovulation
Combined pill	Inhibition of ovulation
Mini pill	Alteration in cervical mucus, endometrium & fallopian tube

CLINICAL QUESTIONS

1. **A 35 years old nulliparous woman complains of menorrhagia and mass per abdomen. On examination, the positive findings are: she is anaemic, has a pelvic mass of 16-18 weeks size, firm in consistency, which moves with the movement of cervix. What is the most likely clinical diagnosis?**

   A. Leiomyoma

   B. Adenomyosis

   C. Endometrial carcinoma

   D. Ovarian tumour

   Uterine fibroids are leiomyomata of the uterine smooth muscle. As other leiomyomata, they are benign, but may lead to excessive menstrual bleeding (menorrhagia), often cause anemia and may lead to infertility.

   Answer: A i.e., Leiomyoma

2. **A 58 years old woman, post menopausal for last 8 years, comes with history of spotting per vaginum. What is the most likely cause?**

   A. Endometrial hyperplasia

   B. Endometrial carcinoma

   C. Atrophic endometritis

   D. Estrogen replacement therapy

   Atrophic endometritis is the most common cause of postmenopausal bleeding (66.67%), followed by endometrial carcinoma (13. 6%) and endometrial polyp (11.6%).

   Answer: C i.e., Atrophic endometritis

3. **A diabetic obese patient comes with history of post-menopausal bleeding. On examination, there is a supra pubic mass and per vagina there is purulent discharge. The probable diagnosis is:**

   A. Carcinoma cervix

   B. Carcinoma endometrium

   C. Uterine myoma

   D. Ovarian carcinoma

   Approximately 40% of cases of endometrial carcinoma are related to obesity. Endometrial cancer is also associated with excessive estrogen exposure, high blood pressure and diabetes. Whereas taking estrogen alone increases the risk of endometrial cancer, taking both estrogen and a progestogen in combination, as in most birth control pills, decreases the risk.

   Answer: B i.e., Carcinoma endometrium

4. **For a woman who has had unprotected intercourse two days ago, which one of the following emergency contraceptive methods *cannot* be suggested?**

   A. LNG IUD (LNg IUD)

   B. Ulipristal acetate

   C. Levonorgestrel 150 mg

   D. Yuzpe regimen

   Methods of emergency contraception/ post-coital contraception include hormones (morning-after pills: levonorgestrel, 0.75 mg, two doses given at 12 hours interval; two tablets (150 mg) can be taken as a single dose also), copper IUCD, combined hormonal regimen (Yuzpe method), anti-progesterone (RU 486-Mifepristone) and ulipristal acetate.

   Answer: A i.e., LNG IUD (LNg IUD)

5. **A 35 years old married woman with no risk factors for cervical cancer is having Pap smear showing 'atypical squamous cells of undermined significance (ASCUS)' for the first time. What is the further step in the management?**

   A. Repeat Pap immediately

   B. Cryotherapy

   C. Large loop excision of the transformation zone

   D. To follow up with Pap test at 6 months

   Atypical squamous cells of undetermined significance (ASCUS): Squamous cells are thin and flat and grow on the surface of a healthy cervix. In the case of ASCUS, the Pap smear reveals slightly abnormal squamous cells, but the changes don't clearly suggest that precancerous cells are present, so repeat pap smear.

   Answer: D i.e., To follow up with Pap test at 6 months

6. For a primary amenorrhoea individual having an XY karyotype, normal infantile female external and internal genitalia fibrous bands in place of gonad, lack of development of secondary sexual characters, what is the most probable diagnosis?

A. Testicular feminization syndrome

B. Mixed gonadal dysgenesis

C. Swyer syndrome

D. Defective anti-mullerian hormone

Swyer syndrome, or XY gonadal dysgenesis, is a type of hypogonadism in a person whose karyotype is 46, XY. The person is externally female with streak gonads, and if left untreated, will not experience puberty. Such gonads are typically surgically removed (as they have a significant risk of developing tumors) and a typical medical treatment would include hormone replacement therapy.

Answer: C i.e., Swyer syndrome

7. A lady who is using oral contraceptive pills comes with a complaint of vaginal discharge and pruritus vulvae. On local examination, there is curdy white discharge from the vagina. What is the most likely clinical diagnosis?

A. Trichomonal vaginitis B. Monilial vaginitis

C. Gardnerella vaginalis D. Atrophic vaginitis

Candidial infection of the vagina or vulva may cause severe itching, burning, soreness, irritation, and a whitish or whitish-gray cottage cheese-like discharge.

Answer: B i.e., Monilial vaginitis

8. A 30 years old female has severe dysmenorrhoea and dyspareunia. On examination, uterus is 8 weeks size, uniformly enlarged and there is tenderness in posterior fornix. What is the most probable diagnosis?

A. Fibroid uterus

B. Dysfunctional uterine bleeding

C. Adenomyosis

D. Endometrial carcinoma

Patients with adenomyosis often present with painful menses (dysmenorrhea), profuse menses (menorrhagia, or both. Other possible symptoms are pain during sexual intercourse (dyspareunia), chronic pelvic pain and irritation of the urinary bladder.

Answer: C i.e., Adenomyosis

9. A infertile woman presents with yellow or green vaginal discharge, bartholin cyst and proctitis. What is the most probable diagnosis?

A. Syphilis B. Trichomoniasis

C. Gonorrhoea D. Candidiasis

Symptoms of gonorrhea in women include vaginal discharge, dysuria, intermenstrual bleeding, dyspareunia and abdominal pain. In men, gonorrhea causes anterior urethritis. Many people with gonococcal proctitis don›t have any symptoms. In a small fraction of men, ascending urethritis progresses to epididymitis. Discharge is usually described as thin, purulent, and mildly odorous; however, many patients have minimal or no symptoms from gonococcal cervicitis

Answer: C i.e., Gonorrhoea

10. A 28 years old P1L1 presents with severe pain in her abdomen and is taken for laparotomy. On opening the abdomen, pseudomyxoma of the peritoneum is present. What should be the probable reason?

A. Mucinous cystadenoma of ovary

B. Serous cystadenoma of ovary

C. Rupture of dermoid tumor

D. Endometriosis

Pseudomyxoma peritonei (PMP) is a clinical condition caused by cancerous cells (mucinous adenocarcinoma) that produce abundant mucin or gelatinous ascites. This disease is most commonly caused by an appendiceal primary cancer (cancer of the appendix); mucinous tumors of the ovary have also been implicated, although in most cases ovarian involvement is favoured to be a metastasis from an appendiceal or other gastrointestinal source.

Answer: A i.e., Mucinous cystadenoma of ovary

11. In a 40 years old woman, pap smear shows atypical glandular cells. The next step of management should be:

A. Repeat pap smear after three months

B. Colposcopic directed cervical biopsy

C. Colposcopy, cervical biopsy, endocervical curettage and endometrial biopsy

D. Hysteroscopy and directed endometrial biopsy

The Papanicolaou test (abbreviated as Pap test, also known as Pap smear, cervical smear, or smear test) is a method of cervical screening used to detect potentially pre-cancerous and cancerous processes in the cervix. Abnormal findings are often followed up by more sensitive diagnostic procedures, and, if warranted, interventions that aim to prevent progression to cervical cancer. Thorough evaluation of endocervix, ectocervix and endometrium is required.

Answer: C i.e., Colposcopy, cervical biopsy, endo-cervical curettage and endometrial biopsy

12. A 50 years old P4L4 has a simple left ovarian cyst of 10 cm. CA-125 is 30 u/ml. Treatment of choice would be:

A. TAH + BSO (Total abdominal hysterectomy + Bilateral salpingo-oophorectomy)

B. Laparoscopic cystectomy

C. Laparoscopic oophorectomy

D. Medical management with oral contraceptives

CA-125 is useful in differential diagnosis and in follow up of the disease of ovarian tumours. CA-125 levels in premenopausal people over 200 U/mL may indicate ovarian cancer, as may any elevation in CA-125 above 35 U/mL in post-menopausal people. If a tumor in a premenopausal woman is determined to be a low malignant potential tumor during surgery, and it is clearly stage I cancer, only the affected ovary is removed. For postmenopausal women with low malignant potential tumors, hysterectomy with bilateral salpingo-oophorectomy is still the preferred option.

Answer: A i.e., TAH + BSO (Total abdominal hysterectomy + Bilateral salpingo-oophorectomy)

13. A seven years old girl with precocious puberty is found to be having a 10 cm. ovarian cyst on USG. The most likely etiology is:

A. Benign cystic teratoma

B. Brenner tumour

C. Choriocarcinoma

D. Granulosa cell tumour

Granulosa cell tumours (or granulosa-theca cell tumours or folliculoma) are is a ovarian stomal tumour which produces estrogen. So, in a pre-pubertal girl, it might lead to precocious puberty.

Answer: D i.e., Granulosa cell tumour

14. A 17 years old girl presents with an ovarian cyst of 5 cm. The cyst is echo free, unilocular and CA 125 of 8U/ml. What is most appropriate management?

A. Laproscopy for cyst removal

B. Laparotomy for cyst removal

C. Conservative with follow up ultrasound

D. Medical treatment

Follow-up imaging in women of reproductive age for incidentally discovered simple cysts on ultrasound is not needed until 5 cm, as these are usually normal ovarian follicles. Simple cysts 5 to 7 cm in premenopausal females should be followed yearly. Simple cysts larger than 7 cm require further imaging with MRI or surgical assessment. Because they are large, they cannot be reliably assessed by ultrasound alone because it may be difficult to see the soft tissue nodularity or thickened septation at their posterior wall due to limited penetrance of the ultrasound beam.

Answer: C i.e., Conservative with follow up ultra-sound

15. The contraceptive choice for a 38 years old P1L1 woman having chronic hypertension, dysmenorrhoea and menorrhagia is:

A. Copper intrauterine device

B. Sterilization

C. Levonorgestrel intrauterine device

D. Combined oral contraceptive pills

Intrauterine device (IUD) with progestogen, sold under the brand name Mirena among others, is a intrauterine device that releases the hormone levonorgestrel. It is used for birth control, heavy menstrual periods (menorrhagia), and to prevent excessive build of the lining of the uterus in those on estrogen replacement therapy. It is one of the most effective forms of birth control with a one-year failure rate around 0.2%. The device is placed in the uterus and lasts three to five years. Following removal fertility returns quickly.

Answer: C i.e., Levonorgestrel intrauterine device

16. **A woman presents with heavy foul smelling discharge with sharply demarcated ulcers without induration on the perineum and the labia majora. Inguinal lymphadenopathy is also present. What is the most probable diagnosis?**

A. Gonorrhoea B. Tuberculosis

C. Chancroid D. Trichomoniasis

The ulcer of chancroid characteristically: (1) ranges in size dramatically from 3 to 50 mm (1/8 inch to two inches) across; (2) is painful; (3) has sharply defined, undermined borders; (4) has irregular or ragged borders; (5) has a base that is covered with a gray or yellowish-gray material; (6) has a base that bleeds easily if traumatized or scraped; (7) painful swollen lymph nodes occurs in 30 to 60% of patients and (8) dysuria (pain with urination) and dyspareunia (pain with intercourse) in females.

Answer: C i.e., Chancroid

17. **A 28 years old woman develops amenorrhoea after having dilatation and curettage. The most likely diagnosis is:**

A. Kallmann syndrome B. Asherman syndrome

C. Anorexia nervosa D. Turner syndrome

Asherman's Syndrome/ AS which is also referred to as intrauterine adhesions (IUA) or intrauterine synechiae, is an acquired uterine condition that occurs when scar tissue (adhesions) form inside the uterus and/or the cervix. It is characterized by variable scarring inside the uterine cavity, where in many cases the front and back walls of the uterus stick to one another. AS can be the cause of menstrual disturbances (amenorrhoea), infertility, and placental abnormalities etc.

Answer: B i.e., Asherman syndrome

18. **A 26 years old woman P_1L_1 reports with High Grade Squamous Intraepithelial Lesion (HGSIL) on Pap smear (Papanicolaou smear). Further management for her is:**

A. VIA, VILI

B. Colposcopy and directed biopsy

C. LEEP

D. Conisation

Colposcopy is a medical diagnostic procedure to examine an illuminated, magnified view of the cervix and the tissues of the vagina and vulva. It is done using a colposcope, which provides an enlarged view of the areas, allowing the colposcopist to visually distinguish normal from abnormal appearing tissue and take directed biopsies for further pathological examination.

Answer: B i.e., Colposcopy and directed biopsy

19. **A 16 years old girl presents with primary amenorrhea with absent vagina, cervix and uterus in the presence of normal secondary sexual characteristics. Ovaries are present on USG. The most probable diagnosis is:**

A. Klinefelter's syndrome

B. Androgen Insensitivity syndrome

C. Mayer Rokitansky Kuster Hauser syndrome

D. Prader Willi syndrome

Müllerian agenesis, also known as Mayer–Rokitansky–Küster–Hauser syndrome (MRKH) or vaginal agenesis, is a congenital malformation characterized by a failure of the Müllerian duct to develop, resulting in a missing uterus and variable degrees of vaginal hypoplasia of its upper portion. Müllerian agenesis (including absence of the uterus, cervix and/or vagina) is the cause in 15% of cases of primary amenorrhoea. Because ovaries do not develop from the Müllerian ducts, affected women might have normal secondary sexual characteristics but are infertile due to the lack of a functional uterus.

Answer: C i.e., Mayer Rokitansky Kuster Hauser syndrome

20. **A 50 years old post menopausal woman comes with complaints of bleeding per vaginum. Which one of the following investigations is NOT required?**

A. Endometrial biopsy

B. Diagnostic laparoscopy

C. Hysteroscopy

D. Pap smear

Evaluation of post-menopausal bleeding: (1) Abnormal endometrium may have to be investigated by a hysteroscopy with a biopsy or a dilation and curettage; (2) Pap smear is done to rule out carcinoma cervix

Answer: B i.e., Diagnostic laparoscopy

21. **In the process of MTP (Medical Termination of Pregnancy) done by suction and evacuation, it was realized that perforation of uterus occurred with cannula. The next step should be:**

A. Laparotomy with exploration of bowel

B. Manual vacuum aspiration

C. Wait and watch

D. Complete the evacuation with curette

If perforation is caused by suction cannula, diagnostic laparoscopy is helpful to assess the size and site of perforation and the amount of hemorrhage. Operative laparoscopy or Laparotomy may be needed to tackle the situation. One should not forget to inspect the intestine or omentum for evidence of injury.

Answer: A i.e., Laparotomy with exploration of bowel

22. **An 18 years old unmarried girl comes with complaints of heavy, prolonged bleeding during menses. Which among the following investigations is NOT usually advised?**

A. Urine pregnancy test

B. Ultrasound uterus and adnexa

C. Coagulation profile

D. Dilatation and curettage

In adolescent dysfunctional uterine bleeding, D & C is rarely needed only if bleeding fails to stop or is severe in nature.

Answer: D i.e., Dilatation and curettage

23. **A 58 years old woman with suspected ovarian cancer was operated for surgical staging. On laparotomy and subsequent histopathological examination of the specimen it was found that both ovaries were involved, capsule was ruptured, ascites was present containing malignant cells. Uterus and tubes were normal and there were no peritoneal implants. The FIGO stage for this patient would be:**

A. Stage I B. Stage II

C. Stage III D. Stage IV

In stage 1, the cancer has not spread beyond the ovaries. Stage 1A means the cancer is only in one ovary. In stage 1B, the cancer is in both ovaries. Stage 1C means that one or both ovaries contain cancer cells and one of the following are also found: the outer capsule broke during surgery, the capsule burst before surgery, there are cancer cells on the outside of an ovary, or cancer cells are found in fluid washings from the abdomen.

Answer: A i.e., Stage I

24. **A 22 years old woman comes with complaints of pain and discomfort in vaginal region. On examination there is unilateral tender swelling in the posterior half of labium minus, overlying skin is red and edematous. What is the most probable diagnosis?**

A. Utero vaginal prolapse B. Inversion of uterus

C. Bartholin's abscess D. Trichomoniasis

On examination of bartholin's abscess, there is a unilateral tender swelling beneath the posterior half of the labium majus expanding medially to the posterior part of the labium minus. The overlying skin appears red and oedematous.

Answer: C i.e., Bartholin's abscess

25. **A 29 years old woman is noted to have three consecutive first trimester spontaneous abortion. Examination reveals fibroid uterus. Which of the following types of uterine fibroids would most likely lead to recurrent abortions?**

A. Submucosal B. Intramural

C. Subserosal D. Cervical

Uterine fibroids, especially the submucosal type, are associated with increased risks of spontaneous abortion, preterm delivery, abnormal presentation in labor, pelvic outlet obstruction, postpartum hemorrhage, and puerperal sepsis

Answer: A i.e., Submucosal

26. **A 25 years old infertile woman is noted to have blocked fallopian tube on Hysterosalpingography/HSG. Which of the following is the best next step for this woman?**

A. Clomiphene citrate therapy

B. Gonadotropin therapy

C. Laparoscopy

D. Intrauterine insemination

The results of HSG and those of laparoscopy are complementary in tubal infertility evaluation. While HSG seems to be reliable when the tubes are patent, laparoscopy helps to reveal false tubal obstructions observed with HSG, and also helps in the diagnosis of pelvic adhesive bands and endometriosis.

Answer: C i.e., Laparoscopy

27. **The contraceptive choice for a 38 years old woman with chronic hypertension and history of dysmenorrhea and menorrhagia (malignancy ruled out) is:**

A. Copper intrauterine device

B. Levonorgestrel intrauterine device

C. Combined oral contraceptive pills

D. Sterilization

The levonorgestrel (LNg) intrauterine device releases small amounts of levonorgestrel, a form of progesterone, into the uterus each day. This type of IUD reduces cramping and heavy menstrual bleeding. And it is a highly effective method of birth control.

Answer: B i.e., Levonorgestrel intrauterine device

28. **A 60-year old woman presents with postmenopausal bleeding. On endometrial curettage she is diagnosed as endometrial carcinoma/EC. Which one of the following is a risk factor for endometrial cancer?**

A. Multiparity B. Oral contraceptive use

C. Smoking D. Diabetes mellitus

Major risk factors for EC are obesity, diabetes, and hypertension.

Answer: D i.e., Diabetes mellitus

29. **A 40-year old woman presented to the gynecologist with complaints of profuse vaginal discharge. There was no discharge from the cervix on the speculum examination. The diagnosis of bacterial vaginosis was made based upon all the following findings on microscopy EXCEPT:**

A. Abundance of gram variable coccobacilli

B. Absence of lactobacilli

C. Abundance of polymorphs

D. Presence of clue cells

Bacterial vaginosis is characterized by malodorous vaginal discharge. The term vaginosis is preferred as there is no vaginal inflammation.

Answer: C i.e., Abundance of polymorphs

30. **A 36 years old woman has absence of menses for the last 4 months. Pregnancy test is negative. Serum levels of LH & FSH are raised. Serum estradiol level is low. These findings suggest:**

A. Bilateral tubal obstruction

B. PCOD

C. Premature menopause

D. Exogenous estrogen administration

Diagnosis of premature ovarian insufficiency include a history of amenorrhea in less than 35 years of age, serum gonadotropin level (FSH >40 mIU/ml) is high and serum E_2 level is low (<20 pg/ml)

Answer: C i.e., Premature menopause

31. **In a woman presenting with amenorrhea, headache, blurred vision & galactorrhea, the appropriate investigation is:**

A. Prolactin level B. LH

C. FSH D. HCG

Hyperprolactinemia inhibits ovarian steroidogenesis. Hyperprolactinemia causes secondary amenorrhea in about 30% of women. Hyperprolactinemia is commonly due to pituitary adenomas (microadenoma or macroadenoma). Visual field examination is essential to detect any compression effect on the optic nerves.

Answer: A i.e., Prolactin level

32. A patient presented with primary amenorrhoea with developed secondary characters and a bulging at hymen. Most probable diagnosis is:

A. PCOS

B. Rokitansky-Kuster-Hauser syndrome

C. Imperforate hymen

D. Kallmann's syndrome

The chief complains of imperforate hymen are periodic lower abdominal pain, which may be continuous, primary amenorrhoea and urinary symptoms, such as frequency, dysuria or even retention of urine. Vulval inspection reveals a tense bulging membrane of bluish coloration.

Answer: C i.e., Imperforate hymen

33. A 46 years old lady has abnormal uterine bleeding with simple hyperplasia of endometrium. The treatment of choice would be:

A. Total Hysterectomy

B. Progesteron

C. Estrogen + progestogen

D. Estrogen

In perimenopausal and postmenopausal women with hyperplasia without atypia, continuous progestin therapy may be considered. However, hysterectomy with bilateral salpingo-oophorectomy is done as an alternative as the risk of carcinoma increases with age.

Answer: A i.e., Total Hysterectomy

34. A female with primary amenorrhoea has normal breast and normal pubic hairs. USG showed absent uterus, absent cervix and short vaginal pouch but normal ovaries. Most likely diagnosis:

A. Klinefelter's syndrome B. Mullerian agenesis

C. Gonadal dysgenesis D. Turner's syndrome

An individual with mullerian agenesis/ MRKH syndrome is hormonally normal; that is, they will enter puberty with development of secondary sexual characteristics including thelarche and adrenarche (pubic hair). Their chromosome constellation will be 46, XX. Ovaries are intact and ovulation usually occurs. Typically, the vagina is shortened and intercourse may, in some cases, be difficult and painful. Medical examination supported by gynecologic ultrasonography demonstrates a complete or partial absence of the cervix , uterus , and vagina.

Answer: B i.e., Mullerian agenesis

35. A 10 years old girl presented with primary amenorrhea, absent breasts, malformed uterus. The most likely diagnosis is:

A. Mayer Rokitansky Kuster Hauser syndrome

B. Turners syndrome

C. Swyer's syndrome

D. Mixed gonadal dysgenesis

Turner's syndrome cases usually present as primary amenorrhea with delayed secondary sex characters. Vagina, uterus and fallopian tubes are present. The uterus is small but is responsive to exogenous estrogen.

Answer: B i.e., Turners syndrome

CHAPTER 15

DERMATOLOGY

RAPID REVISION NOTES

Tzanck smear findings in bullous disorder

Pemphigus	Acantholysis
Bullous pemphigoid	Predominantly eosinophils
Varicella zoster infection	Multinucleated giant cells
Herpes simplex infection	Multinucleated giant cells
Toxic epidermal necrolysis	Necrotic cells

BASIC DERMATOLOGY

Skin

- Skin is stratified squamous keratinized epithelium
- Skin doubling time/ normal turnover time of epidermis is: 4 weeks
- Correct sequence of cell cycle: G0-G1-S-G2-M

Layers of skin

- Stratum germinativum/ Malpighian layers:
  - o Basal cell layer: Melanocytes present
  - o Prickle cell layer/ stratum spinosum
- Stratum granulosum (granular cell layer)
- Stratum lucidum (Clear cell layer) &
- Stratum corneum (horny cell layer): Most superficial layer

Keratin

- Keratinization causes dehydration of cells
- Keratin filaments are hallmark of epidermal cells

Melanocyte

- Melanocyte (& also merkel cells) is immigrant cells
- Melanocyte are present in: Stratum basale

Stratum lucidum

- It is sandwiched between S. corneum & S. granulosum
- It contains degenerated cells
- It is underdeveloped in very low birth weight infants within first 7 days

Macule

- Skin lesion which is neither raised nor depressed
- Flat discoloration of skin of 1 cm

Acantholysis

- Loss of coherence between epidermal cells
- Seen in Pemphigus

Hair

- Anagen phase of hair indicates: Phase of activity & growth

Sweat glands

- Sweat gland of palm can be differentiated from others by: Secretion stimulated by emotional stimuli
- Hypothalamic pre-optic nuclei have key role in sweating
- Miliaria is due to disruption of: Eccrine sweat ductal integrity

Apocrine gland

- Modified sweat gland
- Present in groin & axilla
- Infection of apocrine gland is known as: Hidradenitis suppurativa

Fordyce spots

- Ectopic sebaceous gland
- Mainly involves: Lips & buccal mucosa
- Common in adult woman

Rhinophyma/ potato nose

- Glandular form of acne rosacea
- Sebaceous gland hypertrophy

Phases of growth of hair

- Anagen: Growing
- Catagen: Transitional phase
- Telogen: Resting phase

Structure blocked & Disease

- Eccrine sweat glands: Crystalline miliaria
- Apocrine sweat glands: Hidradenitis suppurativa (Fox-Fordyce disease)
- Sebaceous glands: Fordyce disease

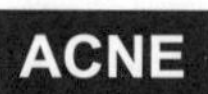

ACNE

Acne

- Causative factors for acne: Hypercornification of duct, androgen, lipophilic yeast, bacterial contamination
- Management of acne is by: 13-cis-retinol/ isotretinoin, minocycline, erythromycin

Acne vulgaris (AV)

- Comedones are characteristic of: Acne vulgaris
- Comedones are:
  - o Small cysts
  - o Formed in hair follicles
  - o Due to blockage of the follicular orifice
  - o By the retention of sebum & keratinous material
- AV is caused by: Obstruction of pilosebaceous duct
- AV present as: Multiple papulopustular erythematous lesions on face & neck in young age group
- Used for treating AV are: Minocycline, tetracycline, cryotherapy, UV rays, estrogen
- Treatment of choice for AV: Minocycline (for inflammatory acne; adverse effect is blue black/ blue-gray/ muddy hyperpigmentation) & Retinoids (for comedonal acne)

Nodulocystic acne (NA)

- Treatment of NA: Isotretinoin (synthetic retinoic acid)

Retinoids

- Drug used to treat recalcitrant acne: Retinoid
- Most common side effect of retinoid: Skin rashes

Terminology

Macule	Flat, circumscribed discolored area of any size
Papule	Elevated solid area of less than 5 mm
Plaque	Elevated flat topped area of more than 5 mm
Vesicle	Fluid filled raised area less than 5 mm
Bulla	Fluid filled raised area more than 5 mm
Blister	Any bulla/ vesicle is known as blister
Pustule	Discrete pus filled raised area
Lichenification	Thickened rough skin characterized by prominent skin markings
Scale	Dry horny plate like excrescences
Hyperkeratosis	Thickened stratum corneum, non-horny layer

Parakeratosis	Keratinization characterized by the retention of nuclei in the stratum corneum
Acanthosis	Thickened prickle cell layer
Dyskeratosis	Faulty development of epidermis (abnormal keratinization occurring prematurely within individual cells or groups of cells below the stratum granulosum e.g. pemphigus)
Acantholysis	Loss of intercellular connections resulting in loss of cohesion between keratinocytes, leading to bullae, vesicles etc. e.g. pemphigus
Pautrier's microabscess	Present in the histopathologic examination of mycosis fungoides; they consist of mycosis cells located within intra-epidermal vesicles

ALOPECIA

- Telogen effluvium: Diffuse hair loss after 3 months of prolonged, high grade fever of any cause (typhoid) or difficult & prolonged child birth
- Time period between the psychic emotional stress & the hair loss is about: 3 months
- Female pattern baldness: Man with diffuse hair loss involving crown & frontal scalp with maintenance of frontal hair line
- Drug contraindicated in androgenic alopecia: Testosterone

Cicatricial alopecia (CA)/ pseudopelade

- Scarring alopecia
- Causes of CA: Lichen planus, discoid lupus erythematosus, lupus vulgaris, SLE

Alopecia areata (AA)

- Non-cicatricial/ non-scaring alopecia
- Thought to be autoimmune in origin
- Exclamation mark sign is characteristic
- Clinical presentation: Single or multiple circumscribed smooth patchy hair loss, most obviously on scalp but frequently involving any hair bearing skin like beard, eyebrows, eyelashes, with pathognomic "exclamation marks" & "going gray overnight" phenomenon
- AA is treated by: Minoxidil

Type of alopecia

- Alopecia universalis: When hair has been lost over the entire body
- Alopecia areata: Patches of smooth area with loss of hair. At the periphery of patches is exclamation hair
- Alopecia totalis: Total loss of scalp hair

Special form

- Kerion celsi: Is a boggy indurated area exuding pus
- Black dot: Areas of alopecia studded with black dots representing hair broken off at surface of the scalp caused by endothrix fungi
- Gray patch: Characterized by scaly patches with stubs of broken hair and easy pluckability of hair. Caused by ectothrix fungi

NAIL

Nail disorder

- Pterygium of nail is seen in: Lichen planus
- Onycholysis is seen in: Psoriasis
- Mees lines is seen in: Arsenic poisoning
- Oil drop, pitting of nails is seen in: Psoriasis
- Tinea unguium affects: Nail plate
- Koilonychia: Iron deficiency anemia
- Koenen's periungual fibroma: Tuberous sclerosis

STD & CAUSATIVE ORGANISM

- Chancroid: H. ducreyi (multiple painful ulcers without induration), Herpes hominis
- LGV: Chlamydia trachomatis (serotype L2)
- Donovanosis: Calymmatobacterium granulomatosis (pseudo-bubo)
- Pinta: T. carateum
- Yaws: T. portune

SCABIES

- Incubation period: 4 weeks

- Pathogenesis lesion of scabies: Burrows
- Location of burrow (layer of skin): Stratum corneum
- MC site of scabies in infants: Scalp, Face
- Most severe form of scabies: Norwegian scabies
- Drug used orally for scabies: Ivermectin

Types of scales

Silvery scales	Psoriasis
Tack like scales	Chronic discoid lupus erythematosis
Fine cigarette paper like scales	Pityriasis rosea
Fish paper like scales	Ichthyosis
Sandpaper like scales	Solar keratosis

PSORIASIS

- MC on: Extensor aspect
- Koebner's phenomenon/ KP: Traumatized lesions develop psoriatic lesion (Lesion at the site of injury)
- KP is also seen with: Lichen planus, Lichen sclerosus, Vitiligo etc.
- Histopathological lesion in psoriasis: Micro-Munro abscesses (St. corneum)
- Rare but severe form of psoriatic arthritis: Arthritis mutilans
- Auspitz sign seen in psoriasis is: Rubbing of skin leading to removal of scales resulting in pin-point bleeding
- Treatment of choice for psoriasis: PUVA

Diseases & immunofluorescent findings

Pemphigus vulgaris	Intracellular IgG in epidermis in fish net pattern
Bullous pemphigoid	C3 & IgG linear band at dermo-epidermal junction (basement membrane)
Dermatitis herpetiformis	IgA, granular band at the dermal papillary tip along the basement membrane (dermo-epidermal junction)

PEMPHIGUS

- MC form of pemphigus: P. vulgaris
- Etiopathology of pemphigus: Autoimmune disease
- Antibodies against intercellular substance (antibodies attacks Desmoglein 3)
- Features of pemphigus:
  - o Intraepidermal (flaccid) Acantholytic bullae
  - o Oral mucosal lesion
- Acantholysis is seen in epidermis (breaking apart of epidermal cells)
- Tense subepidermal bullae are seen in Pemphigoid (NOT pemphigus)
- Nikolsky sign is positive
- Definitive diagnosis of pemphigus: Demonstration of Anti-desmoglein autoantibodies by Direct immuno-fluorescence on Skin biopsy

Pemphigus

- Nikolsky sign present
- Bullae are intraepidermal and flaccid
- Mucosa involved
- Acantholysis present
- Involves upper part of body
- Age-40-60
- Prognosis poor

Nikolsky sign

- Sliding of superficial layers of skin on the deeper layer when a tangential force is applied with the pulp of thumb, especially over bony prominences
- Positive in:
  - o Pemphigus
  - o Staphylococcal scalded skin syndrome
  - o Toxic epidermal necrolysis
  - o Epidermolysis bullosa congenital

Pemphigoid

- Nikolsky sign Absent
- Bullae are subepidermal and tense
- Mucosae are NOT involved
- Acantholysis Absent
- Involves Lower part of body
- Age 60-80
- Prognosis good

HAILEY-HAILEY DISEASE

- Also known as: Familial benign pemphigus
- Feature of Hailey-Hailey disease: No sub-epidermal blistering

LICHEN PLANUS

- Features of lichen planus:
    - o Flat topped papules
    - o With white lacy markings on mucosa (Wickham's striae)
    - o Civatte bodies &
    - o Basal cell degeneration

PITYRIASIS ROSEA

- Terms associated with pityriasis rosacea:
    - o Herald patch/ mother patch
    - o Collarette of scales

TINEA

- Dermatophyte: Parasitic fungus/ mycosis, that infects the skin
- It involves the imperfect fungi of the genera (epidermophyton, microsporum, trichophyton)
- Trichophyton can infect all the 3 structures: Skin, hair & nails
- Dermatophytes are anamorphic (asexual/ imperfect)
- Dermatophytes cause infection of skin, hair & nails due to their ability to obtain nutrients from keratinized material
- Athlete's foot/ Tinea pedis presents as (Does NOT affect only athletes):
    - o Severe itching
    - o Hyperhidrosis
- Onycho-mycosis/ Tinea unguium / Ringworm of the nail affects: Nail plate
- Dhobi itch or jock itch is also known as: Tinea cruris
- Tinea versicolor/ versatile colour
    - o Caused by Malassezia furfur (Dimorphic, lipophilic organism)
    - o Griseofulvin is ineffective (Ketoconazole & Itraconazole are systemic therapy)

Tinea & regions

- Tinea capitis: Scalp
- Tinea cruris: Affects groin
- Tinea corporis: Affects trunk
- Tinea manuum: Affects only the palms with scaling

Special tinea

- Tinea Pedis /athlete's foot: T. mentagrophytes causes vesicular or bullous lesions in web spaces
- Tinea imbricata / Jock itch/ Crotch itch/ Dhobi's itch: Concentric rings of scales forming extensive patches with polycyclic borders. Caused by tinea concentricum
- Trichophytic granuloma / Majocchi's granuloma: Perifollicular granuloma which is annular, raised and crusty, seen on wrists, and shin, caused by tinea rubrum and T. mentagrophytes

ATOPIC DERMATITIS

- Also known as: Itch disease
- Childhood & adolescent pattern of atopic dermatitis is marked by:
    - o Flexural skin dermatitis
    - o Particularly in the ante-cubital fossa/ popliteal fossa
- Other features of AD:
    - o Perioral pallor
    - o Dennies line
    - o Increased palmar markings etc.
- Best test to diagnose AD: Clinical evaluation
- Berloque dermatitis is due to: Cosmetics

Signs of atopy

- Extra crease line just below the lower eyelid, exceeding midline (pupil)
- Dennie Morgan folds (Extra fold beneath the eyelid is called the Dennie Morgan fold)

- White dermographism
- Triple response is replaced by blanching of skin
- Keratosis pilaris
- Hertoghe's sign

SKIN TUMOURS

- Basal cell carcinoma does NOT show lymphatic spread
- Conditions predisposing to Squamous cell carcinoma:
    - o Actinic keratosis
    - o DLE

MYCOSIS FUNGOIDES

- Mycosis fungoides is also known as: Cutaneous T cell lymphoma
- Special features:
    - o MC skin lymphoma
    - o Pautrier's microabscesses
    - o Presents with diffuse erythroderma

DERMATITIS HERPETIFORMIS

- DH is associated with: Gluten sensitive enteropathy (subclinical)
- DH is associated with HLA:
    - o HLA-B8, DR3
    - o HLA-DQ2, DQ8
- Direct immunofluorescence microscopy of normal appearing perilesional skin in DH shows: Granular deposits of IgA
- DOC for DH: Dapsone

ACANTHOSIS NIGRICANS

- Characteristic of acanthosis nigricans:
    - o Dark
    - o Thick
    - o Velvety skin (in body folds & creases)
- MC endocrinal cause of acanthosis nigricans: Type 2 DM (overall obesity)
- Internal malignancies associated with acanthosis nigricans:
    - o Adenocarcinoma lungs
    - o Carcinoma GIT etc.

DERMATOLOGIC CHANGES IN SYSTEMIC DISEASES

- HIV: Reactivation of herpes zoster/ shingles (DOC: Acyclovir/ Famciclovir; Foscarnet for acyclovir resistant cases)
- Secondary syphilis:
    - o Rashes
    - o Moth eaten alopecia
    - o Periostitis

Polar types of leprosy

Tuberculoid	*Lepromatous*
Less severe	More severe
Minimally infectious	Maximally infectious
HLA-DR2	HLA-MT1, HLA-DQ1
Asymmetric skin lesions	Symmetric distribution
Less lesions	More lesions
Confined to skin & peripheral nerves (Ulnar)	All organs affected (except lungs & CNS)
Nerve involvement due to external compression by granuloma	Nerve involvement due to direct invasion of bacilli
Few hypopigmented, hypoesthetic macule/ plaque	Multiple skin nodules/ skin plaques
Acid Fast Bacilli/ AFB are generally absent	Many bacilli in histiocytes (leprae/ Virchow cells)
Cell Mediated Immunity/ CMI present	Cell Mediated Immunity/ CMI absent
Normal humoral response	Exaggerated humoral response
Lesions have granulomatous inflammation	Lesions have non-granulomatous inflammation
Lepromin test positive	Lepromin test negative
Antibodies to M. leprae phenolic glycolipid-1/ PGL-1 are less common	Antibodies to M. leprae phenolic glycolipid-1/ PGL-1 are 95%

LEPROSY

- Associated cells: Virchow cells
- 1st line of drugs:
  - o Rifampicin
  - o Clofazimine
  - o Dapsone
- DOC in neuritis: Steroids
- Treatment of nerve abscess: Incision & drainage
- MC nerve involved: Ulnar nerve
- Organs NOT involved in leprosy (warmer areas of body are not involved): Uterus
- MC type of leprosy in India: TT
- Infective form of leprosy: lepromatous leprosy
- Lepromin test indicates: Strong immunity
- Lucio's phenomenon: M. leprae may be associated with cutaneous ulcerations in patients with lepromatous leprosy

Lepromatous leprosy

- Features:
  - o Gynaecomastia
  - o Madarosis
  - o Collapse of nasal bridge
- Histology: Dermis contains characteristic highly vacuolated cells (Foam cells) (ABSENT/ few non-caseating granuloma)

Lepra reaction

- Type II (ENL):
  - o Type III hypersensitivity reaction
  - o Thalidomide is effective
- Type I:
  - o Type IV hypersensitivity reaction
  - o DOC for type I lepra reaction: Corticosteroids

Type of Leprosy & features

- LL: Bilaterally symmetrical, small oily lesion. Sensations present
- BB: Inverted saucer appearance
- BT: Satellite lesions are seen
- TT: Sensations are absent

WOOD'S LAMP

- Light generated in Wood's lamp: 360 nm ultraviolet/ black light
- Wood's lamp filter is made of: Nickel & silica
- Appearance of erythrasma in wood's lamp: Coral red colour

Wood's lamp Examination (Disease & Appearance)

- Albinism: Bright-white /blue-white
- Tuberous sclerosis: Blue white
- T. versicolor: Golden yellow
- P. aeruginosa: Aqua green
- Leprosy: Blue- white
- Vitiligo: Bright- white /blue -white
- Tinea capitis: Green fluorescence

TB SKIN

- Lupus vulgaris is: Skin TB with no underlying active focus
- Skin TB secondary to involvement of underlying structure i.e. joint, lymph node is: Scrofuloderma
- MC type of cutaneous TB: Lupus vulgaris
- Form of post primary TB with good resistance: TB verrucosa cutis (TB bacillus are inoculated into skin; seen in TB patient, pathologists, veterinary surgeons)

Features of ulcers

- Syphilitic ulcer: Wash leather slough
- Tuberculous ulcer: Apple jelly granulation tissue, pale scanty granulation tissue base
- Spreading ulcer: Necrotic tissue with slough

PYODERMAS

- Predominantly caused by S. aureus (localized and follicular infections) or

- S. pyogenes (spreading infections like erysipelas and cellulitis)
- Staph aureus can cause:
  - Bullous impetigo
  - Impetigo contagiosa (sometimes)
  - Ecthyma (more)
  - Follicular infections (folliculitis, furuncles, carbuncles)
- S. pyogenes can cause:
  - Spreading infections (erysipelas & cellulitis)
  - Sometimes impetigo contagiosa & ecthyma

STAPH AUREUS & DERMATOLOGY

- SSSS (Staphylococcal scalded skin syndrome)
- Bullous impetigo/ Impetigo contagiosa
- Furuncles/ Boils
- Sycosis barbae & Sycosis nuchae

REITER'S SYNDROME

- Reiter's syndrome is secondary to:
  - Chlamydial infection (genital tract)
  - Infectious dysentery (caused by shigella, salmonella, ureaplasma urealyticum)
- Features of Reiter's syndrome:
  - Urethritis
  - Conjunctivitis
  - Arthritis (acute ascending asymmetric oligoarthritis)
  - Keratoderma blennorrhagicum
- HLA associated with Reiter's syndrome: HLA B27

CONDITIONS & IMPORTANT FINDINGS

- Tuberous sclerosis:
  - Ash leaf spot
  - Adenoma sebaceum
  - Shagreen patches
- Urticaria pigmentosa: Darrier's sign
- Amyloidosis: Pinch purpura
- Lichen planus:
  - Wickham's striae
  - Civatte bodies
- Atopic dermatitis: Dennie Morgan folds
- Pityriasis rosacea:
  - Herald patch, Mother patch
  - Annular collarette of scales

DERMATOLOGICAL SIGNS & CONDITIONS

- Casal's necklace: Pellagra
- Berloque dermatitis: Cosmetics
- Calcinosis cutis: Scleroderma
- Crocodile skin: Ichthyosis
- Iris pearls: Leprosy
- Obstruction of pilo-sebaceous glands: Acne vulgaris
- Micro-Munro abscess: Psoriasis
- Pautrier microabscess: Mycosis fungoides
- Max Joseph space: Lichen planus
- Basal layer degeneration/ Hydropic degeneration/ Liquefaction degeneration: Lichen planus (also in DLE, pemphigus etc.)
- Asboe Hansen sign (bulla spread sign): Pemphigus
- Dubois sign: Congenital syphilis
- Ollendorff sign: Secondary syphilis

KEYWORDS & CONDITIONS

- Well defined annular lesion, Central scarring: Lupus vulgaris
- Oval, scaly, hypopigmented macule over chest & back: Pityriasis versicolor

- Flaccid bullae in skin, Oral lesions, Intra-epidermal acantholytic blister (on histopathology): Pemphigus vulgaris
- Multiple grouped vesicular lesion on T10 segment dermatome, Pain: Herpes zoster
- Multiple grouped papulovesicular lesions, Elbows, knees & buttocks, Severe itching: Dermatitis herpetiformis (DH)
- Child, Multiple, Itchy, Papular lesions, Genitalia & fingers, Other family member also affected: Scabies
- Multiple blisters over trunk & extremities, Direct immunofluorescence shows linear IgG deposits: Bullous pemphigoid
- Adult male, Burning micturition, Urethral discharge, Followed by joint pains: Reiter's syndrome
- HIV positive, Indurated ulcer over tongue, Growth on corneal agar at 20 degree C, Growth in human serum at 37 degree C shows budding yeast, Microscopy shows hyphae: Candida albicans
- 8 years old boy, from Bihar, 6 months history of ill-defined, Hypopigmented, slightly Atrophic macule on face: Indeterminate leprosy
- Pain in joints, Silvery scaling plaques on his elbows & knees: Psoriasis vulgaris
- Young female, Koilocytes in cervical biopsy: Human papilloma virus infection

Some conditions & feature

Eczema/ boil over	Pathogenesis is itch – scratch – itch cycle
Urticaria/ hives	Histology shows dermal oedema Angioedema is edema of the dermis & subcutaneous fat Treatment is by hydroxyzine, cyproheptadine, anti-histaminics
Molluscum contagiosum	Viral etiology (poxvirus) Umbilicated papules containing molluscum bodies
Impetigo	Caused by streptococcus/ staphylococcus Honey coloured crusts
Ecthyma	Ulcerated impetigo
Milia	Distended sebaceous glands appearing as white dots on nose and face, in neonates
Mongolian spots	Bluish macules on buttocks and trunk of infants Disappear spontaneously Not related to mongolism (Down syndrome)
Erythema toxicum	Discrete erythematous papules on trunk and face, appearing on the 2nd and 3rd day of life Disappear spontaneously
Erythema multiforme	Iris lesions Target lesions are characteristic

CLINICAL QUESTIONS

1. **A 50 years old patient presented with erythematous scaly plaques over trunk and extremities for last 10 years. Lesions are occasionally itchy. There is history of remission and relapse with exacerbation during winters. Most likely diagnosis:**

A. Pityriasis rosea B. Lichen planus

C. Contact dermatitis D. Psoriasis vulgaris

Psoriasis is characterized by a course of remission and relapse and presence of silvery white scaly papules on erythematous base. Lesions are mildly pruritic or non-pruritic. The condition is aggravated in winters.

Answer: D i.e., Psoriasis vulgaris

2. **A 30 years old sexually active male presented with painful, grouped vesicular eruption on penile shaft for 4 days. He gave past history of similar lesions four times in the past one year. Such lesions are associated with:**

A. Herpes simplex virus-2

B. Treponema pallidum

C. Chlamydia trachomatis serotype L2

D. Hemophilus ducreyi

In males, the lesions of HSV-2 occur on the glans penis or shaft of penis. Classically, it consists of macular or popular skin and mucous membrane lesions occurring about 5-7 days after a sexual contact. These lesions then progress to multiple vesicles, which are often very painful. The characteristic feature of herpes genitalis is that it tends to recur.

Answer: A i.e., Herpes simplex virus-2

3. **24 years old male complains of mild urethral discharge after sexual contact with a sex-worker. Drug used to treat such a patient:**

A. Azithromycin 1 mg single dose

B. Azithromycin 1 mg for 3 weeks

C. Azithromycin 500 mg single dose

D. Azithromycin 1 gram single dose

Chlamydia trachomatis non-gonococcal urethritis is managed by Azithromycin 1 g single stat dose, which also take care of mycoplasma.

Answer: D i.e., Azithromycin 1 gram single dose

4. **A 30 years old male presented with pruritic, flat topped, polygonal, shiny violaceous papules with flexural distribution. The most likely diagnosis is:**

A. Psoriasis B. Pityriasis rosea

C. Lichen planus D. Lichenoid dermatitis

Cutaneous lesions of lichen planus present as purplish, plain topped, pruritic, polygonal, papules on peripheral parts of body with mild scaling in a bilateral symmetrical manner.

Answer: C i.e., Lichen planus

5. **A 50 years old man has a 2 years old history of facial bullae & oral ulcers. Microscopic smear from skin lesions is most likely to disclose:**

A. Tzanck cells B. Acantholytic cells

C. Necrosis D. Koilocytes

Tzanck smear is prepared in pemphigus vulgaris. The scrapings from floor of blister are smeared on a microscopic slide and examine under light microscope after staining with Leishman's stain. Acantholytic cells are seen as large round cells lying free with no attachment with other epidermal cells.

Answer: B i.e., Acantholytic cells

6. **A 23 years old lady presents with vesicular lesions in the buccal mucosa & flaccid blisters on the skin. The possible diagnosis is:**

A. Pemphigus vulgaris

B. Pemphigus foliaceous

C. Pemphigoid

D. Dermatitis herpetiformis

Oral lesions are present in 50-70% of patients of pemphigus vulgaris. Cutaneous lesions erupt in crops and consists of flaccid blisters filled with fluid.

Answer: A i.e., Pemphigus vulgaris

7. A six years old boy presents with generalized seizure disorder and hypo pigmented skin lesions. On examination he has tiny red nodules over the nose and cheeks. The most likely diagnosis is:

A. Tuberous sclerosis

B. Sturge Weber disease

C. PHACE Syndrome

D. Neurofibromatosis

Tuberous sclerosis complex (TSC) is a rare multisystem genetic disease that causes benign tumours to grow in the brain and on other vital organs such as the kidneys, heart, liver, eyes, lungs, and skin. A combination of symptoms may include seizures, intellectual disability, developmental delay, behavioural problems, skin abnormalities, and lung and kidney disease. TSC is caused by a mutation of either of two genes, TSC1 and TSC2, which code for the proteins hamartin and tuberin, respectively. These proteins act as tumour growth suppressors, agents that regulate cell proliferation and differentiation.

Answer: A i.e., Tuberous sclerosis

8. A 7 years old child with history of asthma has developed itching and rashes in the axilla, groin and popliteal region. Most likely diagnosis:

A. Seborrheic dermatitis B. Contact dermatitis

C. Atopic dermatitis D. Irritant dermatitis

Childhood and adolescent form pattern of atopic dermatitis presents with intensively pruritic lesions on flexural areas (popliteal fossa, antecubital fossa, axilla and groin). There is a personal or family history of other atopic conditions like asthma, hay fever, allergic rhinitis or conjunctivitis.

Answer: C i.e., Atopic dermatitis

9. A lady has family history of asthma. She presented with itching in cubital fossa and popliteal fossa. Most likely diagnosis:

A. Xeroderma pigmentosum

B. Psoriasis vulgaris

C. Contact dermatitis

D. Atopic dermatitis

Adult phase of atopic dermatitis is characterised by itchy lesions, which are lichenified. These lesions are present in flexural (cubital and popliteal fossa). One of the very important feature of atopic dermatitis is the presence of personal or family history of other atopic conditions like asthma.

Answer: D i.e., Atopic dermatitis

10. A patient presented with recurrent oral aphthous ulcers with genital ulcers, Ophthalmologic examination show uveitis. History of fever is present. Most likely diagnosis:

A. Measles

B. Henoch-Schonlein purpura

C. Behçet's disease

D. Ankylosing spondylitis

Behçet's syndrome is characterized by genital ulcers, aphthous (oral) ulcers and uveitis.

Answer: C i.e., Behçet's disease

CHAPTER 16

ANESTHESIA

RAPID REVISION NOTES

Anesthetic agent of choice

Condition	*Agent*
Cleft palate, antrostomy, Caldwell luc operations	**GA (general anesthesia)**
Ludwig angina	**LA (local anesthesia)**
Antral puncture	**LA**
Shock	**Ketamine**
Intermittent anesthesia in labor	**Ether**
Pheochromocytoma	**Enflurane**
Cardiac surgery	**Fentanyl**
Self medication in labor	**Trichloro-ethylene**
Hemorrhagic shock	**Cyclopropane**
Caesarean section	**Cyclopropane**
Thoracic surgery	**Cyclopropane**
Treatment of contraction ring & internal podalic version	**Halothane**
Bronchial asthma	**Halothane**

INTRAVENOUS ANAESTHETIC AGENTS (IVA)

- IVA used in shock: Ketamine
- IVA used in porphyria:
  - Ketamine
  - Propofol
- IVA which causes post-operative vomiting: Ketamine
- IVA with high incidence of venous thrombosis: Propofol
- IVA which precipitates porphyria:
  - Thiopentone
  - Methohexitone

Spinal anesthesia

Feature	*Remarks*
Spinal hypotension	Give I/V fluids, keep in head low position
Respiratory paralysis	Due to decreased cardiac output
Rarely involved nerve	Phrenic nerve
Physiological effects of SA are due to	Sympathetic paralysis
Order of paralysis of fibres	Preganglionic sympathetic, somatic sensory, somatic motor

SPINAL ANAESTHESIA

- Site of SA in adults: L2-L3/ L3-L4 space
- Site of SA in children: L4-L5 space

- Site of action of SA: Nerve roots of cauda equine
- Fibres which are blocked earliest: Autonomic pre-ganglionic fibres (sympathetic)
- Percentage of xylocaine used in SA: 5%
- Features of high spinal anaesthesia:
  - o Hypotension &
  - o Bradycardia

Order of sensation loss in spinal anaesthesia

- Preganglionic beta fibres
- Cold
- Warm
- Pin prick
- Pain
- Touch
- Pressure
- Motor
- Vibration /proprioception

Contraindications to spinal anesthesia

- Vertebral abnormalities
- Local sepsis
- Hypotension and hypovolemia
- Uncooperative and mentally ill person
- Infants

RELATED ANATOMY

- Extent of trachea: C6-T4; diameter is 1.2-1.6 cms
- Level of carina: T4
- Angle of right main bronchus with vertical: 25 degree
- Features of infant larynx:
  - o Long & leafy epiglottis
  - o Subglottic region is narrowest &
  - o Large tongue
- Anatomical dead space: Air which remains in conducting airways & not available for exchange
- Anatomical space is increased by: Inspiration, atropine & halothane

IDEAL GAS OBEYS

- Charles law (Volume is directly proportional to temperature)
- Boyles law (Volume is inversely proportional to pressure) &
- Avogadro's law

MUSCLE RELAXANTS

- Depolarizing muscle relaxants (Succinylcholine):
  - o Usually short acting
  - o No tetanic fade
  - o No post tetanic facilitation
- Non-depolarizing muscle relaxant (Mivacurium):
  - o Post tetanic facilitation seen
  - o Diaphragm is resistant to non-depolarizing agents
  - o Train of four fade present
  - o Muscle fasciculation absent

Shortest acting muscle relaxant (Order)

- Succinylcholine
- Mivacurium

Longest acting muscle relaxant

- Doxacurium > Pipecuronium > Pancuronium > d- Tubocurarine

SUCCINYLCHOLINE/ SCH

- Depolarizing muscle relaxant
- Shortest acting depolarizing MR
- Shortest acting MR
- Dual/ biphasic block
- Rapidly hydrolyzed by pseudocholinesterase
- Pressure increased by SCh:
  - o Intra-cranial pressure
  - o Intra-ocular pressure
  - o Intra-gastric pressure

- SCh causes:
  - o Muscle pain
  - o Hyperkalemia
  - o Vagal stimulation
- Predisposing factors SCh induced hyperkalemia:
  - o Massive trauma (rhabdomyolysis)
  - o Burns
  - o Stroke/ encephalitis etc.

ATRACURIUM

- Undergo spontaneous non-enzymatic degradation (Hoffman's elimination)
- Can be used safely in:
  - o Renal &
  - o Liver disease
- Can be used in patient with high serum creatinine
- Laudanosine is the metabolite, responsible for seizure activity

Conditions & Muscle relaxants

- Carcinoid tumour: Vecuronium
- In renal failure: Vecuronium /Atracurium
- In hepatic failure: Atracurium
- Myasthenia gravis: $1/10^{th}$ atracurium
- Short cases: Atracurium/ Rapacuronium / Mivacurium
- Obstetrics: All except Gallamine
- Asthmatics: Pancuronium (avoid Metocurine and Succinylcholine)
- Arterial surgery: Pancuronium
- To reduce blood pressure: Tubocurarine

Concentration of lignocaine as LA

Block	*Concentration*
Topical surface anesthesia	**2%**
Epidural	**1-2%**
Nerve block	**0.5-2%**
Infiltration anesthesia	**0.5%**

LOCAL ANAESTHETICS

- Generally blocks: Sodium channels
- Potency of LA depends on: Lipid solubility
- Susceptibility of fibres to LA: Type B > type C > type A
- Amide linked LA:
  - o Lidocaine
  - o Bupivacaine etc.
- Ester linked LA:
  - o Cocaine
  - o Procaine etc.

Order of sensation loss in Local anaesthesia

- Temperature
- Pain
- Touch
- Deep pressure

Shortest acting anaesthetist

- Chloroprocaine

Longest acting local anaesthetist

- Dibucaine > Tetracaine > Bupivacaine

LIGNOCAINE

- Amide linked LA
- Concentration used in subarachnoid space: 5%
- Maximum dose with adrenaline is: 7 mg/ kg
- Adverse effects:
  - o Convulsions
  - o Cardiac failure etc.

Lignocaine maximum dose without adrenaline

- 3mg/kg = 200 mg (average adult)

Lignocaine maximum dose with adrenaline

- 7 mg/ kg = 500 mg (average adult)

BUPIVACAINE

- Amide with duration of action more than 2 hours
- C/I for: Bier's block/ Intravenous regional anaesthesia/ IVRA
- It is highly cardiotoxic
- Cardiotoxicity is not easily reversible
- Levo-bupivacaine is used by epidural/ intrathecal route

KETAMINE

- Is a phencyclidine
- Causes dissociative anaesthesia
- Causes:
  - o Hallucination
  - o Delusion &
  - o Illusion
- Causes profound analgesia
- Increases all pressures:
  - o Intracranial Tension
  - o Intraocular pressure
  - o BP
- C/I in: Intracerebral mass/ hemorrhage etc.

THIOPENTONE

- Ultra short acting barbiturate (because of rapid redistribution)
- Lacks analgesic effect
- First sign on intra-arterial injection:
  - o Cyanosis &
  - o White hands
- I/V injection presents as:
  - o Pain
  - o Hypotension etc.
- C/I in: Porphyria (may precipitate porphyria)

PROPOFOL

- Agent of choice for day care anaesthesia
- Causes pain on I/V administration
- Contains egg extract
- Safer in porphyria
- Antiemetic
- Cerebroprotective:
  - o Decreases cerebral blood flow
  - o Decreases intracranial tension & intraocular tension
- Causes dose dependent fall in BP, due to:
  - o Vasodilation &
  - o Myocardial depression

ETOMIDATE

- Minimal effects on CVS
- Causes adrenocortical suppression
- It inhibits:
  - o 11-beta hydroxylase &
  - o 17 alpha hydroxylase
- So C/I in adrenal insufficiency

GUEDEL'S STAGES OF ANAESTHESIA

- 4 stages
- Based on ether
- Surgical anaesthesia: Stage III
- Lacrimation occurs in: Stage III

HALOTHANE

- Sensitizes heart to adrenaline
- Adverse effects:
  - o Post partum hemorrhage (relaxes uterine muscle)
  - o Bronchodilation (used in asthma)
  - o Causes severe liver dysfunction

DESFLURANE

- Fluorinated congener of isoflurane
- Low blood & tissue gas partition coefficient
- Fastest acting
- Less soluble

SEVOFLURANE

- Agent of choice for induction in: Paediatric age group
- Fast acting (but not that much as desflurane)
- Causes respiratory depression

NITROUS OXIDE

- Discovered by: Priestly
- Cylinder colour: Blue
- PIN index (code): 3,5
- Also known as: Laughing gas
- Adverse effects:
  - o Megaloblastic anemia
  - o Bone marrow suppression
- Second gas effect/ diffusion hypoxia
- C/I in:
  - o Pneumothorax
  - o Air embolism etc.

Colour coding of gas cylinders

- Oxygen: Black body with white shoulders
- Carbon dioxide: Grey
- Cyclopropane: Orange
- Air: Grey body, black and white quartered shoulders

Anesthetic agent

Feature	*Agent*
Produces megaloblastic anemia	**Nitrous oxide**
With good muscle relaxation	**Ether, cyclo-propane, methoxyflurane**
Depresses CVS	**Halothane**
Contraindicated in close circuit	**Trichloroethylene**

NITRIC OXIDE/ NO

- Produced from: Arginine (by enzyme NO synthetase)
- Acts via: cGMP pathway
- It prevents platelet aggregation
- Drugs forming NO: Sodium nitroprusside

SPINAL ANAESTHESIA/ CENTRINEURAXIAL BLOCKADE

- Site of SA administration in children: L4-L5
- Earliest fibres to be blocked: Sympathetic (autonomiic preganglionic fibres)
- Vasopressor agent of choice: Ephedrine
- C/I:
  - o Patients refusal
  - o Severe hypovolemia
  - o Marked coagulopathy
  - o Blood dyscrasia

POST DURAL PUNCTURE HEADACHE/ PDPH

- Occurs due to low CSF pressure/ CSF leak
- Lasts 7-10 days
- Risk reduction is by using: Sprotte needle/ whitacre needle

LARYNGEAL MASK AIRWAY

- Used for: Airway maintenance
- Indicated in: Difficult airway management during CPR

BRAIN DEATH

- Widespread cortical destruction
- Manifested as:
  - o Deep coma
  - o Unresponsiveness to all forms of stimulation
  - o Absent brain stem reflexes
  - o Absent motor activity
  - o Pupillary dilation

SUMMARY

Enflurane

- Contraindicated in epilepsy

Propofol

- Day care surgery

Fentanyl / Droperidol

- Neurolept analgesia
- Used in endoscopy

Trilene

- Not to be used with soda-lime

Etomidate

- Causes adrenal cortex suppression & pain on injection
- Preferred in porphyria
- No analgesic effect

Atracurium

- Undergoes Hoffman elimination
- Used in hepatic and renal failure

Sevoflurane

- Fastest induction
- Used in pediatric surgery
- Not used in closed circuit with soda-lime.

Nitrous oxide

- It inactivates cobalt in vitamin B_{12};
- Irreversibly inactivates enzyme methionine synthetase
- Megaloblastic anaemia occurs after exposure for periods of more than 3-12 hours
- It can be prevented by pretreatment with Folinic acid
- Second gas effect
- Diffusion hypoxia
- Only analgesic effect

Halothane

- Useful in Asthmatics, version, uterine relaxation (hence not used in post partum hemorrhage as relaxant effect increases bleeding)
- Increases ICT (intracranial tension)
- Sensitizes heart to Catecholamines
- Adverse effects:
  - o Hepatitis
  - o Malignancy
  - o Hyperthermia
  - o Shivering
- Should not be used again in next three months

Thiopentone sodium

- Highly lipid soluble
- Contraindicated in acute porphyria

Ether

- Inflammable
- Causes increased blood glucose levels in diabetics

Ketamine

- Dissociative anaesthesia
- Used in head, and neck surgery, angiography, Cardiac catheterization, burn dressing
- Preferred in asthmatics, Porphyria
- Avoided in – MI, hypertension

Cocaine

- Naturally occurring
- Produces vasoconstriction
- Peripheral sympathomimetic action

Prilocaine

- Safest local anaesthetic agent
- Produces methemoglobinemia

Succinylcholine

- Used during intubation
- Non- competitive muscle relaxant
- Produces fasciculations & biphasic block

- Significant hyperkalemia with Succinylcholine is seen in Burns, Paraplegia, tetanus

Isoflurane

- Decreases intracranial tension
- Used in myocardial infarction, neurosurgery, alcoholic cirrhosis.

Anesthesia

Purpose of color of gas cylinder	**For easy identification**
Intermittent flow machines	**Lucy-baldwin machine, Walters apparatus**
Continuous flow machines	**Boyle's apparatus, foregger apparatus, heat brink ohio machine**
Neuroleptic anesthesia	**Fentanyl (1 part) + droperidol (50 parts)**
Commonly used I/V anesthesia	**Thiopentone**
Agent contraindicated, where electrocautery is used	**Cyclopropane & ether**
Never give neostigmine after	**Halothane**
Safest anesthetic agent	**Nitrous oxide & ether**
Gas pockets (pneumothorax, intestinal obstruction) is a contraindication to use of	**Nitrous oxide**
Most widely used anesthetic agent	**Nitrous oxide**
General anesthesia is contraindicated if	**Patients airway is cannot be assured**
Overdose of anesthesia is measured by	**Heart rate & blood pressure**

CLINICAL QUESTIONS

1. **A 20 years old patient presented with early pregnancy for medical termination of pregnancy (MTP) in day care facility. What will be the induction agent of choice?**

A. Thiopentone B. Ketamine

C. Propofol D. Diazepam

Because of propofol's (i) early induction (ii) early and smooth recovery (iii) inactive metabolites and (iv) antiemetic effects it is, the I/V agent of choice for day care surgery.

Answer: C i.e., Propofol

2. **Administration of succinylcholine to a paraplegic patient led to the development of dysrhythmia, conduction abnormalities & finally cardiac arrest. The most likely cause is:**

A. Hypercalcemia B. Hyperkalemia

C. Anaphylaxis D. Hypermagnesemia

Succinylcholine is contraindicated for up to 2-3 months after trauma, up to 6 months after hemiplegia/paraplegia and up to 1 year after burns (the greatest risk is between 1 week to 2 months). In these conditions denervated/ regenerating nerve develops extrajunctional receptors which can produce hyperkalemia.

Answer: B i.e., Hyperkalemia

3. **A patient was undergoing surgical procedure under general anesthesia. Suddenly he developed tachycardia, sweating, hypertension and tachypnea. Best step to manage such a condition would be:**

A. Intravenous beta-blockers

B. End the surgical procedure

C. Wait and watch

D. Deepen the plane of anesthesia

Signs of light anesthesia/ intra-operative awareness include tachycardia, sweating (perspiration), hypertension, tachypnea, lacrimation, coughing (preserved reflexes) etc. In such cases, anesthesia should be deepened immediately.

Answer: D i.e., Deepen the plane of anesthesia

4. **A 10 years old child was undergoing surgery for squint. During surgery, there was a sudden fall in heart rate from 140 bpm to 40 bpm (beats per minute). As an anesthetist, how will you manage this situation?**

A. Wait and watch

B. Ask the surgeon to stop surgery for some time

C. Deepen the plane of anesthesia

D. Give I/V beta-blockers

Sudden and sudden bradycardia during an ophthalmic surgical procedure suggest the possibility of oculo-cardiac reflex. As soon as the oculo-cardiac reflex is noticed, the ophthalmic surgeon should relieve the traction on the rectus muscles till the episodes ends and there is an increase in heart rate. Otherwise, intravenous atropine needs to be given.

Answer: B i.e., Ask the surgeon to stop surgery for some time

5. **While assessing the adequacy of mouth opening preoperatively in a patient, only soft palate was visible. This is which grade as per Mallampati grading:**

A. I B. II

C. III D. IV

In class III of Mallampati grading, only soft palate is visible.

Answer: C i.e., III

6. **A 55 years old hypertensive male is on ACE inhibitors. There is a past history of CABG (coronary artery bypass grafting) done 3 years back. Now he is planned for hernia surgery. He has good effort tolerance. What should be the initial plan of preoperative evaluation of this patient?**

A. Routine pre-operative examination plus stress testing

B. Routine pre-operative examination plus clinical examination

C. Routine pre-operative examination plus clinical examination plus angiography

D. Routine pre-operative examination plus clinical examination plus ventilation-perfusion scan

Initial step in investigating such a patient would be general pre-operative examination and clinical examination. If everything is good, he can be planned for non-cardiac surgery. If there are some abnormal findings on clinical examination, then only he needs to be evaluated further with 2D-Echocardiography or angiography.

Answer: B i.e., Routine pre-operative examination plus clinical examination

7. **During abdominal surgery under local anaesthetic, patient suddenly felt sharp pain. Injury to which structure is likely:**

A. Liver parenchyma

B. Large gut

C. Small gut

D. Parietal peritoneum

The parietal peritoneum is supplied by nerves (e.g., phrenic and thoraco-abdominal) to the adjacent body wall, and most of it is very sensitive to pain. Painful stimuli to the central part of the diaphragmatic peritoneum are referred to the shoulder. The visceral peritoneum is insensitive to pain.

Answer: D i.e., Parietal peritoneum

CHAPTER 17

RADIOLOGY

RAPID REVISION NOTES

Ultrasonography

Mode	*Remarks*
Grey scales	For contrast studies (improvement over B scales)
B-scope	For 2-dimensional view (obstetrics & abdominal masses)
A-scope	For cerebral lesions, shift of midline structures
M-mode	For moving parts e.g. valves of heart etc.

X RAYS

- X-rays were discovered by: William Roentgen
- X-rays are modified: Electrons (uses principle of linear accelerator)
- X-rays differ from light in: Energy status
- Target material used in X-rays: Tungsten
- Effect of filters used in radiology: Beam of greater intensity
- Device used to reduce scattered radiation: Grid
- Contrast in X-ray depends upon: kV

Expiratory chest films are preferred in

- Small pneumothorax
- Early interstitial lung disease
- Along with an inspiratory film in obstructive emphysema

Condition & minimum collection for X-ray detection

- Pleural effusion: 250 ml
- Pericardial effusion: 200 ml
- Pneumoperitoneum: 1 ml

TERMS

- Atomic number: Number of protons
- Atomic weight: Protons + neutrons
- Isotopes:
  - Same atomic number
  - Different atomic weight
- Isobars:
  - Same atomic weight
  - Different atomic number
- Isomers:
  - Same atomic weight
  - Same atomic number
  - Different energy state in nuclei

Radiation emitted

Rays	*Substance*
Both beta and gamma	Iodine (mainly beta)
Beta	Strontium, gold, phosphorous
Gamma	Cobalt, cesium, technitium

IONIZING RADIATION

- Gamma rays are predominantly emitted by:
    - Cesium-137
    - Cobalt &
    - Radium
- Rays having maximum penetration power: Gamma rays
- Most ionizing rays: Alpha rays
- Phosphorous 32 emits: Beta particles

ULTRASOUND

- Frequency of USG commonly used in medical practice: 1 MHz to 20 MHz
- USG probe is made of:
    - Quartz (previously)
    - Lead zirconate titanate (nowadays)

Remember

- USG is non-ionizing
- Radiation hazard is NOT a feature of MRI/ Doppler USG

USG

- Activity of transducer of USG are based on the principle of piezoelectric effect
- Absolute barrier to USG is air
- Ultrasound in obstetrics can induce changes in cell migration at an early stage of development

Various modes of USG

- A mode (Amplitude): Measures axial length of eyeball
- B mode (Brightness): Main mode used for ultrasound imagine
- M mode (Movement): Echocardiography

CT SCAN

- CT scan was invented by: Hounsfield
- Hounsfield number in CT scan depends upon: Mass density
- Value of water in CT: Zero
- Tissue having highest density on CT: Bone
- CT scan rooms are shielded by:
    - At least 1/16 inch lead shielding
    - Walls, doors, floors, ceilings & operators barrier

CT SCAN APPEARANCES

- Central stellate scar on renal CT indicates: Renal oncocytoma
- Crescentic hyperdense lesion on skull CT indicates: Subdural haemorrhage
- Lentiginous appearance of brain on CT indicates: Medulloblastoma

MRI

- MC contrast agent used in MRI: Gadolinium DTPA
- C/I to MRI:
    - Cardiac pacemakers
    - Aneurysmal clips etc.
- Faradays cage: MRI rooms are shielded by continuous sheets of copper or aluminium from interference by external electromagnetic radiation

Remember

- MRI is non-ionizing
- No radiation exposure

Contraindications to MRI

- Pacemakers
- Intracranial clips
- Size and weight above machine limits
- First trimester of pregnancy
- Claustrophobia

POSITRON EMISSION TOMOGRAPHY (PET SCAN)

- Substance used in PET scan: 2-fluoro-2-deoxy-D-glucose (FDG)
- Uses of PET scan:
  - o Differentiating radiation necrosis from active neoplasm following therapy
  - o Investigation of recurrent GIST tumours etc.

Procedures & dye used

Procedure	*Dye*
Fetography	Ethiodol
Hysterosalpingography	50% diodone with 6% polyvinyl alcohol in water
Splenoportography	Sodium metrizoate
Cholecystography	Indapamide, meglumine, ioglyconate
Myelography	Myodil
Ventriculography	Metrizamide & iophendylate
Esophagus	Barium swallow
Intestinal obstruction	Gastrografin
Lymphangiography	Methylene blue & lipiodol
Intravenous pyelography	Sodium diatrizoate
Urethrography	Ambrodil viscous
Sialography	Neohydriol
Bronchography	Dionosil

MYELOGRAPHY

- Dye used in myelography: Metrizamide
- MC complication of myelography: Headache (MC complication of dural puncture & myelography)

Contrasts used in various studies

- Oral cholecystography: Iopanoic acid
- Intravenous cholecystography: Biligraffin (Meglumine)
- Esophageal atresia: Dionosil
- Intravenous Pyelogram: Conray 420
- Myelography: Myodil (Iodophendylate), Iohexol (Omnipaque)
- Vertebral angiography: Conray 280

CARDIOLOGY

- Right border of heart is formed by:
  - o SVC/ Right brachiocephalic vessels
  - o IVC &
  - o Right atrium
- Left border of heart is formed by:
  - o Left atrial appendage
  - o Left ventricle
  - o Aortic arch &
  - o Pulmonary artery
- Fallot's tetralogy: Boot shaped heart
- Transposition of great arteries: (2nd HS is greater in intensity)
  - o Egg on side heart
  - o Apple on a string
- Total Anomalous Pulmonary Venous Connection (TAPVC): Snowman heart
- Mitral stenosis: Double shadow
- Hydatid cyst: Water lily sign
- Ebstein's anomaly:
  - o Cardiomegaly
  - o Pulmonary oligemia
- Radiological features of heart failure:
  - o Cardiomegaly
  - o Prominent upper lobe veins
  - o Kerley B lines

Radiological signs in cardiovascular system

- Coeur en sabot / Dutch shoe / Boot-shaped heart: Fallot's tetralogy
- Egg on end appearance: TGA
- Cottage loaf heart: Supracardiac total anomalous pulmonary, Venous return, wide mediastinum
- Box-shaped cardiomegaly: Ebstein's anomaly
- Snowman or figure of 8: Supracardiac TAPVC

- '3' sign: Aortic coarctation, due to stenosis of aorta
- Leather bottle or flask shaped heart: Pericardial effusion
- Double atrial shadow: Left atrial enlargement

RESPIRATORY SYSTEM

- Causes of miliary mottling on chest radiography:
  - TB
  - RA
  - Sarcoidosis
  - Fungal infections:
    - Blastomycosis
    - Histoplasmosis
    - Coccidioidomycosis
  - Pneumoconiosis
  - Varicella pneumonia
  - Amyloidosis &
  - Pulmonary edema
- Ground glass appearance on chest radiography:
  - Hyaline membrane disease
  - Pneumonia
  - Pneumocystis pneumonia etc.
- Kerley B lines are seen in: Basal zone (early change of pulmonary edema)
- Hampton's hump is seen in: Pulmonary embolism
- IOC for minimal bronchiectasis: High Resolution CT scan
- Calcification in benign pulmonary hamartoma: Popcorn/ Bulls eye

Radiological signs in respiratory system

- Butterfly/ batwing pattern: Pulmonary edema
- Moustache /Antler sign: Prominence or upper lobe veins due to increased left atrial pressure in case of Mitral stenosis
- Dirty chest: Chronic bronchitis
- Pneumatoceles: Infection due to Staphylococcus and Klebsiella
- Egg shell calcification: Silicosis, Sarcoidosis, Histoplasmosis, Blastomycosis, Scleroderma, Amyloidosis
- Bulging fissure: Klebsiella pneumonia
- Crescent sign: Fungal ball within a cavity

Kerley's lines

- Kerley's A lines: Seen near the apex
- Kerley's B lines: Seen near the base perpendicular to the pleural surface
- Kerley's C lines: Near the center, interlacing, leading to spider web appearance

Kerley's lines are seen in:

- Pulmonary edema
- Mitral valve prolapse
- Pneumoconiosis
- Lymphatic metastatic disease

Radiological signs of pulmonary embolism

- Westermark: Pulmonary oligemia
- Hampton's hump: Peripheral wedge-shaped density
- Palla's sign: Enlarged right descending pulmonary artery

GASTROINTESTINAL TRACT & HEPATOBILIARY SYSTEM

- Single bubble sign: Pyloric stenosis
- IOC for acute cholecystitis: HIDA scan
- Features of cholecystitis:
  - Thick gall bladder wall
  - Peri-gall bladder halo etc.
- Double bubble sign:
  - Annular pancreas
  - Duodenal atresia etc.
- Chain of lake appearance: Chronic pancreatitis
- Fox sign: Acute pancreatitis
- Widening of duodenal C loop: Ca head of pancreas
- Bird of prey sign: Sigmoid volvulus
- Thumb printing sign: Ischemic colitis

Radiological signs of Hypertrophic pyloric stenosis

- String sign: Due to narrowed pyloric canal
- Beak sign: Due to an abrupt cut off of barium point in the pyloric canal
- Tram track sign: Double track of barium

Radiological signs in hepatobiliary system

- Floating membrane/ Water lily of Camalote sign: Ruptured hydatid cyst.
- Rising sun/ Serpent sign: Dry hydatid cyst with crumpled membrane
- Bull's eye lesion in USG of liver: Metastases
- Mercedes benz sign / sea gull sign: Radiolucent gas in triradiate/ biradiate fissure in a gallbladder
- Pad sign in barium meal: Carcinoma pancreas
- Scrambled egg appearance in ERCP: Carcinoma pancreas
- Reversed 3 sign of Frostberg: Carcinoma head of pancreas
- Beading of bile duct seen in ERCP: Sclerosing cholangitis
- Chain of lakes appearance seen in ERCP: Chronic pancreatitis
- Double duct sign seen in ERCP: Pancreatic carcinoma in conjunction with bile duct obstruction or stricture

Radiological signs in gastrointestinal system

- Concertina or stack of coins appearance: Dilated jejunum
- Coffee bean sign: Intestinal obstruction with strangulation
- Cobblestone appearance: Crohn's disease
- Raspberry thorning/Rose thorn ulcers of intestine: Crohn's disease
- Inverted umbrella sign(broad base triangular appearance of ileocecal valve with base towards cecum): Ileocecal junction tuberculosis]
- Sterling's sign (lack of retention of barium in inflamed segment of ileum, caecum and ascending colon): Ileocecal junction tuberculosis, Crohn's disease
- String sign of Kantor (Persistent narrow steam of barium indicating stenosis and strictures): Ileocecal junction tuberculosis, Crohn's disease
- Thumb printing appearance (Due to ulcers and edema): Ulcerative colitis
- Lead pipe appearance (Blunting of haustral folds): Ulcerative colitis
- Omega sign on plain X-ray abdomen: Sigmoid volvulus
- Inverted U appearance of Sigmoid colon: Volvulus
- Twisted bird's beak /Ace of spade Deformity in barium enema: Sigmoid volvulus
- Bent inner tube or Omega loop Sign on straight X-ray of abdomen: Volvulus
- Inverted 3 sign in barium swallow: The impression of aorta on esophagus
- Bird's beak appearance: Achalasia cardia
- Rat tail appearance: Carcinoma esophagus
- Apple core deformity: Carcinoma esophagus
- Cup and spill stomach: Volvulus stomach
- Leather bottle appearance/ Linitis plastica: Carcinoma, Corrosive gastritis, Cohn's disease, Tuberculosis, Syphilis, Eosinophilic gastritis, Lymphoma
- Double bubble sign: Duodena atresia
- Triple bubble sign: Jejunal atresia
- Barber pole sign/ Corkscrew Sign/Spiral sign in barium studies: Midgut volvulus due to spiraling of superior mesenteric artery
- Whirl sign or peacock tail sign in CT/ MRI:
- Midgut volvulus due to spiraling of superior mesenteric artery
- String of beads sign: Small bowel obstruction
- Moulage sign/ Molten wax appearance of intestine in barium studies: Malabsorption

Radiological signs of Intussusception

- Coiled spring appearance
- Empty Quarter sign (due to empty right iliac fossa)
- Pseudo-kidney sign (Seen on USG)
- Claw sign (in barium meal X-ray)

URINARY SYSTEM

- Flower vase appearance: Horse shoe kidney
- Fish hook bladder: BPH
- Dropping flower sign: Ectopic ureter
- Cobra head appearance: Ureterocele
- Adder head appearance: Ureterocele
- Rim sign: Hydronephrosis
- Crescent sign: Hydronephrosis
- Golf hole bladder: TB urinary bladder
- Thimble bladder: Chronic TB
- Bilateral spider leg pattern: Polycystic kidneys
- Bilateral spider leg pattern: Polycystic kidney
- Thimble bladder: Chronic TB
- Rim sign: Hydronephrosis
- Cobra head appearance: Ureterocele
- Adder head appearance: Ureterocele

IVU

- Goblet sign: Filling defect in the ureter due to tumour
- Hourglass bladder: Bladder duplication
- Stipple sign on retrograde pyelography: Transitional cell carcinoma
- Pear shaped bladder: Pelvic lipomatosis
- Fir tree appearance of bladder in X-ray: Upper motor neuron disease
- Pencil like curvilinear calcification in bladder wall: Bilharziasis
- Fish hook appearance of ureters: Prostatic enlargement

Radiological signs of urinary system

- Crescent sign/ Rim sign in Nephrogram: Acquired hydronephrosis
- Mathe's sign (absence of downward displacement of kidney that normally occurs in erect position): Perinephric abscess
- Beak sign in renal arteriogram: Renal cyst
- Flower vase ureters: Horse-shoe kidney
- Spider leg calyces: Polycystic kidney
- Pencil line / Tram line appearance: Acute cortical necrosis
- Egg in cup appearance: Renal papillary necrosis
- Air pyelogram: Emphysematous diabetic pyelonephritis
- Pancake kidney: Failure of both kidney to ascend from the pelvis
- Spoke wheel appearance on angiography: Oncocytoma
- Onion layer appearance on USG: Angiomyolipoma
- Saw toothed, beaded or pipe stem: Ureteric tuberculosis
- Cobra head deformity /Adder head sign: Ureterocele

MUSCULOSKELETAL SYSTEM

- Polka dot in vertebra: Haemangioma
- Champagne glass pelvis: Achondroplasia
- Pencil thin cortex: Scurvy
- Onion skin appearance: Ewing's sarcoma
- Fallen fragment sign: Aneurysmal bone cyst
- Codman's triangle & Sunray appearance: Osteosarcoma
- Cotton wool/ Ground glass appearance: Fibrous dysplasia
- Earliest radiological sign in acute osteomyelitis: Soft tissue swelling
- Water's view/ Occipitomental view is done for:
  - o Maxillary
  - o Frontal
  - o Sphenoid sinus (only with open mouth view)
- Odontoid view is done to visualize: C1, C2 vertebrae

Radiological signs in osteoarthritis

- Osteophytes
- Decreased joint space
- Sclerosis of bone ends forming joints

Commonly involved joints in osteoarthritis

- Major joints of lower limb
- Distal interphalangeal joint
- Proximal interphalangeal joint
- 1st metacarpal joint

Vertebral signs & conditions

- Scotty dog appearance: Normal vertebra
- Scotty dog wearing collar: Spondylosis
- Beheaded Scottish terrier: Spondylolisthesis

Radiological signs in rheumatoid arthritis

- Increased joint space
- Peri-articular erosion and osteoporosis
- Syndesmophytes
- Bamboo spine
- Tram track sign

Radiological signs in musculoskeletal system

- Looser's zone (an area of stress fracture repaired by osteoid in the absence of normal mineralization): Osteomalacia
- Cord fish vertebrae (biconcave): Osteomalacia
- Triradiate pelvis: Osteomalacia
- Pepper pot skull appearance: Hyperparathyroidism
- Aneurysmal sign: Erosion of the anterior surface of vertebral body by tuberculous abscesses, resembling erosions due to aortic aneurysm
- Hot cross bun skull: Congenital syphilis
- Sutural diastases (In children it is the first and the most prominent sign): Raised ICT
- Silver beaten appearance: Raised ICT
- Champagne glass pelvis: Achondroplasia
- Tombstone iliac blades: Achondroplasia
- Saw tooth metaphysis: Congenital syphilis
- Lace work Periostitis: Congenital syphilis
- Wimberger's sign (bilateral symmetrical): Perichondritis and osteitis of tibia Upper growth plate medially): Congenital syphilis
- Dots and commas / Rings and broken Rings calcification: Enchondroma or chondrosarcoma
- Tufting of terminal phalanges of fingers and toes: Acromegaly
- Doughnut appearance on radionuclide scan: Avascular necrosis
- Picture frame vertebra: Paget's disease
- Dural tail sign: Meningiomas
- Licked candy stick appearance (neuropathic resorption of bone): Leprosy

CNS

- IOC for subarachnoid hemorrhage (SAH): Non contrast CT
- Intracranial calcification is seen in:
  - Cysticercosis
  - Pineal & dural calcification
- Basal ganglia calcification is seen in: Hypoparathyroidism
- Suprasellar calcification is seen in:
  - Craniopharyngioma
  - Meningioma
- Rail road/ Tram track calcification: Sturge Weber syndrome
- Periventricular calcification is seen in: CMV infection
- Bracket calcification in skull is seen in: Corpus callosum lipoma
- Separation of sutures in a child is radiological sign of: Raised intra-cranial tension

Structures, which calcify physiologically, are

- Pineal gland
- Habenular commissure
- Falx cerebri
- Choroidal plexus
- Dura
- Petroclinoid ligament
- Interclinoid ligament

Intracranial pathologies, which calcify, are:

- Gliomas
- Haematomas
- A-V malformations/ Aneurysms
- Tuberculomas
- Cysticercosis
- Hydatid disease
- Sturge- Weber syndrome
- Tuberous sclerosis

General facts radiotherapy

Radioactive phosphorous is useful in diagnosis of	**Eye cancers, esophageal cancers**
Radioactive phosphorous is useful in management of is useful in diagnosis of	**Polycythemia vera, multiple myeloma, secondary's in bones, carcinoma prostate after priming with androgen, malignant ascites**
For permanent insertion into cavities	**Colloidal gold, yttrium, phosphorus 32**
Substances used as permanent implant for radiation	**Gold grains, radon seeds**
Machine used for electron therapy	**Betatron**
Most used material for external radiation	**Cobalt 60, cesium 137**
Isotopes	**Elements with same atomic number; number of proton is same, number of neutron value**

BASICS OF RADIOTHERAPY

- Background radiation is present in:
  - o Everywhere in nature
  - o Usually NOT detrimental to life
- Maximum permissible dose of radiation (in a year) should NOT exceed: 5 rad/ year
- Stochastic effects of radiation:
  - o Probability that a particular effect will increase
  - o With increase in dose of radiation
  - o Often show up years after exposure

MEASURE OF RADIATION

- Measure of activity of radiation: Becquerel
- Measure of absorbed dose: Gray, (1 gray = 100 rads)
- Measure of radioactivity: Curie
- Radioactivity was discovered by Curie (1896)

Half-lives

Radio-isotope	*Duration*
Iodine 132	**2.3 hours**
Iodine 123	**13 hours**
Iodine 131	**8 days**
Technetium	**6 hours**
Thallium chloride	**3.1 days**
Gallium	**3.2 days**
Radon	**3.8 days**
Cobalt	**5.2 years**
Strontium 90	**28 years**
Cesium 137	**30 years**
Radium	**1622 years**

HALF LIVES

- I-131: 8 days
- Rn-222: 3-6 days
- Co-60: 5.2 years

USES

- Hot spot in MI is detected by: Technetium scan
- Pancreatic scanning is done by: Selenium 75
- Scan used for parathyroid gland: Sestamibi scan
- Scan for measurement of renal GFR: Tc99-DTPA scan
- Vesicoureteral reflex (VUR) is seen by: MAG3-tc99 scan
- Isotope used in thyroid scan: I-131
- 99Tc scan shows hot spot in: Adenolymphoma (Salivary gland tumour)
- PACS/ picture archiving & communication system: New system (completely computerized network) to replace conventional analogue film & paper clinical request forms & reports

- Brachytherapy: Radiation therapy in which sources are placed within or near tumour for therapy
- Gamma knife (using gamma rays) is used in: Stereotactic surgery (cuts tumour in different location/ 3D)
- Mantle irradiation is done in: Hodgkin's disease
- Hyper-fractionation radiotherapy is used to treat: Lung cancer
- Intra-operative radiotherapy is used to treat: Pancreatic Ca
- Stereo-tactic radiosurgery is: A form of radiotherapy
- Emergency radiotherapy is given in:
  - o SVC syndrome
  - o Pericardial tamponade
- RAIU/ (RadioActive Iodine Uptake test) is done mostly using: I-123
- Photodynamic therapy with hematoporphyrins & light is used in the treatment of:
  - o Colon & skin Ca

RADIOSENSITIVITY

- Most radiosensitive cell: Lymphocytes
- Most radiosensitive cell structure: DNA
- Phase of cycle most sensitive to radiation: G2M
- Most radiosensitive brain tumour: Medulloblastoma
- Cartilage is: Radioresistant

RADIATION SYNDROMES

- MC manifestation in skin is: Erythema
- Papillary Ca of thyroid in infancy develops due to: Radiation exposure

DRUGS

- Amifostine is: Cytoprotective/ radioprotective agent (a thiophosphate)
- Hydroxyurea, 5 FU are: Radio-sensitizers

Radio-isotope scans

Scan for	*Isotope used*
Renography (measures renal output of radio-active isotope)	**Iodine 131 labelled hippuran**
Cisternography (for communicating hydrocephalus)	**Radioactive iodinated serum albumin**
Placental position	**Radioactive sodium**
Thyroid function	**Iodine 131**
Thyroid malignancy	**Selenium**
Pancreas scan	**Selenomethionine**
Tumour/ abscess	**Gallium citrate**
Myocardial perfusion	**Thallium chloride**
Myocardial infarction	**Technetium pyrophosphate**
Myocardial function	**Technetium labeled albumin**
Brain, bone	**Technetium pertechnetate**
Kidney	**Technetium 99**
Lung ventilation	**Xenon gas or krypton 81**
Lung	**Technetium 99 macroaggregates**
Spleen, marrow	**Technetium 99 Sulphur colloid**
Liver & biliary function	**Technetium 99 glucoheptonate**

CLINICAL QUESTIONS

1. **There is consolidation in middle lobe of right lung. Which of the heart border will be obliterated on chest X-ray?**

   A. Right heart border B. Left heart border

   C. Anterior heart border D. Posterior heart border

   As the right middle lobe of lung lies adjacent to the right cardiac border, diseases like consolidation of the right middle lobe will obliterate the right cardiac border.

   Answer. A i.e., Right heart border

2. **A 7 weeks pregnant lady is accidentally exposed to chest X-ray in a hospital. What needs to be done next?**

   A. Continue pregnancy

   B. Terminate pregnancy

   C. Chromosomal checking

   D. Amniocentesis

   In first trimester of pregnancy, any radiation exposure of more than 5 rads needs consideration for continuing pregnancy. Single exposure rarely causes such a large exposure so pregnancy can be continued.

   Answer. A i.e., Continue pregnancy

CHAPTER 18

PSYCHIATRY

RAPID REVISION NOTES

Substance abuse

Feature	*Substance*
Paranoid hallucinatory syndrome	**Amphetamine**
Bad trip, flash back	**LSD**
Delirium tremens, morbid jealousy, Mac-ewen's sign	**Alcohol**
Run amok, flash back, amotivational syndrome	**Cannabis**
Tactile hallucination/ cocaine bugs/ magnan symptom	**Cocaine**
Flashback phenomenon	**Cannabis, LSD, psilocybin**
Formication (tactile hallucination in the form of bugs crawling under the skin)	**Cocaine, chronic amphetamine use, methyl-phenidate, alcohol withdrawal**
Bad trip (acute panic reaction with loss of control on oneself)	**LSD**
Black pigmentation of tongue & teeth	**Cocaine**
NO/ MINIMAL withdrawal symptoms	**LSD, cannabis**
Brown sugar or smack	**Heroin**

PSYCHIATRY & NEUROTRANSMITTERS

- Schizophrenia: Increased dopamine
- Depression: Decreased serotonin
- Epilepsy: Decreased GABA
- Obsessive Compulsive Disorder:
    - o Decreased serotonin &
    - o Decreased noradrenaline
- Mania & anxiety: Increased noradrenaline
- Dementia: Decreased acetylcholine

SIGMOND FREUD

- Associated with:
    - o Psychoanalysis (founder)
    - o Concept of free association
    - o Concept of id, ego & superego
    - o Oedipus complex
    - o Analysis of properties of cocaine

Id, Superego & Ego

- Id: Selfish, primitive, childish and pleasure-oriented part of the personality with no ability to delay gratification

- Superego: Internalised societal and parental standards of good, bad, right and wrong behavior
- Ego: Moderator between the Id and Superego, which compromises to pacify both

TERMS & SCIENTISTS

- Classical conditioning: Pavlov
- Schizophrenia: Bleuler
- Ambivalence: Bleuler
- Father of attachment theory: John Bowlby
- Adolescent turmoil: Ericson
- Catatonia: Kahlbaum

Delirium & dementia

Feature	*Delirium*	*Dementia*
Onset	Acute	Insidious
Consciousness	Clouded	Usually normal
Orientation	Grossly disturbed	Disturbed only in late stages
Memory	Immediate & recent disturbed	Immediate in normal, recent & remote disturbed
Attention & concentration	Grossly disturbed	Usually normal
Perception	Visual illusion and hallucination common	Hallucination may occur
Diurnal variation	Marked (sun-downing present i.e. worsening of symptoms in evening & night)	Usually absent

DELIRIUM

- Also known as acute confusional state
- Memory registration & retention impaired
- Clouding of consciousness
- Disorientation
- Attention & concentration disturbed
- Marked diurnal variation

DEMENTIA

- No disturbance of consciousness
- Cognitive impairment
- Impaired judgement &
- Personality alteration

Causes of reversible dementia

- Hypothyroidism
- Hypoparathyroidism
- Hyperparathyroidism etc.

Causes of irreversible dementia

- Alzheimer's dementia (MC cause)
- Multi-infarct dementia etc.

ALZHEIMER'S DEMENTIA

- Cortical (NOT subcortical) dementia
- Progressive
- Associated with Apo E gene
- Neurofibrillary tangles are seen &
- Donepezil is used in management

AUTISM

- Difficulty in concentration & communication
- Lesion in frontal & temporal lobe and cerebellum
- Delayed speech & language development
- Problems in forming social relationships in early childhood
- Stereotyped movements
- Poor speech
- Lack of social interaction

Asperger's syndrome

- It is a variant, but without any delay in language or cognitive development
- Better prognosis

ATTENTION DEFICIT HYPERACTIVITY DISORDER/ ADHD

- Easy distractibility/ poor attention span
- Impulsivity
- Methylphenidate & Atom-oxetine are used in management

DELUSION, HALLUCINATION & ILLUSION

Delusion

- Disorder of thought
- FALSE unshaken belief NOT amenable to reasoning

Hallucination

- Disorder of perception
- Perception in the absence of external stimuli
- Not dependent of will of observer

Illusion

- Misinterpretation of external stimuli

Delusions

- De Clerambault: Delusion that someone from higher socioeconomic
- Othello syndrome: Delusion of infidelity
- Capgras's syndrome: Delusion of doubles
- Cotard's syndrome/ Nihilism: Delusion that one has lost everything, including possessions, status, strength and body orgAnswer:

Formal thought disorder (disorders of thought process)

Thought	*Condition*
Racing thought	Anxiety, schizophrenia
Retarded thought	Depression
Circumstantiality	Mania, schizophrenia
Thought blocking	Schizophrenia, severe anxiety
Perseveration	Organic brain disease, schizophrenia
Neologism, word salad, echolalia	Schizophrenia
Clubbing and pubbing	Mania, schizophrenia
Flight of ideas	Mania
Loosening of association	Schizophrenia

SCHIZOPHRENIA

- 1st rank symptoms of schizophrenia:
  - o Hallucination
  - o Thought alienation phenomenon:
    - ♦ Thought insertion
    - ♦ Thought withdrawal
    - ♦ Thought broadcasting
  - o Delusional perception
  - o Passivity phenomenon
- Bleuler's criterion for schizophrenia:
  - o Association disturbance
  - o Affect disturbance
  - o Autism &
  - o Ambivalence
- 1st symptom to go with treatment: Auditory hallucination
- Amphetamines causes: Paranoid schizophrenia
- Late onset schizophrenia: More than 40 years
- Good prognostic factors:
  - o Acute onset
  - o Late onset etc.

Catatonic schizophrenia

- Defect of conation
- Negativism
- Echolalia (repetition of words/ phrases)
- Echopraxia
- Mannerism & grimacing
- Automatic obedience
- Cataplexy etc.

Eugen Bleuler's cardinal symptoms of schizophrenia (four A's)

- Blunted Affect
- Loosening of Association
- Ambivalence
- Autism

Kurt Schneider's first rank symptoms of schizophrenia

- Hearing one's thoughts aloud
- Auditory hallucinations commenting on one's behaviour.
- Thought withdrawal, insertion and broadcasting
- Somatic hallucinations or the experience of one's thoughts as being controlled or influenced from outside

Types of schizophrenia

- Paranoid schizophrenia: Delusions of persecution, late onset and progressive course
- Hebephrenic: Marked thought disorder, severe loosening of association, Emotional disturbances, Progressively worse course
- Catatonic: Acute onset in 2nd to 3rd decade Episodic and complete recovery; Clinical features include - Mutism, rigidity, negativism, posturing, stupor, echolalia, Echopraxia, waxy flexibility, ambitendency, automatic obedience, verbigeration
- Pseudo neurotic: Initially, there are predominant neurotic symptoms. Three classical features are pan anxiety, pan neurosis, and pan Sexuality
- Oneiroid: Subtype of schizophrenia with acute onset, clouding of consciousness, disorientation, dream like state and perceptual disturbances with rapid shifting
- Van Gogh syndrome: Schizophrenia with self-mutilation
- Prove syndrome: Schizophrenia with mental retardation

SOMATIZATION DISORDER

- Patient presents with multiple physical complaints (referable to different organ systems)
- Formal diagnostic criteria require the recording of at least 4 pains:
    - o 2 gastrointestinal
    - o 1 sexual &
    - o 1 pseudo-neurologic symptom

CONVERSION DISORDER

- La belle indifference is seen
- Primary & secondary gains are associated

HYPOCHONDRIASIS

- Essential feature: Belief of serious medical illness that persists despite reassurance & appropriate medical evaluation
- Abnormal pre-occupation of normal body functions

IMPULSE CONTROL DISORDERS

- Dipsomania: Irresistible desire for alcohol drinks
- Trichotillomania: Need to pull out hair
- Pyromania: Irresistible desire to set things on fire
- Kleptomania: Irresistible desire to steal articles

PHOBIC DISORDERS

- Marked & persistent fear of objects/situations, exposure to which results in immediate anxiety reaction
- Agoraphobia: Fear of open spaces
- Claustrophobia: Fear of closed spaces
- Management of phobia: Cognitive behavioural therapy (best) & SSRI

Types of phobias

- Acrophobia: Fear of high places
- Zoophobia: Fear of animals
- Xenophobia: Fear of strangers
- Claustrophobia: Fear of closed spaces
- Thanatophobia: Fear of death

LSD

- Flash back/ bad trips are seen
- Treatment NOT required for LSD withdrawal

DEPRESSION

- MC psychiatric disorder in India: Depression
- Neurotransmitter involved in depression:
  - o Serotonin
  - o Norepinephrine
- MC cause of suicide: Depression
- MC type of post puerperal psychosis: Depression
- Nihilistic ideas are seen in: Depression
- Risk factors for suicide in depression:
  - o Endogenous type of depression
  - o Psychotic depression etc.

MANIA

- Inflated self-esteem
- Grandiosity
- Flight of ideas &
- Distractibility

ALCOHOL & PSYCHIATRY

- Wernicke's encephalopathy involves: Mammillary bodies
- Korsakoff's syndrome presents as:
  - o Profound & persistent anterograde amnesia &
  - o Confabulation
- Feature of alcoholic paranoia: Hallucination
- Questionnaire used: CAGE
- Alcohol withdrawal:
  - o Visual & tactile hallucination (hangover)

Delirium tremens

- MC severe symptom of alcohol withdrawal
- Disorientation
- Anxiety
- Perceptual defect
- Chlordiazepoxide is used for management

SLEEP

- Delta waves: Deep sleep
- Night terrors are seen in: NREM sleep
- Sleep walking/ somnambulism is seen in: NREM sleep (stage 3/ 4)
- Sleep terror/ pavor nocturnus:
  - o Seen in NREM sleep (stage 3/ 4)
  - o Treated by diazepam

EEG waves and sleep cycles

- Awake and alert: Beta waves
- Awake, result, eyes closed: Alpha
- NREM-1: Theta
- NREM-2: Theta
- NREM-3: Delta
- NREM-4: Delta
- REM: Beta

DISSOCIATIVE DISORDER

- Dissociative amnesia: Patchy impairment of personal memory
- Dissociative identity disorder: Person is dominated by 2 or more personalities
- Depersonalization disorder: It is detachment from self, social situation or environment (derealization)

DRUGS IN PSYCHIATRY

- Naltrexone:
  - o Used in opioid dependency:
    - ♦ For rapid detoxification
    - ♦ Maintenance therapy
  - o To prevent relapse
  - o Used to reduce craving &
  - o Prevent relapse in heavy alcohol drinking (alcohol dependence)

- Lithium:
  - o Therapeutic serum level is 0.8-1.2 mmol/L
  - o Lithium is C/I in pregnancy (causes CVS defects)
  - o Liver is NOT affected in lithium toxicity
  - o ECG changes of lithium toxicity are: Sinus tachycardia/ bradycardia, Flattened/ inverted T waves, AV block & A prolonged QT interval
- Drugs used in Maniac Depressive Psychosis/ MDP:
  - o Lithium
  - o Valproate
  - o Carbamazepine
  - o Levothyroxine
- Agent of choice for prophylaxis in mania: Lithium (mood stabilizer)
- Drugs causing depression:
  - o OCP
  - o Bromocriptine etc.
- TCA:
  - o Amitriptyline
  - o Clomipramine etc.
- Tetracyclic antidepressant:
  - o Maprotiline
  - o Mianserin etc.
- SSRI:
  - o Fluoxetine
  - o Fluvoxamine etc.

Lithium

- Therapeutic level of blood lithium: 0.8-1.2 mEq/L
- Prophylactic blood lithium: 0.6-1.2 mEq/L
- Side effects: >2 mEq/L
- Life threatening toxicity: >3.5 mEq/L

Drugs of choice for psychiatric disorders

- Generalized anxiety: Benzodiazepines
- Panic attack: Fluoxetine
- Nocturnal enuresis: Imipramine
- Opioid withdrawal: Methadone →2nd DOC →Clonidine
- Opioid intoxication: Naloxone/Naltrexone
- Alcohol withdrawal: Chlordiazepoxide → 2nd DOC → Diazepam
- Alcohol abstinence; Disulfiram
- Benzodiazepines intoxication: Flumazenil
- Obsessives compulsive disorder: Fluoxetine
- Attention deficit hyperactivity disorder: Amphetamine → 2nd DOC→ Methylphenidate
- Tic disorder: Haloperidol
- Bulimia nervosa: Fluoxetine
- Alcoholic hallucinations: Diazepam
- Neuroleptic induced urinary retention: Bethanechol
- Neuroleptic induced hyperprolactinemia: Amantadine
- Akathisia: Propranolol

ELECTROCONVULSIVE THERAPY/ ECT

- Used in:
  - o Delusional depression
  - o Severe psychosis
  - o Severe catatonia etc.
- Absolute C/I for ICT: Raised ICT
- MC side effect of modified ECT is: Retrograde amnesia (antegrade amnesia also occurs but with decreased frequency)
- Effect of ECT on intra-ocular tension: Decrease

COGNITIVE BEHAVOURAL THERAPY/ CBT

- CBT is based on: Learning theory/ operant conditioning
- Flooding is a type of CBT
- CBT is used in:
  - o Phobia
  - o Eating disorders etc.

OBSESSIVE COMPULSIVE DISORDER/ OCD

- Neurotransmitter implicated: Serotonin

- Features of OCD:
  - o Obsessive thoughts & compulsive behaviors that impair everyday functioning
  - o Shows perfectionism,
  - o Repetitive thoughts/ images etc.
- Obsession is ego alien (conscious about disorder)
- Group A streptococci are associated with OCD
- Management of OCD:
  - o Fluoxetine (DOC)
  - o Fluvoxamine
  - o Exposure & response prevention

Intelligence quotient

Label	*IQ score*
Genius	>145
Very superior	>130
Superior	120-130
Bright normal	110-120
Normal	90-110
Dull normal	80-90
Borderline retardation	70-80
Mild retardation	50-70
Moderate retardation	35-50
Severe retardation	20-35
Profound retardation	<20

MENTAL RETARDATION

- Normal IQ: 100
- IQ is calculated as: (Mental age/chronological age) X 100
- Mental ill health is usually due to: Social maladjustment
- Chromosomal abnormality causing MR:
  - o Down syndrome (MC)
  - o Fragile X syndrome (2nd MC)
- Mild MR: 50-70

Personality types

- Schizoid personality type: introverted, withdrawn, solitary and distant
- Paranoid personality: Interprets the action of others as deliberately threatening. Untrusting, unforgiving, guarded, and prone to aggression. Perceive others as jealous, deceitful and condescending
- Schizotypal personality: Odd and eccentric manners of dressing and speaking. Strange, paranoid beliefs. Have difficulties forming relations and extreme anxiety in social situations. Display sign of magical thinking
- Antisocial personality: Impulsive, irresponsible, callous and aggressive. No respect for others and no remorse. High risk for alcohol and substance abuse
- Borderline personality: Abrupt and extreme mood changes. Unstable Disorder and fluctuating self-image. Unpredictable and self-Destructive. Fears of abandonment. Excessive Dependency, self-mutilation or recurrent suicidal gestures. Impulsive, chronic feeling of boredom, bouts of intense Anger
- Avoidant personality: Hypersensitive to rejection, excessive social Disorder discomfort, timidity fear of criticism, avoidance of social work
- Dependent personality: Dependent and submissive behavior, feel fear No respect, lack self confidence
- Compulsive personality: Compulsive personalities, high levels of aspirations, strive for perfection never satisfied with achievements. Reliable, dependable, orderly, methodical and highly cautious
- Histrionic personality: Self-dramatization, exaggerated expressions suggestibility Attention seeking attitude Seductiveness, concerned with Physical appearance

Neuroleptic malignant syndrome

- Muscle rigidity autonomic dysregulation and hyper-thermia
- Idiosyncratic reaction to inhibition of central dopamine receptors that results in increased heat production and failure of heat dissipation
- Management:
  - o Rapid physical cooling
  - o Administration of an antipyretic or bromocriptine with acetaminophen and

- o Dantrolene

Anorexia nervosa & bulimia nervosa

Feature	*Anorexia nervosa*	*Bulimia nervosa*
Onset	Mid-adolescence	Late adolescence/ early adulthood
Female: male	10:1	10:1
Prevalence in women	0.5%	1-3%
Weight	Markedly decreased	Usually normal
Menstruation	Absent	Usually normal
Binge eating	25-50%	Required for diagnosis
Mortality	5%	Low
Skin/ extremities	Lanugo, acrocyanosis, edema	
CVS	Bradycardia, hypotension	
GIT	Salivary gland enlargement, slow gastric emptying, constipation, elevated liver enzymes	Salivary gland enlargement, dental erosion
Hematopoietic	Normocytic - normochromic anemia, leukopenia	
Fluid/ electrolyte	Increased BUN, creatinine, hyponatremia	Hypokalemia, hypochloremia, alkalosis
Endocrine	Hypoglycemia, low estrogen/ testosterone, low LH & FSH, normal TSH, increased cortisol	
Bone	Osteopenia	

CLINICAL PRESENTATIONS

- Patient with increased sweating, lacrimation, diarrhea, rhinorrhea: Heroin withdrawal
- Female patient with anxiety, palpitation, breathlessness, feeling of impending doom but a normal physical examination: Panic attack
- Young female with episodes of excessive eating followed by laxative use: Bulimia nervosa
- A patient after a car accident was admitted in ICU for 6 months. After discharge, she often gets up at night & feels terrified. She has fear to sit in car again: Post traumatic stress disorder
- Patient with pneumonia was admitted in hospital. He suddenly ceases to recognize hospital staff. He is in altered sensorium, thinks he is in jail & complains of scorpion attacking him: Acute delirium
- A child is restless all the time, so that all the other students are unable to concentrate in class. He hardly sits on his own seat & roams around in hall: ADHD
- Female patient feels that dirt hung on him, whenever she passes through dirty street. This thought causes distress & anxiety. She knows that there is actually no such thing after she had cleaned once but she is NOT satisfied & compelled to think so: OCD
- Female patient had headache for 7 months. She had taken several consultations. All the investigations are also normal. She still insists that there is something wrong: Hypochondriasis
- Alcoholic patient is talking irrelevantly. He has stopped taking alcohol 4 days back. He is disoriented (to time, place & person). Also having visual illusions & hallucination: Delirium tremens
- 2-year-old boy with delayed speech & poor concentration. He has difficulty in communication & is NOT making any friends: Autism
- Male patient with decreased sleep, excitement & spending excessive money for last 7 days: Mania
- Male patient having auditory hallucinations saying that people staying upwards are talking & conspiring about him. Allegations proved to be wrong: Schizophrenia
- Female patient complains of having deformed nose & thinks that nobody likes her because of this. She consulted cosmetic surgeons but everyone said that there is nothing wrong with her nose: Delusional disorder

- Female patient with feeling low, lack of interest in activities, multiple body aches, disturbed sleep with early morning awakening: Depression

Drug producing dependence

Feature	*Substance*
Drugs withdrawal NOT causing suicidal tendency	LSD, cannabis
Drug NOT causing significant withdrawal symptoms	LSD, cannabis
Drug causing significant withdrawal symptom	Alcohol, opioids, nicotine, amphetamine, cocaine, barbiturates, benzodiazepines
NO/ MINIMAL physical dependence	LSD, cannabis, cocaine, phencyclidine (ketamine)
Only psychological dependence	Cannabis (marijuana), cocaine
Both physical & psychological dependence	Opioids, alcohol, amphetamines, barbiturates, nicotine

CLINICAL QUESTIONS

1. **1. Lallu, an occasional alcoholic has got a change in his behavior. He has become suspicious that people are trying to conspire against him though his father says that there is no reason for his fears. He is having hallucinations of voices commenting on his actions. Most likely diagnosis is:**

   A. Delirium tremens

   B. Alcohol induced psychosis

   C. Schizophrenia

   D. Delusional disorder

   Schizophrenia is characterized by disturbances in thought and verbal behavior, perception, affect, motor behavior and relationship to the external world. The diagnosis is entirely clinical.

   Answer: C i.e., Schizophrenia

2. **A 40 years old female had headache for last 6 months. She had several consultations. All her investigations were normal. She still insists that there is something wrong & seeks another consultant. Most likely diagnosis is:**

   A. Phobia B. Psychogenic headache

   C. Hypochondriasis D. Depression

   Hypochondriasis is defined as a persistent preoccupation with a fear (or belief) of having one (or more) serious diseases (s), based on person's own interpretation of normal body function or a minor physical abnormality.

   Answer: C i.e., Hypochondriasis

3. **A patient is depressed for last 3 years, do not go out of his house much & is isolated from the society. He is having normal weight & normal sleep. Most probably, he is having:**

   A. No psychiatric illness

   B. Chronic fatigue syndrome

   C. Dysthymia

   D. Major depression

   If the symptoms consist of persistent mild depression, the disorder is called as dysthymia; and if symptoms consist of persistent instability of mood between mild depression and mild elation, the disorder is called as cyclothymia.

   Answer: C i.e., Dysthymia

4. **A young patient with self-mutilating behaviour & impulsivity is having:**

   A. Paranoid personality disorder

   B. Adjustment disorder

   C. Borderline personality disorder

   D. Dependent personality disorder

   The borderline type of personality is also known as borderline personality disorder (DSM-IV-TR), the characteristic features of which include impulsivity, deliberate self-harm (in the form of self-mutilation, suicidal gestures, or accident proneness) etc.

   Answer: C i.e., Borderline personality disorder

5. **A 16 years old male is found to have a mental age of 9 years on IQ testing. He has:**

   A. Mild mental retardation

   B. Moderate mental retardation

   C. Severe mental retardation

   D. Profound mental retardation

   IQ of 50-70 is categorized as mild MR.

   Answer: A i.e., Mild mental retardation

6. **A 30 years old lady complained of sudden onset of breathlessness, anxiety, palpitation & feeling of impending doom. Physical examination is normal. What is the diagnosis?**

   A. Panic attack B. Schizophrenia

   C. Conversion disorder D. Acute psychosis

   Panic disorder is characterized by discrete episodes of acute anxiety. The onset is usually in early third decade with often a chronic course. The episode is usually sudden, lasts for a few minutes and is characterized by very severe anxiety.

   Answer: A i.e., Panic attack

7. **Female patient presented with acute restlessness & fear of impending doom. Most probable diagnosis is:**

A. Schizophrenia B. Delirium

C. Anxiety neurosis D. MDP

Anxiety is a 'normal' phenomenon, which is characterized by a state of apprehension or unease arising out of anticipation of danger.

Answer: C i.e., Anxiety neurosis

8. **A 30 years old male presented with symptoms of palpitations & sweating on meeting seniors & on making public presentations. This makes him avoid such situations. The diagnosis is:**

A. Panic reaction B. Social phobia

C. Avoidance personality D. Adjustment disorder

Social phobia is an example of irrational fear of activities of social interaction, characterized by an irrational fear of performing activities in the presence of other people or interacting with others. The patient is afraid of his own actions being viewed by others critically, resulting in embarrassment or humiliation.

Answer: B i.e., Social phobia

9. **A girl with normal milestones spends her time seeing her own hand & do not interact with others. Likely diagnosis is:**

A. ADHD

B. Autism

C. Asperger's syndrome

D. Rett's syndrome

Autism is characterized by stereotyped behaviours such as head banging, body spinning, hand-flicking, lining-up objects, rocking, clapping, twirling etc. and marked impairment in making friends.

Answer: B i.e., Autism

10. **A 10 years old child is very restless & hyperactive. His activities & running in school are very disturbing to his friends. Likely diagnosis is:**

A. Schizophrenia

B. Attention deficit hyperactivity disorder

C. Autistic disorder

D. Conduct disorder

ADHD is commonest type of attention deficit disorder/ ADD which is characterized by poor attention span with distractibility (does not seem to listen), hyperactivity (moving about here and there and difficulty in sitting still at one place for long) and impulsivity (acts before thinking, on the spur of the moment).

Answer: B i.e., Attention deficit hyperactivity disorder

CHAPTER 19

ORTHOPEDICS

RAPID REVISION NOTES

Bony tumours and their common site

Tumour	*Common sites*
Giant cell tumour	Lower end of femur, upper end of tibia and fibula
Synovial sarcoma	Knee, ankle, wrist
Osteosarcoma	Lower end of femur, upper end of tibia and fibula
Aneurismal bone cyst	Upper end of humerus
Osteoid osteoma	Femur, tibia
Peripheral chondrosarcoma	Flat bones, scapula
Central chondrosarcoma	Femur, tibia

RADIOLOGICAL FEATURES OF BONY TUMOURS

- Codmans triangle: Osteosarcoma
- Soap bubble appearance: Osteoclastoma
- Onion skin appearance: Ewing's sarcoma
- Sunray appearance: Osteosarcoma
- Linear striations: Vertebral haemangioma
- Cotton wool/ ground glass appearance: Fibrous dysplasia

Malignancy features

- Codman's triangle: Triangular area of subperiosteal new bone at the tumor host junction seen in osteosarcoma.
- Sunray appearance: New bone laid along the blood vessels within the tumor growing centrifugally seen in osteosarcoma.
- Onion peel appearance: New bone formation in layers, seen in Ewing's sarcoma.

TERMINOLOGY

- Orthopaedics was coined by: Nicholas Andry
- Greenstick fracture:
  - o Children's
  - o Bending force
  - o Distraction of cortex on convex side &
  - o Compression on the concave side (cortex intact)
- MC fracture in childhood: Distal humeral fracture
- Bennet's fracture: Intra-articular base of 1st metacarpal
  - o Extra-articular involvement is Rolando's fracture
- Chauffer's fracture: Fracture radial styloid process
- Jefferson's fracture: Burst fracture of C1 (atlas)
- Monteggia fracture: Proximal ulna fracture with dislocation of head of radius
- Galeazzi fracture: Fracture distal radius with dislocation of distal radio-ulnar joint

- March fracture: Stress fracture of shaft of 2nd or 3rd metatarsal (commonly)
- Pott's fracture: Bimalleolar fracture
- Burst fracture: Compression fracture of vertebrae
- Crescent fracture: Fracture iliac bone with sacro-iliac disruption

Fracture eponyms

- Barton's fracture: Distal radius, intra articular
- Colle's: Distal radius, extra articular with dorsal tilt
- Smith's: Distal radius, extra articular with volar tilt
- Galeazzi's: Distal ½ radius, with dislocation of distal radio-ulnar joint.
- Monteggia: Proximal ½ of ulna with dislocation of radial head
- Chauffeur's: Radial styloid
- Night stick: Shaft ulna
- Bennett's: Base of 1st metacarpal, intra articular
- Rolando: Base of 1st metacarpal, extra articular (T/Y configuration)
- Boxer's fracture: Neck 5th metacarpal
- Mallet: Avulsion tendon from distal phalanx
- Hangman's: Second cervical vertebra
- Malgaigne's: Pelvic disruption, injury on one side
- Bumper: Lateral condyle of tibia
- Cotton: Trimalleolar ankle fracture
- Pott's: Bimalleolar ankle fracture
- Aviators: Neck of talus fracture
- March: Fracture shaft of 2nd metatarsal
- Jone's: Fracture bases of 5th metatarsal
- Side sweep fracture/ Baby car facture: Elbow injury sustained when one puts one's elbow projecting out of a car
- Massonaise's fracture: Fracture of neck of fibula
- Pilon fracture: Comminuted intra articular fracture of the neck of fibula
- Clay shoveler's fracture: Avulsion fracture of the spinous process of vertebra
- Straddle fracture: Bilateral ischiopubic rami fracture

IMPORTANT FACTS

- Most important factor for fracture healing: Degree of immobilization
- MC bone fracture in body: Clavicle
- MC bone fracture during birth: Clavicle
- Infrapatellar bursitis: Clergyman's knee
- Dinner fork deformity: Colles fracture

Stage of fracture heading

- Stage of hematoma: Less than 1 week
- Stage of granulation tissue formation: 2-3 weeks
- Stage of callus: 4-12 weeks
- Stage of remodeling: 1-2 years
- Stage of modeling: Many years

Bone grafts

- Autogenous graft: Graft is taken from the patient himself, from sites like iliac crest, upper end of tibia, fibula
- Allogenous graft: Can be obtained from cadavers (Cadaveric graft) – Allogenous grafts from the mother are used when a child's bone reserves are not enough to fill a big gap. Also the bone preserved by deep freezing, by decalcifying or formalin preservation can be used for allogenous bone grafting
- Xenografting: Bone grafts from some other species are used
- Artificial bones: Hydroxyapatite derived from corals

CAST & BRACES

- Milwaukee brace: Scoliosis
- Boston brace: Scoliosis
- Tube/ cylindrical cast: Fractures around knee

SPLINTS

- Cock up splint: Radial nerve injury
- Aeroplane splint: Brachial plexus injury

- Von Rosen splint: Congenital Dislocation of Hip/ Developmental Dysplasia of Hip (CDH/ DDH)

Splints used in nerve injuries

- Axillary nerve: Shoulder abduction splint
- Radial nerve palsy: Cock-up splint
- Sciatic nerve palsy: Foot drop splint

OSTEOTOMY

- McEwan's osteotomy: Genu valgum
- Pemberton's osteotomy: DDH/ CDH

Bony injury & nerve injured

Injury	*Nerve involved*
I/M injection in deltoid region	**Axillary**
I/M injection in gluteal region	**Sciatic**
Posterior dislocation of hip	**Sciatic**
Lunate dislocation	**Median**
Fracture neck of fibula	**Common peroneal**
Fracture upper tibia	**Tibial nerve**
Fracture shaft of femur	**Sciatic**
Fracture head of radius	**Posterior interosseous (branch of radial nerve)**
Fracture medial epicondyle humerus	**Ulnar**
Fracture lateral epicondyle humerus	**Ulnar (tardy ulnar nerve palsy)**
Fracture lower third humerus/supracondylar	**Anterior interosseous (branch of median nerve)**
Fracture mid humerus	**Radial**
Fracture neck humerus	**Axillary**
Crutch palsy	**Radial**

NEUROPATHIES

- Neuropraxia:
  - o Anatomical continuity normal
  - o Physiological cessation of activity
  - o Complete recovery is possible
- Meralgia paresthetica involves: Lateral cutaneous nerve of thigh
- Winging of scapula involves: Long thoracic nerve of Bell
- Foot drop: Common peroneal nerve (Related to neck of fibula)
- Supracondylar fracture humerus: Median (Anterior interosseous nerve)
- Tarsal tunnel syndrome: Posterior tibial nerve entrapment

Nerve injuries

- Neurapraxia: Physiological disruption of nerve conduction in the absence of structural changes, complete spontaneous recovery occurs
- Axonotmesis: Axons are damaged but the internal structure is preserved. Spontaneous recovery possible
- Neurotmesis: Structure of the nerve is damaged by actual cutting Nerve repair is required, no spontaneous recovery

Nerve degeneration

- Proximal part undergoes primary or retrograde degeneration
- Part of the neuron distal to point of injury undergoes secondary or Wallerian degeneration
- The rate of recovery of axon is 1 mm / day
- Motor march –the nearest to the site of injury recovers first followed by others form proximal to distal

NERVES & RELATED TERMS

- Ulnar nerve:
  - o Positive card test
  - o Ulnar claw hand
- Median nerve:
  - o Carpal tunnel syndrome
  - o Pointing index
- Radial nerve: Crutch palsy
- Axillary nerve:
  - o Anterior dislocation of shoulder
  - o Fracture surgical neck humerus

Nerve palsies

- Wrist drop: Radial nerve palsy
- Foot drop: Common peroneal nerve palsy
- Winging of scapula: Paralysis of serratus anterior in long thoracic never palsy
- Main-en-griffe/ Claw hand: Paralysis of lumbricals in ulnar nerve palsy
- Ape thumb: Paralysis of opponens pollicis in median nerve palsy
- Pointing index: Paralysis of flexor digitorum superficialis in median nerve palsy
- Crutch palsy/ Saturday night: Radial nerve
- Honeymoon palsy: Median nerve palsy

Muscle wasting in nerve injuries

- Flat shoulder: Axillary nerve
- Flat thenar eminence: Median nerve
- Flat hypothenar eminence: Ulnar nerve
- Hollowing between metacarpals: Ulnar nerve
- Thigh washing: Femoral nerve
- Calf wasting: Sciatic nerve

CARPAL TUNNEL SYNDROME

- CTS is associated with:
    - o C: Compressed median nerve
    - o A: Acromegaly
    - o R: Rheumatoid arthritis
    - o P: Pregnancy
    - o A: Amyloidosis
    - o L: Low thyroid (hypothyroidism)

SCAPHOID

- Only carpal bone to undergo fracture as well as AVN: Scaphoid
- Fragment undergoing necrosis in fracture scaphoid: Proximal
- MC site of fracture scaphoid: Waist

Common sites of avascular necrosis

- Fracture neck femur: Necrosis femoral head
- Fracture Scaphoid waist: Necrosis of proximal pole of Scaphoid
- Fracture neck talus: Necrosis of body of talus

COLLE'S FRACTURE

- Colle's fracture is the commonest fracture in adults above 40 years
- Dinner fork deformity is seen in malunited Colle's fracture
- Sudeck's osteodystrophy: Colle's fracture is its commonest cause in the upper limb

FRACTURES AROUND ELBOW

- Commonest complication of supracondylar fracture is cubitus varus deformity
- Fracture of lateral condyle of humerus, results in cubitus valgus deformity, leading to tardy ulnar nerve palsy

Carrying angle of elbow

- Normal in males: 11 degrees
- In females: 14 degrees

Three bony relationship

- Three points relationship in elbow is formed by: Medial epicondyle, Lateral epicondyle & Tip of olecranon
- Tip of radius is considered as fourth point
- When elbow is flexed to 90 degree, these points form a near isosceles triangle, whereas on extension, they lie in a straight line
- They are important in diagnosing injuries around elbow joint
- Maintained in supracondylar fractures & disturbed in posterior dislocation of elbow

Injury & common complication

Injury	*Common complication*
Extracapsular fracture neck femur	**Malunion**
Intracapsular fracture neck femur	**Nonunion**
Colles fracture	**Malunion**
Fracture lower end femur	**Stiffness**
Fracture neck of femur with dislocation hip	**Avascular necrosis**
Dislocation hip	**Avascular necrosis**

DISLOCATION SHOULDER

- MC type: Subcoracoid type (anterior) dislocation
- Rare type: Posterior dislocation (associated with epilepsy)
- Reduction of dislocated shoulder: Kocher's manoeuvre
- Term's related to shoulder dislocation:
  - o Hamilton ruler test
  - o Dugas test
  - o Callaway test
- Recurrent dislocation shows:
  - o Bankart's lesion (glenoidal labrum)
  - o Hill Sach's lesion (humeral lesion)

Shoulder dislocation

- Shoulder dislocation: Commonest joint to dislocate
- Bankart's lesion: Stripping of the glenoidal labrum and periosteum from the anterior surface of glenoid and scapular neck
- Hill-Sach's lesion: Depression on the humeral head in its posterolateral quadrant due to impingement by anterior edge of the glenoid on the head

CONGENITAL DISLOCATION OF HIP/ DEVELOPMENTAL DYSPLASIA OF HIP

- Associated with: Oligohydramnios
- MC in: Western race
- Predisposing factor: Shallow acetabulum
- Clinical tests done: Ortolani (click of entrance)
- Radiological sign: Shenton's line is broken
- Splint used: Von Rosen splint

HIP DISLOCATION

- MC type: Posterior dislocation
- Attitude of limb in posterior dislocation:
  - o Flexion
  - o Adduction
  - o Internal rotation
- Dislocation, which can be felt of per rectal examination: Posterior type

CTEV

- Incidence of clubfoot: 1/1000
- Associated with: Arthrogryposis multiplex congenital
- Manipulation should begin: Immediately after birth (by mother)
- PMSTR (Posteromedial Soft Tissue Release) is done at: 2 years
- Treatment of chronic cases: Triple arthrodesis

Management of clubfoot by age

- 0-1 months: Manipulation by mother
- 1-6 months: Manipulation with plaster cast (Ponseti casting)
- ½ -3 years: Posterolateral soft tissue release
- 4-8 years: Evan's surgery (posteromedial soft tissue release with calcaneocuboid fusion
- 8-11 years: Wedge tarsectomy
- > 12 years: Triple arthrodesis
- Already operated: Ilizarov technique

Older method of manipulation in CTEV (Kites method; NOT used nowadays)

- A - Adduction
- I - Inversion
- E - Equinus

- If not corrected in this order then it can lead to Rocker bottom feet

OSTEOCHONDRITIS

- Perthes disease:
  - o Osteochondritis of femoral head
  - o Adduction is unaffected
  - o IOC for Perthes disease: MRI
- Osteochondritis of lunate: Kienbock's disease
- Osteochondritis of tibial tubercle: Osgood-schlatter disease
- Osteochondritis of calcaneum: Sever's disease

BONE TUMOURS

- Benign tumours of cartilage origin:
  - o Enchondroma
  - o Osteochondroma
  - o Chondroblastoma
- Benign tumour of bony origin:
  - o Osteoid osteoma
  - o Osteoblastoma
- Location:
  - o Epiphyseal: Osteoclastoma
  - o Metaphyseal: Osteosarcoma

Premalignant bone lesions

- Paget's disease
- Diaphyseal aclasis
- Enchondromatosis
- Post-radiation

Remember

- Most common bone tumour: Secondary's (metastasis) from other regions
- Most common benign bone tumor: Osteochondroma
- Most common true benign bone tumour: Osteoid osteoma
- Most common primary bone malignancy: Multiple myeloma, followed by osteosarcoma

EWING SARCOMA

- Location: Diaphysis
- Age group: 2nd decade
- X-ray appearance: Onion peel
- May mimic: Osteomyelitis
- Presence of fever, anemia, raised WBC, raised ESR & raised LDH suggests: Poor prognosis

OSTEOSARCOMA

- Location: Metaphysis
- MC site in body: Lower end of femur
- X-ray appearances:
  - o Sunburst appearance
  - o Codman's triangle
- Special feature: Secondary's in lungs
- Treatment:
  - o Chemotherapy
  - o Limb salvage surgery

MULTIPLE MYELOMA

- Calcium levels: Raised
- X-ray appearance: Geographic/ punched out (lytic lesion)
- Special features:
  - o MC primary malignant bony neoplasm
  - o Bence Jones proteins in urine
  - o Russel bodies

UNICAMERAL BONE CYST

- Presentation:
  - o Single cavity
  - o Connective tissue lining
- In children present as: Lytic lesion

CHONDROBLASTOMA

- Location: Epiphyseal
- X-ray appearance: Dense punctate/stippled or mottled calcification with sclerotic rim

PAGET'S DISEASE

- Commonly involved bones:
  - o Pelvis (MC)
  - o Tibia
  - o Skull
- Complication: Osteosarcoma

FIBROUS DYSPLASIA

- Special features:
  - o Developmental in origin
  - o Hormone dependent
- X-ray appearances: Shepherd's crook deformity (femur)

OSTEOMYELITIS

- Earliest site of involvement: Metaphysis
- Diagnosis of acute OM: Blood culture (positive in 65% cases)
- Periosteal reaction seen in acute OM appears after: 10 days
- MC organism in acute OM: Staph. aureus
- Brodies abscess:
  - o Equilibrium between host & organism
  - o Abscess cavity remains without further enlargement

Acute osteomyelitis

- Treatment within 48 hours off onset of symptoms: Conservative (antibiotics)
- Beyond 48 hours: Surgical exploration
- Sequestrum: Dead bone, surrounded by infected granulation tissue
- Involucrum: Dense sclerotic bone overlying sequestrum

SKELETAL TB

- MC site of skeletal TB: Vertebrae
- In Spine, TB starts in: Vertebral body
- MC region involved in spinal TB: T9-L1
- Earliest symptom of spinal TB: Pain
- Earliest X-ray sign in Pott's disease: Narrowing of disc space
- Tuberculosis of knee/Rheumatoid arthritis of knee: Triple Subluxation and external rotation
- Spina ventosa: Tubercular dactylitis (phalanges)

Tubercular arthritis of hip joint

- Stage 1/ Stage of synovitis or stage of apparent Lengthening: Flexion, abduction, external rotation
- Stage 2/ Stage of arthritis or stage of apparent: Flexion, adduction, internal rotation shortening
- Stage 3/ Stage of erosion or stage of true shortening: Flexion, adduction, internal rotation

RICKETS

- Pathology: Defective mineralization of osteoid/ bones & cartilage
- Features:
  - o Craniotabes
  - o Wide open fontanelle
  - o Rachitic rosary (Enlargement of costochondral junction)
- X-ray appearances:
  - o Widening & thickening of epiphysis
  - o Cupping & fraying of metaphysis

Clinical features of rickets

- Craniotabes (earliest manifestation of rickets)
- Bossing of frontal and parietal bones
- Delayed closure of fontanelle

- Rachitic rosary- prominent costochondral junction
- Harrison's groove horizontal depression along the lower border of chest corresponding to diaphragm
- Pigeon breast –forward projection of sternum
- Pot belly- hypotonia of abdominal muscles
- Ewing's sarcoma is the most radiosensitive tumor, but not most radiocurable tumour

Remember

- Epiphyseal enlargement: JRA
- Epiphyseal widening: Rickets
- Epiphyseal dysgenesis: Hypothyroidism

OSTEOGENESIS IMPERFECTA

- Brittle bone disease
- Basic defect: Lies in collagen type 1
- Mostly inherited as: Autosomal dominant trait
- Ophthalmological finding: Blue sclera (but not in all cases)

Some conditions

- Osteogenesis imperfecta: Tendency for frequent fracture, due to brittleness of bones. Autosomal dominant inheritance. Associated with blue sclera, joint laxity and otosclerosis
- Diaphyseal aclasia: Multiple exostoses, Multiple cartilage capped bony outgrowths from the metaphysic of long bones. Inherited as autosomal dominant. X-ray shows trumpet shaped metaphysic and bony projections.
- Osteopetrosis/ Marble- bone disease/ Albert –Schonberg disease: Dense but brittle bones
- Paget's disease/ Osteitis deformans: Progressive tendency for one or more bones to bend, get thickened and spongy, followed by increased density and hardening. Pathological fractures and malignant change can occur
- Histiocytosis X: Proliferation of histiocytes in the bones, includes Eosinophilic granuloma, Hand-Schuller Christian disease, Littre-siwe disease
- Achondroplasia: Trident hand, Globular skull, Dwarfism & Prognathism

SCURVY

- Barlow's disease
- Reason- Vitamin C deficiency
- Decreased activity of enzymes, prolyl and lysyl hydroxylase required for hydroxylation of lysine and praline, affecting collagen synthesis
- When scurvy and rickets, both are present (Barton's disease), then signs of scurvy dominate because of diminished osteoblastic activity

Radiological signs of scurvy (usually studied in knee joints)

- Wimberger's sign/Signet ring/halo sign: Sclerotic rim around epiphysis
- White line of Frankel: Zones of provisional calcification
- Trummerfeld's zone: Radiolucent cortex proximal to white line
- Pelkan spur/ Corner sign: Marginal metaphyseal infarction with healing
- Pencil thin cortex: Cortical thinning
- Ground glass shaft: Rarification of cortical bone
- Scorbutic rosary: Sharp elevation at costochondral junction
- Raised periosteum: Subperiosteal haematoma

RHEUMATOID ARTHRITIS

- RA is a disease of: Synovium/ synovial membrane
- RA starts in: Synovium
- Body tissue mostly affected in RA: Synovium
- Characteristic features:
    - Persistent inflammatory synovitis
    - Peripheral joint
    - Symmetrical distribution
- Causes:
    - Immunological
    - Familial
    - Infective (implicated)

- Mostly affects: Females (three times)
- Earliest lesion in rheumatoid synovitis:
  - Microvascular injury
  - Increase in number of synovial lining cells
- Joints characteristically involved in RA:
  - MCP
  - PIP (symmetric arthritis)
- Boutonniere deformity:
  - Flexion contracture of the PIP
  - Extension of DIP
- Criteria for diagnosis: Any 4 criteria must be present
- Pathognomonic feature: Rheumatoid nodule
- Extra-articular manifestations are seen in: Individuals with high titres of RF (autoantibodies to the Fc component of IgG)
- Indication of steroids in RA: Mononeuritis multiplex
- Most common cause of Mononeuritis multiplex: polyarteritis nodosa

Diagnostic criteria of rheumatoid arthritis

If four or more criteria are present, it is R.A:

- Morning stiffness
- Swelling of 3 or more specified joints
- Swelling of joints in the hand and wrist
- Symmetric swellings
- Rheumatoid nodule
- Rheumatoid factor [positive]
- Erosion or unequivocal periarticular osteopenia on X-ray

RA associated syndromes

- Felty's syndrome: Rheumatoid arthritis, Splenomegaly, Neutropenia & High titres of rheumatoid arthritis
- Caplan's syndrome: Rheumatoid arthritis & Pneumoconiosis
- Still's disease: Rheumatoid arthritis, Splenomegaly, Leukocytosis, Rash & Rheumatoid factor absent

Joints commonly affected in R.A.

- Metacarpophalangeal joint
- Proximal interphalangeal joint
- Wrist
- Knees
- Elbows
- Ankles

ANKYLOSING SPONDYLITIS

- Associated HLA: HLA B27
- Special features of AS:
  - Enthesopathy
  - Pain improving with exercise
- X-ray shows: Bamboo spine

Neural tube defects

- Spina bifida occulta: Mildest and the commonest. Failure of the fusion of vertebral arches results in bifid spinous process
- Spina bifida aperta: Failure of fusion of not only vertebral arches but also soft tissue, skin and meninges
- Meningomyelocele: Protrusion of meninges through a defect in the neural arch. Contains only CSF
- Meningomyelocele: Protrusion of meninges with some neural element
- Syringomyelocele: Spinal cord with dilated central canal (Syringomyelia) lies within the meningeal sac
- Myelocele: Central canal opens to the exterior

Bony problems and their common site

Condition	*Common sites*
Paget's disease	Pelvis
Pseudogout	Knee (menisci and articular cartilage)
Congenital pseudo-arthrosis	Tibia
Osteochondritis dissecans	Femoral condyles
Ankylosing spondylitis	Sacro-iliac joint

Rheumatoid arthritis	Small joints of the hands
Gout	Metatarso-phalangeal joint of great toe
Osteoarthrosis	Hip (western), knee (India)
Osteoarthrosis in foot	Subtalar & midtarsal joints
Neuropathic arthritis	Knee, ankle, subtalar joint

OSTEOARTHRITIS

- Usually OA involves:
  - o Hip
  - o Knee
- Does not affect MCP joint
- Interphalangeal joints & nodes:
  - o DIP – Heberden's node
  - o PIP - Bouchard nodes
- X-ray shows: Osteophyte formation

Miscellaneous conditions

- Tennis elbow: Lateral epicondylitis; Pain and tenderness at the lateral epicondyle of the humerus due to inflammation at the origin of extensor muscles of forearm
- Golfer's elbow: Medial epicondylitis, pain and tenderness at the medial epicondyle of The humerus due to Inflammation at the origin of flexor tendons of foremen
- De Quervain's tenosynovitis: Pain and swelling over the radial styloid process Inflammation of the common sheath of abductor pollicis longus and extensor pollicis longus tendon's tenderness is elicited by adducting the thumb
- Meralgia paresthetica: Paresthesia in the area of skin supplied by lateral cutaneous nerve of thigh as it gets trapped beneath the fascia
- Gamekeeper's thumb: Tear of ulnar collateral ligament of thumb digital nerve.
- Jumper's knee: Tendonitis of quadriceps apparatus
- Madelung deformity: Development ulnar and volar tilt of distal end of radius with dorsal dislocation of ulna (manus valgus)
- Dupuytren's Contracture: Contracture of palmar aponeurosis Flexion deformity of one or more fingers due to thickening and shortening of the palmar aponeurosis
- Frog hand: Infection of midpalmar space, resulting in deep palmar abscess. Edema of dorsum of hand Interphalangeal joint movements are not painful, while metacarpophalangeal joints movements are painful

VOLKMANN ISCHEMIC CONTRACTURE

- Compartment syndrome: Stretch test is the earliest sign of impending compartment syndrome
- Compartment pressure of > 40 mm of water is indicative of compartment syndrome
- Muscles commonly affected:
  - o FDP
  - o FPL

Degree of sprain

- First: Tear of only few fibers
- Second: From third to almost the fibres of ligaments are disrupted, movements are disrupted, movements are normal
- Third: Complete tear of ligament

SCOLIOSIS

- Associated conditions:
  - o Hemivertebrae
  - o Wedge vertebrae
  - o Block vertebrae
- Braces used:
  - o Boston brace
  - o Milwaukee brace
- Radiological assessment: Cobb's angle

Charcot's joint

- Diabetic arthropathy: Foot joint
- Tabes dorsalis: Knee and hip

- Diabetes mellitus: Foot
- Syringomyelia: Upper limb

SYNONYMS

- Blount's disease: Tibia vara
- Caffey's disease: Osteomyelitis of jaw
- Trevor's disease: Dysplasia epiphysis hemimelica
- Englemann disease: Progressive diaphyseal dysplasia
- Burtons disease: Combination of scurvy & rickets

TEST IN ORTHOPAEDICS

- Barlow test: CDH/ DDH
- Thomas test: Fixed flexion deformity (at hip)
- Allen test: Palmar arch integrity
- McMurray test: Meniscal injury (knee)
- Lachman test, Pivot shift test: Anterior cruciate test
- Apprehension sign/ test: Shoulder dislocation
- Phalen test: Carpal tunnel syndrome
- Lift off test: Subscapularis
- Jerk test: Posterior gleno-humeral instability

Some tests

- Oschner's clasping test: Interlock the digits of both the hands and flex the metacarpophalangeal and interphalangeal joints. In median nerve palsy, lateral part of flexor digitorum profundus, will get paralysed leading to pointing index
- Hook sign: Suppurative tenosynovitis Metacarpophalangeal joint movement is not painful while interphalangeal movement is painful
- Book test/Froment's sign: In ulnar nerve paralysis, adductor pollicis will be paralyzed and the patient will not be able to grasp the book between the thumb and index finger
- Simon's test: Diagnostic of ruptured tendo Achilles
- Kanavel's sign: Seen in ulnar bursa infection point of maximum tenderness is over the part lying between transverse palmar creases

CLINICAL PROBLEMS

- Young male, treated for retinoblastoma at 1 year of age, C/O pain, swelling around knee: Osteosarcoma
- Adult male, trauma & haematoma at elbow, hard calcific mass in muscle belly: Myositis ossificans
- Patient with road traffic accident, multiple injuries, on day 2 develops, tachypnea, tachycardia, reduced pO2 & rash: Fat embolism
- Post Total hip replacement, patient develops chest pain, CVS collapse: PTE (pulmonary thromboembolism)

Circumstances of injury

Injury	*Mechanism*
Fracture vertebrae	**Hyperflexion**
Burst fracture vertebrae	**Axial compression**
Fracture dislocation of dorsal vertebrae	**Collapse of a roof**
Fracture dislocation of dorsolumbar spine	**Flexion-rotation violence**
Fracture talus	**Fall from height**
Meniscal tear	**Twisting force in flexion or semi-flexion**
Anterior cruciate ligament tear	**Hyperextension of knee**
Lateral collateral ligament of knee tear	**Adduction of tibia over femur**
Medial collateral ligament tear	**Abduction of tibia over femur**
Knee injury	**Football players**
Posterior dislocation of hip	**Motorcycle crash injury with femur/ knee in flexed or semiflexed position**
Fracture neck of metacarpals	**Punching**
Dislocation head of radius	**Forced pronation**
Fracture olecranon	**Fall on point of elbow**
Dislocation shoulder	**Forced extension and external rotation of abducted arm**

CLINICAL QUESTIONS

1. **A young patient presented to the Orthopedic OPD with pain and swelling around the shoulder joint after a fall on outstretched hand. After thorough clinical examination, treating doctor suspected it to be a case of fracture clavicle. What is the most common site of fracture clavicle?**

   A. Junction of lateral half and medial half

   B. Junction of medial one-third and lateral two-thirds

   C. Junction of medial two-thirds and lateral one-third

   D. Medial half

   The clavicle (collarbone) is one of the most fractured bones in the body.

   Most common site of fracture clavicle is junction of medial 2/3rd and lateral 1/3rd.

   Answer: C i.e., Junction of medial two-third and lateral one-third

2. **A patient was operated on hand for some pathology, but after the surgery, he was not able to flex the index finger. Which structure is most probably damaged?**

   A. Median nerve B. Ulnar nerve

   C. Radial nerve D. Flexor pollicis longus

   Clinical presentation is suggestive of median nerve palsy.

   The deformity discussed is pointing index.

   "Pointing finger" deformity is caused due to injury to the median nerve in the mid-forearm by paralysis of flexor digitorum superficialis.

   Answer: A i.e., Median nerve

3. **A young male had pain in the right hip joint since few months. He was examined by an Orthopedic surgeon and it was found that there is true shortening of the right lower limb. There is no history of trauma. Most likely diagnosis:**

   A. Stage of synovitis of TB hip

   B. Stage of the arthritis of TB hip

   C. Stage of erosion of TB hip

   D. Avascular necrosis of head of femur

   After the spine, the hip joint is the most common site of involvement for tuberculosis, and constitutes approximately 15% of all cases

   Answer: C i.e., Stage of erosion of TB hip

4. **An alcoholic patient slept at the night keeping his head over the arm. Next morning, when he woke up, his radial nerve was paralysed. This is which kind of injury:**

   A. Neurapraxia

   B. Axonotmesis

   C. Neurotmesis

   D. Wallerian degeneration

   Neurapraxia is a mild form of nerve damage that can lead to temporary motor and sensory loss. Neurapraxia is the mildest form of peripheral nerve injury.

   Answer: A i.e., Neurapraxia

5. **A 24 years old male, a known epileptic, presented to following a seizure with pain in the right shoulder region. Examination revealed that the right upper limb was adducted and externally rotated and the movements could not be performed. Most likely diagnosis:**

   A. Luxatio erecta

   B. Posterior dislocation of the shoulder

   C. Intra-thoracic dislocation of the shoulder

   D. Subglenoid dislocation of the shoulder

   Clinical presentation is suggestive of posterior dislocation of the shoulder

   Answer: B i.e., Posterior dislocation of the shoulder

6. **After falling from a height, a child lands on his fully outstretched hands. On examination, there is pain and swelling over his right elbow. There is S-shaped deformity at elbow. Most likely diagnosis:**

   A. Olecranon fracture

   B. Posterior dislocation of the elbow

   C. Fracture supracondylar humerus

   D. Fracture both bone forearm

Clinical presentation is suggestive of fracture supracondylar humerus

Answer: C i.e., Fracture supracondylar humerus

7. **A 10 years old boy presenting with a cubitus varus deformity and a history of trauma 3 months back. On examination, the three points bony relationship is preserved. Most likely diagnosis:**

   A. Old unreduced dislocation of elbow

   B. Non-union of lateral humeral condylar fracture

   C. Malunited inter-condylar fracture of the humerus

   D. Malunited supracondylar fracture of the humerus

   Clinical presentation is suggestive of malunited supracondylar fracture of the humerus

   Supracondylar fracture malunion usually results in cubitus varus deformity.

   Three points bony relationship is maintained as the fracture line is above the landmarks (line joining medial epicondyle and lateral epicondyle)

   Answer: D i.e., Malunited supracondylar fracture of the humerus

8. **A patient sustained injury to the upper limb 3 years back; he now presents with valgus deformity in the elbow and paresthesia over the medial border of the hand. Most likely diagnosis:**

   A. Supracondylar humerus fracture

   B. Lateral condyle humerus fracture

   C. Medial condyle humerus fracture

   D. Posterior dislocation of elbow

   Clinical presentation is suggestive of old lateral condylar fracture, which has failed to unite, resulting in cubitus valgus deformity and features of ulnar nerve involvement (paresthesia over medial border of the hand).

   Therefore operative fixation of a displaced fracture lateral humeral condyle is a must.

   Answer: B i.e., Lateral condyle humerus fracture

9. **A child is spinned around, by his father holding the hand. Suddenly, the child started crying and did not allow his father to touch the elbow. Most likely diagnosis:**

   A. Supracondylar fracture of humerus

   B. Pulled elbow

   C. Fracture olecranon process

   D. Radial head fracture

   Clinical presentation is suggestive of pulled elbow.

   Pulled elbow is defined as a radial head subluxation caused by axial traction or a sudden pull of the extended pronated arm.

   Answer: B i.e., Pulled elbow

10. **3 days after Colle's fracture, a person is not able to extend the thumb. Most likely diagnosis:**

    A. Rupture of EPL tendon

    B. Osteoarthritis

    C. Compartment syndrome

    D. Shoulder hand syndrome

    Clinical presentation is suggestive of rupture of extensor pollicis longus tendon.

    Function of EPL is to extend the thumb.

    Answer: A i.e., Rupture of Extensor Pollicis Longus tendon

11. **A female with Colle's fracture was treated with below elbow cast, presented with severe pain, numbness and paresthesia. Most likely diagnosis:**

    A. Unreduced fracture

    B. Compartment syndrome

    C. Reflex sympathetic dystrophy

    D. Malingering

    Clinical presentation is suggestive of compartment syndrome

    Acute compartment syndrome is a condition in which there is increased pressure within a closed osteofascial compartment, resulting in ischemia of muscles due to compression of arteries.

    Answer: B i.e., Compartment syndrome

12. **Following anterior dislocation of the shoulder, a patient develops weakness of flexion at elbow and lack of sensation over the lateral aspect of forearm. Which nerve is likely to be damaged?**

A. Radial nerve

B. Musculocutaneous nerve

C. Axillary nerve

D. Ulnar nerve

Clinical presentation is suggestive of injury to musculocutaneous nerve.

Flexors of the elbow (biceps and brachialis) are supplied by musculocutaneous nerve.

Sensory nerve supply on the lateral aspect of the forearm is provided by musculocutaneous nerve.

Answer: B i.e., Musculocutaneous nerve

13. **A two years old child was walking holding her father's hand. She suddenly slipped and fell but did not let go her father's hand. After a while, she started crying and was holding the forearm in pronated position. She was afraid of moving the affected extremity. Most appropriate management:**

A. Supinate the forearm

B. Examine the child under GA

C. Elevate the limb and observe

D. Investigate for shoulder dislocation

Clinical presentation is suggestive of pulled elbow.

It is managed by supination and flexion of the forearm.

Answer: A i.e., Supinate the forearm

14. **A one and a half years old girl has developed painful elbow after being jerked on the forearm, while lifting by her mother. Next thing to be done in such a case:**

A. Cuff and collar sling mobilization

B. Reduction setting and above elbow plaster of Paris cast

C. X-ray and elevation of the limb in posterior slab

D. Fully supinate the forearm

Clinical presentation is suggestive of pulled elbow.

Answer: D i.e., Fully supinate the forearm

15. **A 30 years old male involved in a fist-cuff, injured his middle finger and noticed slight flexion of distal interphalangeal joint. X-ray was normal. Most appropriate management:**

A. Ignore

B. Splint the finger in hyperextension

C. Surgical repair of the flexor tendon

D. Buddy strapping

Clinical presentation is suggestive of mallet finger.

A mallet finger, also known as hammer finger or PLF finger or Hannan finger, is an extensor tendon injury at the farthest away finger joint.

Answer: B i.e., Splint the finger in hyperextension

16. **A 6 years old boy has a history of recurrent dislocation of the right shoulder. During examination, the orthopedician puts the patient in the supine position and abducts his arm to 90 degrees with the bed as the fulcrum and then externally rotates it but the boy does not allow the test to be performed. The test done by the orthopedician is:**

A. Sulcus test

B. Apprehension test

C. McMurray's test

D. Apley's test

Patient is scared that his shoulder joint will dislocate again with the maneuver being carried out by the orthopedician. This test is known as apprehension test.

Answer: B i.e., Apprehension test

17. **A 60 years old male fell in the bathroom and was unable to stand. On right hip region, ecchymosis was found. There is external rotation of the leg and the lateral border of foot is touching the bed. Most likely diagnosis:**

A. Extracapsular fracture neck of femur

B. Anterior dislocation of the hip

C. Intracapsular fracture neck of femur

D. Posterior dislocation of the hip

Clinical presentation is suggestive of extracapsular fracture of femur.

Lateral border of foot is touching the couch means that there is free external rotation (as the fracture line is outside the capsule of hip joint) so that the lateral border of the foot is touching the couch.

Answer: A i.e., Extracapsular fracture neck of femur

18. **An 80 years old female after fall was unable to walk. There was external rotation deformity. On examination SLR (straight leg raising) was not possible. There is broadening of greater trochanter and the lateral border of the foot is touching the couch. Most likely diagnosis:**

A. Intracapsular fracture neck of femur

B. Fracture intertrochanter

C. Fracture subtrochanteric

D. Fracture greater trochanter

Clinical presentation is suggestive of fracture inter-trochanter.

SLR is not possible because of fracture.

Lateral border of foot is touching the couch means that there is free external rotation (as the fracture line is outside the capsule of hip joint)

Answer: B i.e., Fracture intertrochanter

19. **A 30 years old male was brought to the casualty following a road traffic accident. His physical examination revealed that his right lower limb was short, internally rotated, flexed and adducted at the hip. Most likely diagnosis:**

A. Fracture neck of femur

B. Trochanteric fracture

C. Central fracture dislocation of the hip

D. Posterior dislocation of the hip

Clinical presentation is suggestive of posterior dislocation of the hip joint

*FADIR (**F**lexion, **AD**duction, **I**nternal **R**otation) deformity is characteristic*

Answer: D i.e., Posterior dislocation of the hip

20. **A patient with hip in adduction and medial rotation, is unable to move. Most likely diagnosis:**

A. Posterior dislocation of the head of femur

B. Fracture shaft of femur

C. Fracture neck of femur

D. Sciatica

Clinical presentation is suggestive of posterior dislocation of the hip joint.

On X-ray, lesser trochanter is not seen on the affected side.

Answer: A i.e., Posterior dislocation of the head of femur

21. **Patient presented with flexion, adduction and internal rotation of lower limb after a road traffic accident suggest the diagnosis of:**

A. Intracapsular fracture of the femoral neck

B. Extracapsular fracture of the femoral neck

C. Posterior dislocation of the hip

D. Anterior dislocation of the hip

Clinical presentation is suggestive of posterior dislocation of the hip joint

Answer: C i.e., Posterior dislocation of the hip

22. **A women aged 60 years suffers a fall. Her lower limb is extended and mildly externally rotated. Likely diagnosis:**

A. Fracture neck of femur

B. Intertrochanteric fracture

C. Anterior dislocation of the hip

D. Posterior dislocation of the hip

Clinical presentation is suggestive of fracture neck of femur.

Lower limb is mildly externally rotated as the fracture line is within the capsule of hip joint (intracapsular fracture), which prevents free external rotation of lower limb, as we see in intertrochanteric fractures (also known as extracapsular fracture).

Answer: A i.e., Fracture neck of femur

23. If a patient with a suspected fracture of the pelvis has some bleeding from the urethra and is unable to pass urine, what should be done next:

A. He should be encouraged to pass urine after being given antibiotics and analgesics

B. He should be immediately catheterized in the ward

C. A hot water bottle should be followed by injection of carbachol

D. He should be prepared for surgery and catheterization attempted in the operation theatre

Clinical presentation is suggestive of rupture of urethra (as there is fracture of pelvis).

Catheterization is although contraindicated as this might further aggravate the rupture. Suprapubic cystostomy is preferred if a gentle attempt of catheterization fails.

Answer: D i.e., He should be prepared for surgery and catheterization attempted in the operation theatre

24. Femoral neck fracture of three weeks old in a young patient is best managed by:

A. Total hip replacement

B. Reduction of fracture and femoral osteotomy

C. Prosthetic replacement of femoral head

D. Reduction of fracture and fixation with multiple pin or screw

In young patients, chances of fracture union are more (as compared to elderly) so internal fixation is preferred.

Answer: D i.e., Reduction of fracture and fixation with multiple pin or screw

25. Treatment of choice in fracture neck of femur in a 40 years old male presenting after 2 days:

A. Hemiarthroplasty

B. Closed reduction and internal fixation by cancellous screws

C. Closed reduction and internal fixation by Austin Moore pins

D. Plaster of Paris cats

In young patients, chances of fracture union are more (as compared to elderly) so internal fixation is preferred.

Answer: B i.e., Closed reduction and internal fixation by cancellous screws

26. In a 65 years old male with history of 6 weeks old, fracture neck of femur, is best managed by:

A. Smith Peterson nailing

B. McMurray's osteotomy

C. Hemiarthroplasty

D. Total hip replacement

In older patients, chances of fracture union are less (as compared to young) so hemi-replacement arthroplasty is preferred.

Answer: C i.e., Hemiarthroplasty

27. An elderly woman was admitted with a fracture of the neck of right femur, which failed to unite. On examination, an avascular necrosis/ AVN of the head of femur was noted. The condition would have resulted most probably from damage to:

A. Superior gluteal artery

B. Inferior gluteal artery

C. Acetabular branch of obturator artery

D. Retinacular branches of circumflex femoral arteries

Clinical presentation is suggestive of injury to arterial blood supply to head of femur, which are torn during fracture neck of femur. That's why AVN of head of femur may develop despite operative fixation, as operation can fix the bone fragments but there is no surety that arterial supply would be regained.

Answer: D i.e., Retinacular branches of circumflex femoral arteries

28. An 18 years old boy was playing football, when he suddenly twisted his knee on the ankle and he fell down. He got up after 10 minutes and again started playing but next day, his knee was swollen and he could not move it. Most likely diagnosis:

A. Medial meniscus tear

B. Anterior cruciate ligament tear

C. Medial collateral ligament injury

D. Posterior cruciate ligament injury

Clinical presentation is suggestive of medial meniscus tear

Answer: A i.e., Medial meniscus tear

29. A 24 years old college student while playing hockey injured his right knee. This patient presented after 3 months with instability of knee joint in full extension without instability at 90 degrees of flexion. Structure most commonly damaged is:

A. Anteromedial bundle of anterior cruciate ligament

B. Posteromedial bundle of anterior cruciate ligament

C. Posterior cruciate ligament

D. Anterior horn of lateral meniscus

Clinical presentation is suggestive of damage to posteromedial bundle of anterior cruciate ligament

Answer: B i.e., Posteromedial bundle of anterior cruciate ligament

30. Treatment of choice for non-united fracture of lower one-fourth tibia with multiple discharging sinuses and various puckered scar with 4 cm shortening of leg:

A. Plating B. External fixator

C. Ilizarov's fixator D. Intramedullary nail

Clinical presentation is suggestive of non-union of fracture with chronic osteomyelitis and shortening.

Such a case is best managed with Ilizarov's fixator, which allows lengthening as well.

Answer: C i.e., Ilizarov's fixator

31. A person comes with fracture of tibia with swelling of lower leg. Pulse is feeble but palpable. Intra-compartmental pressure was raised. Next step in management:

A. Fasciotomy

B. External fixation

C. Lower limb venography

D. Interlock nailing

Clinical presentation is suggestive of impending compartment syndrome.

It is best managed by fasciotomy.

Answer: A i.e., Fasciotomy

32. A 46 years old, known alcoholic presented with pain in the dorsal spine. On examination, there is tenderness at the dorso-lumbar junction. Radiograph shows destruction of the 11th dorsal vertebra with loss of disc space between D11-D12 vertebra. Most likely diagnosis:

A. Metastatic spine disease

B. Pott's spine

C. Missed trauma

D. Multiple myeloma

Clinical presentation is suggestive of Pott's spine/ Tuberculosis of spine.

Loss of intervertebral disc space is an early sign of TB spine.

Answer: B i.e., Pott's spine

33. A patient presented with chronic discharging sinus through which bone particle comes out occasionally. Most likely diagnosis:

A. Acute osteomyelitis

B. Subacute osteomyelitis

C. Chronic osteomyelitis

D. Garre's osteomyelitis

Clinical presentation is suggestive of chronic OM.

Discharge of bony spicules through the sinuses is diagnostic of chronic OM.

Answer: C i.e., Chronic osteomyelitis

34. An 8 years old boy presents with gradually progressing swelling and pain since, 6 months over the upper tibia. On X-ray, there is a lytic lesion with sclerotic margins in the upper tibial metaphysis. Most likely diagnosis:

A. Osteogenic sarcoma

B. Osteoclastoma

C. Brodie's abscess

D. Ewing's sarcoma

Clinical presentation is suggestive of Brodie's abscess

Answer: C i.e., Brodie's abscess

35. **A 35 years old lady had chronic backache. On X-ray, she had a D12 vertebra collapse, but intervertebral disc space is maintained. All are possible EXCEPT:**

A. Multiple myeloma B. Osteoporosis

C. Metastasis D. Tuberculosis

In TB spine, there is reduction in intervertebral disc space.

Answer: D i.e., Tuberculosis

36. **A 7 years old comes with fever and tibial swelling. X-ray shows periosteal reaction. Laboratory result shows raised ESR and leukocytosis. What is the next step in diagnosis of the patient:**

A. MRI B. Pus culture

C. Bone biopsy D. Blood culture

Clinical presentation is suggestive of acute osteomyelitis.

Blood culture can yield the causative organism in many cases, against which we can start the appropriate antibiotic (as per sensitivity report)

Answer: D i.e., Blood culture

37. **Babu, a 19 years old male has a small circumscribed sclerotic swelling over diaphysis of femur. Most likely diagnosis:**

A. Osteoclastoma B. Osteosarcoma

C. Ewing sarcoma D. Osteoid osteoma

Clinical presentation is suggestive of osteoid osteoma.

An osteoid osteoma is a noncancerous (benign) bone tumor. Each tumor usually measures less than 1 inch across. These tumors don't grow or spread anywhere else.

Answer: D i.e., Osteoid osteoma

38. **A 7 years old child presents with a lesion in the upper tibia. X-ray shows radiolucent area with Codman's triangle and Sunray appearance. Most likely diagnosis:**

A. Ewing sarcoma B. Osteosarcoma

C. Osteoid osteoma D. Chondrosarcoma

Clinical presentation is suggestive of osteosarcoma.

Osteosarcoma is a rare type of bone cancer in which malignant (cancerous) cells produce irregular bone.

Answer: B i.e., Osteosarcoma

39. **A patient presents with pain in the thigh, relieved by aspirin. X-ray shows a radiolucent mass surrounded by sclerosis. Most likely diagnosis:**

A. Osteoma B. Osteoid osteoma

C. Osteoblastoma D. Osteoclastoma

Clinical presentation is suggestive of osteoid osteoma.

Aspirin relieves pain of osteoid osteoma therefore it is also known as aspirin tumor.

Answer: B i.e., Osteoid osteoma

40. **A 10 years old child presented with mid-tibial swelling which X-ray revealed a lytic lesion with sclerotic margins. Most likely diagnosis:**

A. Osteoid osteoma

B. Eosinophilic granuloma

C. Fibro Cortical defect

D. Fibrous dysplasia

Clinical presentation is suggestive of osteoid osteoma.

Answer: A i.e., Osteoid osteoma

41. **A 12 years old girl complains of pain persisting in her right thigh for several weeks with low-grade fever. Radiograph reveals a mass in the diaphyseal region of the left femur with overlying cortical erosion and soft tissue extension. A biopsy of the lesion shows numerous small round cells, rich is PAS positive diastase sensitive granules. Most likely diagnosis:**

A. Osteogenic sarcoma B. Osteoblastoma

C. Ewing's sarcoma D. Chondrosarcoma

Clinical presentation is suggestive of Ewing's sarcoma.

Ewing sarcoma (ES) is an aggressive tumor of adolescents and young adults, which constitutes 10% to 15% of all bone sarcomas.

Answer: C i.e., Ewing's sarcoma

42. **A 15 years old boy is injured while playing cricket. X-rays of the leg rule out possibility of a fracture. But the radiologist reports that the boy has an evidence of an aggressive bony tumour with bone destruction and soft tissue mass. The bone biopsy reveals a bone cancer with neural differentiation. Most likely diagnosis:**

A. Chondroblastoma B. Ewing's sarcoma

C. Neuroblastoma D. Osteosarcoma

Clinical presentation is suggestive of Ewing's sarcoma.

Answer: B i.e., Ewing's sarcoma

43. **A young girl presented with swelling of right thigh, with history of trauma 2 months back. Now she presents with swelling at mid-shaft of femur and low-grade fever. ESR is mildly elevated. X-rays show a laminated periosteal reaction. Next line of investigation:**

A. MRI

B. Biopsy

C. Bone scan

D. Blood count & C-reactive protein

Clinical presentation is suggestive of Ewing's sarcoma

Answer: A i.e., MRI

44. **A 15 years old boy presented with painful swelling over the left shoulder. Radiograph of the shoulder showed an osteolytic area with stippled calcification over the proximal humeral epiphysis. Biopsy of the lesion revealed an immature, fibrous matrix with scattered giant cells. Most likely diagnosis:**

A. Giant cell tumour

B. Chondroblastoma

C. Osteosarcoma

D. Chondromyxoid fibroma

Clinical presentation is suggestive of chondroblastoma.

Chondroblastoma, also called a calcifying giant cell tumor or Codman tumor, is a rare, non-cancerous tumor made up of a mass of cartilage tissue.

Answer: B i.e., Chondroblastoma

45. **A 45 years male presented with an expansile lesion in the centre of femoral metaphysis. The lesion shows endosteal scalloping and punctuate calcifications. Most likely diagnosis:**

A. Osteosarcoma B. Chondrosarcoma

C. Simple bone cyst D. Fibrous dysplasia

Clinical presentation is suggestive of chondrosarcoma.

Chondrosarcomas are a heterogeneous group of malignant bone tumors that share in common the production of chondroid (cartilaginous) matrix

Answer: B i.e., Chondrosarcoma

46. **A 33 years old man presented with a slowly progressive swelling in the middle one-third of his right tibia. X-ray examination revealed multiple sharply demarcated radiolucent lesions separated by areas of dense and sclerotic bone. Microscopic examination of a biopsy specimen revealed island of epithelial cells in a fibrous stroma. Most likely diagnosis:**

A. Adamantinoma

B. Osteofibrous dysplasia

C. Osteosarcoma

D. Fibrous cortical defect

Clinical presentation is suggestive of adamantinoma.

Adamantinoma is a rare low-grade malignant bone tumor of uncertain histogenesis, which occurs commonly in the diaphysis and metaphysis of the tibia.

Answer: A i.e., Adamantinoma

47. **Skull X-ray of a patient shows lytic bevelled lesion. Most likely diagnosis:**

A. Multiple myeloma

B. Eosinophilic granuloma

C. Metastasis

D. Osteosarcoma

Clinical presentation is suggestive of eosinophilic granuloma.

Eosinophilic granuloma of the bone is a rare, noncancerous tumor that tends to affect children.

Answer: B i.e., Eosinophilic granuloma

48. **A 50 years old patient presents with long standing backache. Skiagram shows lesion in the midline involving the sacrum, which is lytic and expansile. Most likely diagnosis:**

A. Chordoma B. Synovial sarcoma

C. Osteoclastoma D. Fibrosarcoma

Clinical presentation is suggestive of chordoma.

Chordoma is a rare slow-growing neoplasm thought to arise from cellular remnants of the notochord.

Answer: A i.e., Chordoma

49. **Ramu, an 11 years old boy presented with pain in the arm. On X-ray, his upper end of humerus demonstrates an expansile lesion in the metaphysis with breach of the overlying cortex. Most likely diagnosis:**

A. Aneurysmal bone cyst

B. Unicameral bone cyst

C. Chondroblastoma

D. Osteoclastoma

Clinical presentation is suggestive of aneurysmal bone cyst.

An aneurysmal bone cyst is a benign, blood-filled lesion in the bone that tends to expand or grow. While it is referred to as a cyst, it is a true benign bone tumor surrounded by a thin wall of bone

Answer: A i.e., Aneurysmal bone cyst

50. **Babloo, a 10 years old boy presented with fracture of humerus. X-ray revealed a lytic lesion at the upper end. Most likely diagnosis:**

A. Unicameral bone cyst

B. Osteosarcoma

C. Osteoclastoma

D. Aneurysmal bone cyst

Clinical presentation is suggestive of unicameral bone cyst.

Unicameral bone cysts are fluid-filled spaces inside bone. The word unicameral means "one chamber" and describes the single fluid-filled chamber in each cyst. It can lead to pathological fracture.

Answer: A i.e., Unicameral bone cyst

51. **A 60 years old male has back pain and vertebral collapse. Most likely diagnosis:**

A. TB spine

B. Ankylosing spondylitis

C. Secondary's in spine

D. Intervertebral disc prolapse

Clinical presentation is suggestive of secondary's/ metastasis to spine.

Spinal metastases form when cancer spreads to the spine from another area in the body (metastasizes)

Answer: C i.e., Secondary's in spine

52. **A patient developed paraplegia. On routine examination and X-ray, it was found that there was osteoblastic lesion in the spine. Most likely cause of such a presentation:**

A. Carcinoma thyroid

B. Carcinoma prostate

C. Carcinoma breast

D. Carcinoma pancreas

Clinical presentation is suggestive of carcinoma prostate.

Osteoblastic metastases develop when cancer cells invade the bone and cause too many bone cells to form. The bone becomes very dense (sclerotic). Osteoblastic metastases often happen when prostate cancer spreads to the bone.

Answer: B i.e., Carcinoma prostate

53. A male patient had expansile, lytic, osseous metastasis in bone. Most likely primary malignancy is in:

A. Kidney B. Bronchus

C. Breast D. Prostate

Clinical presentation is suggestive of bony metastasis from renal cancers.

Osteolytic metastases develop when metastatic cancer cells break down too much of the bone, making it very weak.

Answer: A i.e., Kidney

54. A 60 years old male with bony abnormality at upper tibia associated with sensorineural deafness. On laboratory examination, serum alkaline phosphatase levels are 440 IU/ ml, elevated serum calcium and normal phosphate levels. Skeletal survey shows ivory vertebrae and cotton wool spots on X-ray skull. Most likely diagnosis:

A. Fibrous dysplasia

B. Paget's disease

C. Osteosclerotic metastasis

D. Osteoporosis

Clinical presentation is suggestive of Paget's disease.

Paget's disease of bone disrupts the normal cycle of bone renewal, causing bones to become weakened and possibly deformed.

Answer: B i.e., Paget's disease

55. A patient of leprosy presented with clumsiness of hand. Clumsiness is due to palsy of which muscle:

A. Extensor carpi ulnaris

B. Abductor pollicis brevis

C. Opponens pollicis

D. Interossei muscles

Clinical presentation is suggestive of paralysis of interossei muscles.

All the interossei muscles are supplied by ulnar nerve.

Answer: D i.e., Interossei muscles

56. Following an incised wound in front of the wrist, the subject is unable to oppose the tips of the little finger and the thumb. Nerves involved are:

A. Ulnar nerve

B. Median nerve

C. Musculocutaneous nerve

D. Radial nerve

Clinical presentation is suggestive of paralysis of median nerve.

Muscle paralyzed is opponens pollicis and the movement lost is opposition.

Answer: B i.e., Median nerve

57. A boy presents with complaints of hypoesthesia and wasting of thenar eminence. The nerve most likely to be damaged in this patient:

A. Musculocutaneous nerve

B. Median nerve

C. Ulnar nerve

D. Radial nerve

Clinical presentation is suggestive of median nerve palsy.

The majority of the thenar muscles are innervated by the median nerve (T1). The exceptions are the deep head of flexor pollicis brevis and adductor pollicis muscle that receive their innervation via the ulnar nerve (C8, T1).

Answer: B i.e., Median nerve

58. A 56 years old female presents with nocturnal pain in the right thumb, index and middle fingers for the past 3 months. All the provocative tests can be performed EXCEPT:

A. Finkelstein's test B. Tinel sign

C. Phalen's test D. Tourniquet's test

Clinical presentation is suggestive of Carpal tunnel syndrome

Finkelstein's test is done for DeQuervain's tenosynovitis.

Answer: A i.e., Finkelstein's test

59. **A young boy who was driving motorcycle at a high speed collided with a tree and was thrown on his right shoulder. Though there was no fracture but later on his right arm was medially rotated and pronated. Following facts are correct regarding this patient EXCEPT:**

A. The injury was at Erb's point

B. A lesion of C5 and C6 was present

C. The median and ulnar nerves were affected

D. Supraspinatus, infraspinatus, subclavius and biceps brachii were paralyzed

Clinical presentation is suggestive of Erb's palsy.

Erb's palsy is a paralysis of the arm caused by injury to the upper group of the arm's main nerves, specifically the severing of the upper trunk C5–C6

Answer: C i.e., The median and ulnar nerves were affected

60. **A 30 years old male underwent excision of the right radial head. Following surgery, the patient developed inability to extend the fingers and thumb of the right hand. He did not have any sensory deficit. Most likely diagnosis:**

A. Injury to posterior interosseous nerve

B. Iatrogenic injury to common extensor origin

C. Injury to anterior interosseous nerve

D. High radial nerve palsy

Clinical presentation is suggestive of finger drop, which is due to paralysis of posterior interosseous nerve (branch of radial nerve)

Answer: A i.e., Injury to posterior interosseous nerve

61. **A young female presented with bony pain. She had raised serum alkaline phosphatase and raised parathormone level along with low calcium and low phosphate level. Most likely diagnosis:**

A. Primary hyperparathyroidism

B. Paget's disease

C. Osteoporosis

D. Vitamin D deficiency

Clinical presentation is suggestive of osteomalacia.

Osteomalacia describes a disorder of "bone softening" in adults that is usually due to prolonged deficiency of vitamin D.

Answer: D i.e., Vitamin D deficiency

62. **During a routine check-up, a 67 years old man is found to have a level of serum alkaline phosphatase three times the upper limit of normal. Serum calcium and phosphate concentrations and liver function test results are normal. He is asymptomatic. Most likely diagnosis:**

A. Metastatic bone disease

B. Primary hyperparathyroidism

C. Paget's disease of the bone

D. Osteomalacia

Clinical presentation is suggestive of osteomalacia.

Answer: D i.e., Osteomalacia

63. **A 50 years old man presented with multiple pathological fractures. His serum calcium was 11.5 mg/dl and phosphate were 2.5 gm/ dl. Alkaline phosphate was 940 IU/ dl. Most likely diagnosis:**

A. Osteoporosis
B. Osteomalacia
C. Multiple myeloma
D. Hyperparathyroidism

Clinical presentation is suggestive of hyperparathyroidism (excess of parathormone).

Normal serum calcium level is 9-11 mg/ dl.

Answer: D i.e., Hyperparathyroidism

64. **A young patient presents with enlargement of costochondral junction and with the white line of Frenkel at metaphysis. Most likely diagnosis:**

A. Scurvy
B. Rickets
C. Osteomalacia
D. Hyperparathyroidism

Clinical presentation is suggestive of scurvy.

Scurvy happens when there is a lack of vitamin C, or ascorbic acid. The deficiency leads to symptoms of weakness, anemia, gum disease, and skin problems.

Answer: A i.e., Scurvy

65. A 40 years old man presented with acute onset of pain and swelling of left great toe. Urate crystals could be seen from the joint aspirate. Most likely diagnosis:

A. Gout

B. Rheumatoid arthritis

C. Psoriatic arthritis

D. Reiter's syndrome

Clinical presentation is suggestive of gout.

Gout is characterized by sudden, severe attacks of pain, swelling, redness and tenderness in one or more joints, most often in the big toe.

Answer: A i.e., Gout

66. A 40 years old female present with multiple lytic bone lesions, fracture clavicle, periosteal resorption of 2nd and 3rd metacarpals. Most likely diagnosis:

A. Renal osteodystrophy B. Osteomalacia

C. Hyperparathyroidism D. Hypoparathyroidism

Clinical presentation is suggestive of hyperparathyroidism

Answer: C i.e., Hyperparathyroidism

67. Young male having pain with morning stiffness of spine for 30 minutes and reduced chest movements. Most likely diagnosis:

A. Ankylosing spondylitis B. Rheumatoid arthritis

C. Gouty arthritis D. Osteoarthritis

Clinical presentation is suggestive of AS.

Ankylosing spondylitis is a form of painful, ongoing joint inflammation (chronic inflammatory arthritis) that primarily affects the spine.

Answer: A i.e., Ankylosing spondylitis

68. A lady having flexion at proximal interphalangeal joint and hyperextension at distal interphalangeal joint of index finger is called:

A. Boutonniere deformity B. Swan neck deformity

C. Wind swept deformity D. Z-deformity

Clinical presentation is suggestive of Boutonniere deformity, which is seen in rheumatoid arthritis.

Boutonniere deformity is a deformity of the fingers in which the proximal interphalangeal joint (PIP) is flexed and the distal interphalangeal joint (DIP) is extended.

Answer: A i.e., Boutonniere deformity

69. In a middle-aged male having back pain, syndesmophytes involving 4 continuous vertebrae are seen on X-ray. Most likely diagnosis:

A. Alkaptonuria

B. Ankylosing spondylitis

C. Rheumatoid arthritis

D. Osteoarthritis

Clinical presentation is suggestive of AS

Answer: B i.e., Ankylosing spondylitis

70. 40 years old patient having arthritis of proximal interphalangeal joint and distal interphalangeal joint along with carpo-metacarpal joint of thumb and sparing of wrist and metacarpophalangeal joint. Most likely diagnosis is:

A. Rheumatoid arthritis

B. Psoriatic arthropathy

C. Osteoarthritis

D. Pseudogout

Clinical presentation is suggestive of OA.

Osteoarthritis (OA) is the most common chronic joint condition. OA is also called wear-and-tear arthritis, degenerative arthritis, and degenerative joint disease.

Answer: C i.e., Osteoarthritis

71. A 35 years old male develops involvement of proximal interphalangeal joint, distal interphalangeal joint and metacarpophalangeal joints with sparing of the wrist and carpometacarpal joint. Most likely diagnosis:

A. Psoriatic arthropathy B. Osteoarthritis

C. Rheumatoid arthritis D. Pseudogout

Clinical presentation is suggestive of psoriatic arthropathy.

Psoriatic arthritis is a chronic inflammatory arthritis that develops in at least 5% of patients with psoriasis.

Answer: A i.e., Psoriatic arthropathy

72. **An old lady presented with long standing arthritis of both hands and feet. X-ray feature, which suggests rheumatoid arthritis, rather than seronegative spondyloarthropathies, is:**

A. Loss of joint space

B. Peri-articular erosions

C. Osteophytes

D. Periosteal reaction

RA is a chronic disease that causes joint pain, stiffness, swelling and decreased movement of the joints. Small joints in the hands and feet are most commonly affected.

Answer: B i.e., Peri-articular erosions

73. **A diabetic patient develops swelling of the knee joint, associated with sclerosis without deformity. Loose bodies are seen on aspiration. Most likely diagnosis:**

A. Neuropathic joint

B. Non-specific synovitis

C. Osteoarthritis

D. Septic arthritis of knee

Clinical presentation is suggestive of neuropathic/ Charcot's joint.

Neuropathic arthropathy (Charcot joint) can be defined as bone and joint changes that occur secondary to loss of sensation and is most often associated with diabetes, syphilis, syringomyelia, spina bifida, traumatic spinal cord injury, and leprosy.

Answer: A i.e., Neuropathic joint

74. **A 60 years old man with diabetes mellitus presents with painless, swollen right ankle joint. Radiographs of the ankle show destroyed joint with large number of loose bodies. Most likely diagnosis:**

A. Charcot's joint B. Clutton's joint

C. Osteoarthritis D. Rheumatoid arthritis

Clinical presentation is suggestive of neuropathic/ Charcot's joint

Answer: A i.e., Charcot's joint

75. **A lady presents with right knee swelling. Aspiration was done in which CPPD crystals were obtained. Likely diagnosis:**

A. Osteoarthritis B. Rheumatoid arthritis

C. Gout D. Pseudogout

Clinical presentation is suggestive of pseudogout.

Pseudogout is similar to gout but is generally less painful. It is caused by calcium pyrophosphate (CPP) crystals in the joints.

Answer: D i.e., Pseudogout

76. **A 65 years old man with history of back pain for 3 months. ESR is raised. On examination, marked stiffness and mild restriction of chest movements is found. On X-ray, syndesmophytes were present in vertebrae. Most likely diagnosis:**

A. Ankylosing spondylitis

B. Degenerative osteoarthritis of spine

C. Lumbar canal stenosis

D. Rheumatoid arthritis

Clinical presentation is suggestive of AS

Answer: A i.e., Ankylosing spondylitis

77. **A 68 years old man came with pain and swelling of the right knee. Grade II osteoarthritis changes were found on investigation. Further management:**

A. Arthroscopic washout

B. High tibial osteotomy

C. Total knee replacement

D. Conservative

Grade II OA can be managed conservatively.

Answer: D i.e., Conservative

78. **A newborn child presents with inverted foot and the dorsum of the foot cannot touch the anterior tibia. Most likely diagnosis:**

A. Congenital vertical talus

B. Arthrogryposis multiplex

C. CTEV

D. Flat foot

Clinical presentation is suggestive of clubfoot/ CTEV.

Clubfoot is a deformity in which an infant's foot is turned inward, often so severely that the bottom of the foot faces sideways or even upward.

Answer: C i.e., CTEV

79. A 11 years old, 70 kg child presents with limitation of abduction and internal rotation. There is tenderness in Scarpa's (femoral) triangle. On flexing the hip, the limb is abducted. Most likely diagnosis:

A. Perthes disease

B. Slipped capital femoral epiphysis

C. Observation hip

D. Tuberculosis hip

Clinical presentation is suggestive of SCFE.

Slipped Capital Femoral Epiphysis refers to a fracture through the growth plate (physis), which results in slippage of the overlying end of the femur (metaphysis).

Answer: B i.e., Slipped capital femoral epiphysis

80. A 10 years old male with pain in the left hip and limping on examination, has restricted abduction and internal rotation. Most likely diagnosis:

A. Septic arthritis of the hip

B. Tuberculous arthritis of the hip

C. Congenital dislocation of the hip

D. Perthes disease

Clinical presentation is suggestive of Perthes disease.

Legg–Calvé–Perthes disease (LCPD) is a childhood hip disorder initiated by a disruption of blood flow to the head of the femur.

Answer: D i.e., Perthes disease

81. A 2 years old male child has been limping ever since he has started walking. There is no pain. Examination reveals a short right lower limb with limited abduction at the hip. The Trendelenburg sign is positive however, telescopy is absent. Most likely diagnosis:

A. Congenital dislocation of the hip

B. Congenital coxa vara

C. Perthes disease

D. Slipped capital femoral epiphysis

Clinical presentation is suggestive of congenital coxa vara.

Congenital Coxa vara is a deformity of the hip, whereby the angle between the head and the shaft of the femur is reduced to less than 120 degrees.

Answer: B i.e., Congenital coxa vara

82. A 15 years old with slipped capital femoral epiphysis develops increasing pain and stiffness in the affected hip. Serial X-rays show progressive reduction in the joint space. What complication has the patient developed?

A. Avascular necrosis

B. Coxa vara

C. Secondary osteoarthritis

D. Chondrolysis

Clinical presentation is suggestive of AVN.

Avascular necrosis (AVN), also known as osteonecrosis, is a condition where bone tissue dies due to lack of blood supply.

Answer: A i.e., Avascular necrosis

83. A 7 years old young boy, had fracture of lateral condyle of the femur. He developed malunion as the fracture was not reduced anatomically. Malunion will produce which deformity:

A. Genu valgum
B. Genu varum
C. Genu recurvatum
D. Wind swept deformity

Clinical presentation is suggestive of genu valgum.

Genu valgum, commonly called "knock-knee", is a condition in which the knees angle in and touch each other when the legs are straightened.

Answer: A i.e., Genu valgum

84. A six years old boy presents with a painful limp. Clinical examination reveals tenderness in the femoral triangle and some limitation of hip movements. An X-ray was done which was normal. Next course of action:

A. Wait and watch

B. Ultrasonography

C. Aspiration

D. MRI scan

Clinical presentation is suggestive of transient synovitis of the hip/ observation hip.

Transient synovitis of the hip refers to a self-limiting acute inflammatory condition affecting the synovial lining of the hip.

Answer: A i.e., Wait and watch

85. A 14 years old boy with 78 kg weight and hypothyroidism developed sudden onset of severe pain and tenderness on left hip as a result of minor fall. Most likely diagnosis:

A. Fracture neck of femur

B. Slipped capital femoral epiphysis

C. Perthes disease

D. Hip dislocation

Clinical presentation is suggestive of SCFE

Answer: B i.e., Slipped capital femoral epiphysis

CHAPTER 20

PEDIATRICS

RAPID REVISION NOTES

Paediatric problems, which do not require any intervention

Condition	*Remarks*
Bowed legs	Normal upto 2 years
Umbilical hernia	Seen in 25% upto 3-4 years
Pot belly	Normal upto 3 years
Physiological jaundice	Appears at 36 hours; disappears by 7 days
Breast engorgement	Appears on 3rd to 4th day
Epsteins pearls	Seen on hard palate
Vaginal bleeding	Appears between 3-7 days
Erythema toxicum	Appears at 2-3 day; disappears itself

IMPORTANT MILESTONES

- Copies circle: 3 years
- Crawls:11 months
- Child smiles at familiar persons: 2 months
- Head/ neck control: 3 months
- Sits with support: 6 months
- Transfer object from one hand to other: 6 months
- Says mama dada: 10 months
- Self decisions: 7 years
- Walks alone: 13-14 months
- Knows age & sex: 3 years
- Can draw a rectangle: 4 years
- Can draw a triangle: 5 years

Weight

- Average birth weight: 3 kg
- Newborn gains weight at the rate of 25 grams per day for the first 3 months
- Doubling of weight occurs at 5 months
- Tripling by 1 year
- Quadruples by 2 years

Height

- Average newborn length: 50 cm
- Increases by 25 cm in first year
- Then by 12.5 cm in second year
- Then 6 cm in third year
- Child is 100 cm tall at end of fourth year

Head circumference

- Head circumference at birth is 35 cm
- Circumference of chest is 3 cm less than head circumference at birth
- Equals head circumference by 1 year of age

Other parameters

- At birth the upper segment is to lower segment ratio is 1.7
- Normal temperature of neonate is 36.5-37.5 degrees
- Normal heart rate: 100-160/min
- Normal respiratory rate is: 40-60/min
- Anterior fontanelle: 0.5 cm in diameter

Gross motor (age in months)

- 3: Neck
- 6: Sitting with support
- 8: Sitting without support
- 9: Standing with support
- 11: Crawling
- 12: Standing without support
- 13: Walking with support
- 18: Running
- 24: Walking upstairs
- 36: Riding a tricycle

Fine motor (age in months)

- 3: Grasping
- 3: Intentional reaching with bidextrous grasp
- 7: Palmar
- 9: Pincer

Language (age in months)

- 1: Turns head to sound
- 3: Cooing
- 6: Monosyllables
- 9: Bisyllables
- 12: 2 words with meaning
- 24: Simple sentences
- 36: Story telling

Social (age in months)

- 2: Social smile
- 3: Recognizes
- 6: Smiles at mirror image
- 9: Waves bye-bye
- 12: Plays a simple ball game
- 15: Identifies body parts
- 36: Knows gender

NEONATE

- Perinatal period: 28 weeks gestation to 7 days post natal age
- Early neonatal period: First 7 days of life
- Late neonatal period: 8-28 days after birth

Low Birth weight

- Low birth weight: < 2500 gm
- At risk low birth weight: < 2000 gm
- Very low birth weight: < 1500 gm
- Very very low birth weight/ extremely low birth weight: < 1000 gm

BODY PARAMETERS

- Body weight doubles at: 5 months
- Body weight triples at: 1 year
- Body length increases in 1st year by: 25 cm

WHO growth Charts

- Upper curve: Median for boys – 50th percentile of Boston /Harvard standards
- Lower curve: Median for girls – 3rd percentile of Boston /Harvard standards

Government of India growth chart

- First curve: 50th percentile, i.e., 80 percent
- Second curve: 70 percent
- Third curve: 60 percent
- Fourth curve: 50 percent

Formula for weight

- 3 months to 1 year: (age + 9)/2
- 1-6 years: (2 x age)+8
- 6-12 years: {(7x age) -5}/2

Order of puberty in girls

- Thelarche
- Adrenarche
- Height
- Menarche

INTRAUTERINE GROWTH RETARDATION/ IUGR

- Associated with:
  - o Alcohol
  - o Smoking etc.
- Brain is affected in asymmetrical IUGR
- Propranolol may be associated with IUGR
- Fetal well-being in IUGR is assessed by:
  - o Amniocentesis
  - o NST
  - o Amniotic fluid volume

Gestational age

- Small for gestational age: < 10th percentile for that gestational age
- Appropriate for gestational age: 10th – 90th percentile for respective gestational age
- Large for gestational age: > 90th percentile

Term

- Preterm: < 37 weeks / < 258 days
- Term: 37 - 42 weeks/ 259 - 294 days
- Post-term: > 42 weeks/ > 294 days

Well-come classification, using harvard standards

- Children between 60-80 percent of expected weight without edema: Underweight
- Children between 60-80 percent of expected weight with edema: Kwashiorkor
- Children below 60 percent of expected weight without edema: Marasmus
- Children below 60 percent of expected weight with edema: Marasmic kwashiorkor

IAP grading of PEM

- Grade 1: 70-80: percent of 50th percentile
- Grade 2: 60-70: percent of 50th percentile
- Grade 3: 50-60: percent of 50th percentile
- Grade 4: <50: percent of 50th percentile

Shakir's tape (Colour zone: Mid- arm circumference: Interpretation (for children between 1-5 years)

- Green: > 13.5 cm: Well nourished
- Yellow: 12.5- 13.5cm: Borderline
- Red zone: <12.5 cm: Malnourished

Age independent criteria for malnutrition

Test	*Remarks*
Kanawati index	Mid arm circumference/ head circumference
Rao index	Weight × 100/ $height^2$
Dugdale index	Weight × 100/ $height^{1.6}$
Quac stick test	Compares height to mid arm
Bangle test	Inner diameter 4 cms; slips over forearm in malnourished baby
Mid arm circumference with shakir's tape	Useful between 1-5 years; red zone – malnourished; yellow zone – borderline; green zone – normal

NUTRITION

- Edema is seen in: Kwashiorkor
- Hepatomegaly is seen in: Kwashiorkor
- Acute malnutrition is judged by: Weight for height
- Chronic malnutrition is judged by: Height for age
- Flag sign is seen in: Kwashiorkor

Kwashiorkor

- Flag sign – Alternate bands of hypopigmented and normally pigmented hair
- Flaky paint dermatosis – hyperpigmented patches of skin desquamate to expose raw hypopigmented skin

Breast milk

- 70 cal /100 ml

- Proteins 1.1gm / 100 ml, 7 gm lactate/ 100 ml
- Expressed breast milk can be stored at
    - o Room temperature of 8 hours
    - o In refrigerator for 24 hours
    - o In cold room for 3 months

WHO classification of xerophthalmia

- X1A: Conjunctival xerosis
- X1B: Bitot's spots
- X2: Corneal xerosis
- X3B: Keratomalacia
- XN: Night blindness
- XF: Fundal changes
- XS: Corneal scarring

Treatment of vitamin A deficiency

- **In endemic areas**
    - o 2 lac units immediately
    - o 2 lac units on second day
    - o And 2 lac units after 14 days
- **Infants (less than 1 year)**
    - o Should be given 1 lac IU along with measles vaccine
    - o Water miscible retinol palmitate injection can be given in those with continuous vomiting

Marasmus & Kwashiorkor

Features	*Marasmus*	*Kwashiorkor*
Appetite	Voracious	Poor
Skin		Crazy pavement dermatosis, flaky paint dermatosis
Hair	Texture modified	Sparse, easily pluckable; flag sign
Mental features	Alert & irritable	Apathetic, withdrawn, lethargic
Facies	Monkey facies	Moon facies (baggy cheeks of travelers)
Edema	Absent	Present
Weight	Below 60%	Below 80% (of Harward standard)

RICKETS

- Craniotabes (calvariae are softened)
- Rachitic rosary (prominent costochondral junction)
- Pot belly
- Bow legs etc.
- Biochemical values:
    - o Low S. calcium & phosphate
    - o Raised alkaline phosphatase & PTH

Signs of latent tetany

- Trousseau's sign: Carpal spam is elicited by occluding brachial artery, by inflating pressure cuff for 3 minutes. Carpal spasm is seen as flexion at the wrist and metacarpophalangeal joints, extension of proximal and distal interphalangeal joints, adduction of thumb and fingers
- Chvostek sign: When facial nerve is tapped at the angle of mandible
- Weiss' sign: Facial muscles go into spasm (twitching of nose or lips)
- Peroneal sign: The peroneal sign consists of dorsiflexion and abduction of the foot on tapping the peroneal nerve on the lateral surface of the fibula just before the knee
- Erb sign: Increased electric irritability of motor nerves in tenant

Paediatric diseases and X-ray findings

Condition	*Appearance on radiographs*
Necrotizing enterocolitis	Pneumatosis intestinalis
Thalassemia	Hair on end appearance in X-ray skull
Congenital syphilis	Wimberger sign (knee), bilateral erosion in upper medial end of tibia
Cretinism	Retarded bone age, epiphyseal dysgenesis
Scurvy	Fragmentation – trummerfeld zone, spur – pelkan's sign, marginal cleft – corner sign, thickened provisional zone of calcification around epiphysis – wimberger's sign, ring like epiphysis
Rickets	Cupping & fraying of metaphysic, saucer like epiphyseal end

SCURVY

- Bleeding into skin & joints
- Wimberger sign on X-ray
- Pseudoparalysis etc.

DOWN SYNDROME

- MC trisomy
- Brachycephalic skull
- Hypotonia
- Palpebral fissure slopes upwards
- Marked epicanthic folds
- Brushfield's spots
- Increased nuchal fold thickness
- Iliac index less than 60
- Simian crease (single palmar crease)
- MC associated cardiac lesions: Endocardial cushion defect/ ASD
- Duodenal atresia, CML & transient myeloproliferative disorders are seen
- May be associated with Alzheimer's dementia
- MC cause of down syndrome: Maternal non-disjunction

TURNER SYNDROME

- Lymphedema
- Short stature
- Webbed neck
- Low posterior hairline
- Cubitus valgus (increased carrying angle)
- Finger deformities
- Coarctation of aorta
- Short 4th metacarpal
- 45 XO karyotype

KLINEFELTER SYNDROME

- 47 XXY
- MC cause of hypergonadotropic hypogonadism
- Subnormal intelligence

FRAGILE X SYNDROME

- Large forehead
- Large head
- Macro-orchidism
- Moderately to severely retarded

Ophthalmia neonatorum

- Gonococcal, Chemical: < 48 hours
- Other bacteria: 2-3 days
- H. Simplex: 5-7 days

LATE CONGENITAL SYPHILIS

- Hutchinson's triad:
    - o Hutchinson teeth
    - o 8th cranial nerve deafness &
    - o Interstitial keratitis
- IgM FTA-ABS is best to diagnose congenital syphilis
- Periostitis also seen

Late manifestations of syphilis

Stigmata of initial lesions	*Late hypersensitivity reactions*
Hutchinson's teeth	Interstitial keratitis
Frontal bossing	Nerve deafness
Short maxilla	Clutton's joint
Saddle nose	
High arched palate	
Enlargement of sternoclavicular	
portion of clavicle	
Protuberant mandible	
Radiating perioral scars / Rhagades	
Saber tibia	
Mulberry molars	

Hutchinson's triad - Congenital syphilis

- Hutchinson's teeth

- Interstitial keratitis
- 8th nerve deafness

JAUNDICE

- Causes of unconjugated hyperbilirubinemia:
  - o Crigler Najjar syndrome I & II
  - o Physiological jaundice
  - o Gilbert syndrome
  - o Breast milk jaundice etc.
- Causes of conjugated hyperbilirubinemia: Biliary atresia (extrahepatic/ intrahepatic)
- MC cause of conjugated bilirubinemia in newborn: Idiopathic infantile hepatitis
- Physiological jaundice appears on: 3rd day (lasts upto 10th day in term and 14th day in preterm)
- MC cause of jaundice within 24 hours after birth: Erythroblastosis fetalis
- Breast milk jaundice is due to: Pregnanediol
- Kernicterus: Unconjugated bilirubin, in basal ganglia
- Rise in level of bilirubin in physiological jaundice: Less than 5 mg/dl/day

Unconjugated hyperbilirubinemia

- Crigler- Najjar syndrome UDP glucuronyl transferase deficiency
- Gilbert's syndrome – Decreased activity of UDPGT
- Decreased hepatic uptake of bilirubin

Conjugated Hyperbilirubinemia

- Rotors syndrome and Dubin-Johnson syndrome-deficiency in excretion
- A cardinal feature of Dubin – Johnson syndrome is accumulation in Lysosome of Centrilobular hepatocytes of dark, coarsely granular pigment. As a result, liver may be grossly black in colour; the pigment is derived from epinephrine metabolites that are not excreted normally
- Clinical jaundice in neonate, when bilirubin level is more than 5 mg/dl

Pathological jaundice

- Clinical jaundice appearing in first 24 hours
- Increase in level of total bilirubin by more than 0.5 mg/dl/ hour
- Total bilirubin > 15 mg /dl
- Direct bilirubin >2mg/dl

INFANTILE HYPERTROPHIC PYLORIC STENOSIS

- Appears around 2 weeks after birth
- Hypokalemic metabolic alkalosis
- Compensated by:
  - o Paradoxical aciduria
  - o Hyponatremia &
  - o Hypochloremia

CYSTIC FIBROSIS

- Abnormal sweat chloride test
- Lung is normal at birth
- Causes intractable diarrhea in children

INTUSSUSCEPTION

- MC cause of intestinal obstruction in children (in neonate, it is duodenal atresia)
- Sausage shaped periumbilical mass
- Red currant jelly stools

REYE SYNDROME

- H/O recent viral URTI/ varicella infection
- Commonly caused by:
  - o Adeno
  - o Herpes virus etc.
- Hypoglycemia may be seen

BILIARY ATRESIA

- First sign is: Prolongation of jaundice

- Urine is always yellow
- Stools are acholic (no yellow/ green pigment)
- Conjugated hyperbilirubinemia

HYALINE MEMBRANE DISEASE

- Manifested within first few hours of life
- Hyaline membrane is made of fibrin
- Seen in:
  - o DM
  - o Premature babies
- Ground glass appearance/ reticulonodular/ reticulo-granular pattern on chest radiography

Pneumonia

Cause	*Features*
Mycoplasma	Interstitial pneumonia
Pneumocystis carinii	In immunodeficiency
Staphylococcus	Pneumatocele formation & associated empyema
Pneumococcus	Rusty sputum, lobar pneumonia

BRONCHIOLITIS

- MC Caused by Respiratory Syncytial Virus/ RSV
- MC in boys (less than 2 years)
- Chest X-ray shows:
  - o Hyperinflation with
  - o Multiple areas of interstitial infiltration
- May lead to asthma
- Self-limiting
- DOC is ribavirin
- Oxygen is helpful
- RSV Immunoglobulins has no role in acute attacks
- Antibiotics are NOT used initially

Tachypnoea

- 0-2 months: more than 60 /min
- 2 months to 12 months: more than 50 /min
- 1-5 years: more than 40/min

INHALED FOREIGN BODIES

- MC sign is: Cough
- Indicated by:
  - o Acute onset cough
  - o Stridor,
  - o Dyspnea in a child
- Intrabronchial foreign bodies need:
  - o Bronchoscopy
  - o Thoracotomy etc.

RIGHT TO LEFT SHUNTS

- TOF/ Tetralogy of Fallots
- TGV/ Transposition of great vessels
- Tricuspid atresia

Nada's criteria for diagnosis of heart disease (Presence if 1 major or 2 minor criteria are essential for diagnosis)

Major criteria	*Minor criteria*
Systolic murmur of grade III	Systolic murmur less than or more grade II
Diastolic murmur	Abnormal S2
Cyanosis	Abnormal X-ray
Congestive cardiac failure	Abnormal blood pressure

Conditions in which there can be CCF without cardiac enlargement

- Congenital mitral stenosis
- Cor triatriatum
- Obstructive variety of total anomalous pulmonary venous connection

ATRIAL SEPTAL DEFECT

- Left parasternal heave seen
- Chest X-ray shows enlarged right atrium & ventricle (NOT Left atrium)
- Associated with Holt Oram syndrome

- ASD + Mitral stenosis: Lutembacher syndrome
- ASD + Single atrium: Ellis Creveld syndrome
- ASD + Bony abnormalities: Holt Oram syndrome

Holt-Oram syndrome

- Thumb hypoplasia
- Hypoplasia of clavicle
- ASD
- First degree heart block

VENTRICULAR SEPTAL DEFECT

- Left ventricular failure, Biventricular hypertrophy
- Left axis deviation

PATENT DUCTUS ARTERIOSUS

- Seen in rubella
- Predisposed by:
  - o Hypoxia &
  - o Prematurity
- Differential cyanosis is seen
- Prostaglandin inhibitor stimulate PDA closure

COARCTATION OF AORTA

- MC below origin of left subclavian artery
- Associated with:
  - o Turner's syndrome
  - o Bicuspid aortic valve
  - o Upper extremity hypertension
  - o Lower extremity hypotension
  - o Headache
  - o Dizziness
- Rib Notching with double bulging is seen
- Cause of death is:
  - o Complications of hypertension
  - o Congestive heart failure etc.

TETRALOGY OF FALLOT

- Components:
  - o VSD
  - o Pulmonary stenosis
  - o Over-riding of aorta
  - o Right ventricular hypertrophy
- Chest X-ray: Boot shaped heart/ cour en sabot heart
- Single S2
- Ejection systolic murmur
- Right sided aortic arch

Pentalogy of fallot

- TOF + ASD

Systemic pulmonary shunts

- Blalock-Taussig: Subclavian artery- Pulmonary artery anastomosis
- Pott's shunt: Descending aorta – Pulmonary artery
- Waterson's shunt: Ascending aorta- Right pulmonary artery
- Modified B – T Shunt: Same as above but uses Gore-tex conduit
- Glenn: SVC with right pulmonary artery

HAEMATOLOGY

- 1st recognizable precursor in bone marrow during erythropoiesis: Pronormoblast
- 1st hemoglobin to appear in fetus: Hb Gowers
- Shifting of fetal Hb to adult Hb occurs at: 14 weeks of gestation
- Fetal Hb is completely replaced by adult Hb by: 6 months
- Increased fetal Hb is seen in: CML

IRON DEFICIENCY ANEMIA/ IDA

- MC type of anemia in children: IDA

- Time to start iron supplementation to a term, breast fed baby: 6 weeks
- First indicator of response after iron therapy: Increased reticulocyte count

ANEMIA

- Hypochromic, microcytic anemia with decreased serum iron & raised TIBC: Iron deficiency anemia
- Hypochromic, microcytic anemia with raised serum ferritin & decreased TIBC: Anemia of chronic diseases
- Early indicator of iron deficiency anemia: Serum ferritin

Sickle cell anemia

- Vaso-occlusive crisis/ Painful crisis: Due to blockade of end organ capillaries resulting in ischemia, pain and organ damage
- Aplastic crisis: Acute worsening of anemia producing pallor, tachycardia and fatigue; Precipitated by Parvovirus B 19 infection. Erythropoiesis is stopped for 2-3 days
- Splenic sequestration crisis: Acute painful enlargement of spleen

THALASSEMIA

- Features:
  - o Splenomegaly
  - o Hemolytic facies
  - o Decreased osmotic fragility (NOT increased)
  - o Hair on end appearance (X-ray)
- Diagnostic test: Electrophoresis
- Microcytosis & hypochromia
- Target & tear drop cells

Hb H disease

- Deletion of 3 alpha gene

Loss of alpha gene	*Manifestation*
1	Silent carrier state
2	Alpha thalassemia trait
3	Hemoglobin disease
4 (all)	Hydrops fetalis

VON WILLEBRAND DISEASE

- Autosomal disease
- MC hereditary bleeding disorder
- APTT may be prolonged
- BT prolonged
- Factor VIII levels may be reduced
- Defective platelet aggregation with ristocetin

IDIOPATHIC THROMBOCYTOPENIC PURPURA/ ITP

- Antibodies (IgG) are against: Platelet membrane glycoproteins IIb-IIIa or Ib-IX
- Bleeding Time is prolonged &
- Platelet transfusion are NOT helpful in immunogenic variety

Acute ITP	*Chronic ITP*
4-6 weeks of duration	> 6 months/year
Acute onset	Insidious onset
Antecedent infection is seen	Not so
Spontaneous remission in many	Unlikely

THROMBOTIC THROMBOCYTOPENIC PURPURA/ TTP

- Pentad of TTP:
  - o Fever
  - o Thrombocytopenia
  - o Microangiopathic hemolytic anemia
  - o Neurological symptoms &
  - o Renal failure
- Lab features:
  - o BT prolonged
  - o Normal PT, PTT & complement

VESICO-URETERAL REFLEX/ VUR

- MC cause of renal scarring in children
- Presentation:

- o Straining & dribbling of urine
- o In a male child with
- o Recurrent UTI
- Diagnosis is by: MCUG/ micturating cystourethrogram

NEPHROTIC SYNDROME

- MC of nephrotic syndrome in children: Minimal change disease
- Characterized by:
  - o Proteinuria (more than 3.5 gm/ day)
  - o Hypoalbuminemia
  - o Edema,
  - o Hyperlipidemia
  - o Lipiduria
  - o Hypercoagulability
  - o Low serum calcium is also seen

PAEDIATRIC ONCOLOGY

- MC inherited malignancy: Retinoblastoma
- MC malignant neoplasm in infancy: Neuroblastoma
- MC viral tumour: Warts
- MC malignant tumour (childhood): Leukemia

Most common malignancies in children in descending order

- Leukemia
- Lymphoma
- Brain tumors
- Neuroblastoma
- Retinoblastoma
- Wilm's tumor

Brain tumors in children

- Most common. Subtentorial – Cerebellar astrocytoma: also has best prognosis
- Medulloblastoma – Second most common; most radio-sensitive
- Most common supratentorial – Craniopharyngioma
- Worst prognosis is seen with – Glioblastoma multiforme

NEUROBLASTOMA

- MC presentation: Large abdominal mass
- May present as:
  - o Lytic lesion in skull with
  - o Sutural diathesis
- MC mass in posterior mediastinum (children)
- Metastasizes to bone most commonly
- Associated with hypertension &
- VMA & catecholamines are seen in urine

WILM TUMOUR

- Also known as nephroblastoma
- MC presenting symptom: Palpable abdominal mass
- Involves chromosome 11
- Highest cure rates
- Chemotherapy is with:
  - o Actinomycin-D &
  - o Vincristine

RHABDOMYOSARCOMA

- MC soft tissue sarcomas
- MC tumours of face in children

GLYCOGEN STOARGE DISEASES

- Von gierke's disease is due to deficiency of: Glucose-6-phosphatase deficiency
- Features of Von gierke's disease:
  - o Hyperuricemia
  - o Lactic acidosis etc. (NO muscles involvement)
- Andersen disease is due to deficiency of: Branching enzyme
- McArdle's disease is due to deficiency of: Muscle phosphorylase

- Galactosemia:
  - o It is due to deficiency of GPUT/ galactose-1-phosphate-uridyl transferase
  - o Reducing sugars are seen in urine

PHENYLKETONURIA

- Deficiency of: Phenyl-Alanine Hydroxylase
- Manifests as: Mental retardation, seizures etc.
- Urine: Musty odour
- Tests:
  - o Ferric chloride
  - o Guthrie's test

Classification of mental retardation by IQ

- Mild: 50-70
- Moderate: 35- 50
- Severe: 20-35
- Profound: <20

HOMOCYSTINURIA

- Enzyme deficient in homocystinuria: Cystathionine synthetase
- Most characteristic feature: Subluxation of the ocular lens
- Treatment: Large doses of pyridoxine (100-500 mg/ day)

CONGENITAL HYPOTHYROIDISM

- Large & open posterior fontanelle
- Absent social smile & eyebrows
- Growth retardation
- Delayed puberty
- Cold extremities
- Large tongue
- Prolongation of physiological jaundice &
- Epiphyseal dysgenesis

MENINGITIS

- MC presentation of neonatal meningitis: Poor breast feeding
- MC cause (in neonates) of bacterial meningitis: Group B streptococci
- Causes of aseptic meningitis:
  - o Mumps virus
  - o Polio virus etc.
- Low CSF protein is seen in:
  - o Infants
  - o Pseudotumour cerebri etc.

Causative agents of meningitis

- Neonate: Group B Streptococci
- < 2 months: E.coli
- 2 months to 2½ years: H. influenza
- 2½ years to 20 years: Meningococci
- >20 years: Pneumococcus

NEONATAL SEIZURES

- MC cause of seizure in newborn: Hypoxic ischemic encephalopathy
- MC type of seizure in newborn: Subtle

JUVENILE RHEUMATOID ARTHRITIS/JRA

- MC chronic arthritis in children: JRA
- More common in girls
- 5 or more joints are affected

DUCHENNE MUSCULAR DYSTROPHY

- Disease of sarcolemmal proteins
- Gowers sign (patient tries to climb on himself)

Duchenne muscular dystrophy

- Pseudohypertrophic muscular dystrophy
- Cause by mutation in the gene, located at p 21 that encodes dystrophin
- X-linked recessive disorder

- Valley sign-groove between supraspinatus and teres minor increases on abduction on shoulder

Gower's sign

- The sign describes a patient that has to use his or her hands and arms to "walk" up his or her own body from a squatting position due to lack of hip and thigh muscle strength

There are three Gowers' signs

- Pain along the compressed sciatic nerve on passive dorsiflexion of the foot.
- The irregular contraction of the pupil in early tabes (Argyll Robertson).
- The climbing up the legs signs in Duchenne dystrophy.

Reflexes

Reflex	*Appearance to disappearance*
Parachute reaction	9 months – persists
Neck righting	5 months – 24 months
Lindau reflex	3 months – 24 months
Tonic neck reflex	2 months – 6 months
Plantar grasp	Birth – 10 months
Palmar grasp	Birth – 6 months
Sucking & rooting	Birth – 6 months
Placing reflex	Birth – 6 weeks
Moro reflex	Birth – 3 months

Level of intelligence & IQ range

- Idiot: 0-24
- Imbecile: 25-49
- Moron: 50-69
- Borderline: 70-79
- Low normal: 80-89
- Normal: 90-109
- Superior: 110-119
- Very superior: 120-139
- Near genius: 140 and over

Acute low respiratory tract infection

- 'No pneumonia' is when patient is having cough & cold but NO fast breathing, NO chest indrawing or NO indicators of severe illness
- 'Pneumonia' is said to be present if respiratory rate is 60 or more in less than 2 months of age; 50 or more in 2-12 months & 40 or more in 12-60 months of age (treated by cotrimoxazole at home)
- 'Severe pneumonia' if there is chest indrawing (treated by I/V or I/M penicillin at hospital)
- 'Very severe pneumonia' is indicated by presence of severe chest indrawing & inability to feed (treated by I/V chloramphenicol at hospital)

Common causes

Condition	*Common cause*
Large intestinal obstruction in infancy	**Hirschsprung's disease**
Constant crying	**Hunger**
Bleeding per rectum in infants	**Fissure-in-ano**
Bleeding per rectum in children	**Polyp**
Hemetemesis in infancy	**Acute duodenal ulcer (stress & sepsis)**
Hemoptysis in chil	**Pneumonia**

CLINICAL QUESTIONS

1. **A 6 years old child presents with oliguria, haematuria, puffiness of face, convulsions, B.P. of 200/100 mm Hg and blood urea 80 mg%. What is the most likely diagnosis?**

   A. Haemolytic uraemic syndrome

   B. Nephrotic syndrome

   C. Acute glomerulonephritis with hypertensive encephalopathy

   D. Obstructive uropathy

   Hypertensive encephalopathy (HE) is general brain dysfunction due to significantly high blood pressure. Symptoms may include headache, vomiting, trouble with balance, and confusion. In hypertensive encephalopathy, generally the blood pressure is greater than 200/130 mmHg. Hypertensive encephalopathy is caused by an increase in blood pressure. Several conditions may evoke blood pressure elevation: acute nephritis, eclampsia, crises in chronic essential hypertension, sudden withdrawal of antihypertensive treatment.

   Answer: C i.e., Acute glomerulonephritis with hypertensive encephalopathy

2. **A 3 years old child is brought for sudden inability to walk following fever of two days duration. On clinical examination, sensorium is normal, both the lower limbs are hypotonic with the right limb more affected than the left. Plantar reflex is equivocal and deep tendon reflexes are not elicitable in the lower limbs on both sides. The most probable diagnosis is**

   A. Acute poliomyelitis

   B. Acute rheumatic fever

   C. Acute transverse myelitis

   D. Acute infective polyneuritis

   Poliomyelitis, often called polio or infantile paralysis, is an infectious disease caused by the poliovirus. In about 0.5 percent of cases, there is muscle weakness resulting in an inability to move. This can occur over a few hours to a few days. The weakness most often involves the legs but may less commonly involves the muscles of the head, neck and diaphragm. Many people fully recover. In those with muscle weakness about 2 to 5 percent of children and 15 to 30 percent of adults die. Another 25 percent of people have minor symptoms such as fever and a sore throat and up to 5 percent have headache, neck stiffness and pains in the arms and legs. These people are usually back to normal within one or two weeks. In up to 70 percent of infections, there are no symptoms. Years after recovery post-polio syndrome may occur, with a slow development of muscle weakness similar to that which the person had during the initial infection.

   Answer: A i.e., Acute poliomyelitis

3. **A 4 years old boy diagnosed as a case of sickle cell disease presents with pain and swelling of bones, marked in small bones of hand and feet along with severe pain in abdomen. Investigation reveals necrosis of femoral head and upper third of tibia. The symptoms have resolved after one week. The possible explanation is:**

   A. Aplastic crisis B. Sequestration crisis

   C. Vaso-occlusive crisis D. Hemolytic crisis

   Sickle cell disease (SCD) usually manifests early in childhood. For the first 6 months of life, infants are protected largely by elevated levels of Hb F; soon thereafter, the condition becomes evident. The most common clinical manifestation of SCD is vaso-occlusive crisis. A vaso-occlusive crisis occurs when the microcirculation is obstructed by sickled RBCs, causing ischemic injury to the organ supplied and resultant pain

   Answer: C i.e., Vaso-occlusive crisis

4. **A three years old male child has a poor stream of urine and strains at micturition. After voiding, the bladder is still palpable. The patient should be advised:**

   A. Abdomen X-ray B. Urine examination

   C. Circumcision D. Excretory urogram `

   Presentation of a boy with posterior urethral valve will depend on the severity of obstruction. The boy may present at birth or as late as 3 - 4 years. The symptoms are the same - difficulty in passing urine, straining to pass urine, dribbling of urine, poor stream of urine. There may be distension of the lower abdomen caused by a stretched out filled up bladder. The common mistake that can be made is to diagnose this condition as phimosis and then get a circumcision done. Investigations are done to look for the complications associated with this entity - like electrolyte imbalances and infection of urine and also in the blood stream by sending both blood and urine for Culture studies and treating the infection first before specific therapy for the PUV.

Answer: B i.e., Urine examination

5. **A two years old child has weight less than 3 SD (less than 3 Z score) as per WHO growth chart and mid upper arm circumference (MUAC) less than 11 cm. What is the correct diagnosis for this child?**

A. Acute malnutrition

B. Chronic malnutrition

C. Severe acute malnutrition

D. Moderate acute malnutrition

Severe Acute malnutrition/ SAM is defined as a weight to height ratio less than -3 Standard Deviations on the Z-score for the reference population and MUAC (mid-upper arm circumference) < 110 mm with or without Oedema corresponds to SAM.

Answer: C i.e., Severe acute malnutrition

6. **For a three years old male child, the height for age is 82% of the expected for that age and weight for height is 65% of the expected value. The child is labelled as:**

A. Normal

B. Wasted

C. Stunted

D. Wasted and stunted

Low weight-for-height: Wasting or thinness indicates in most cases a recent and severe process of weight loss, which is often associated with acute starvation and/or severe disease. The definition of stunting according to the WHO is for the "height for age" value to be less than two standard deviations of the WHO Child Growth Standards median

Answer: D i.e., Wasted and stunted

7. **A seven years old child presents with intermittent claudication, pain and weakness of legs and dyspnea on running. Examination shows delayed and weak femorals compared to brachial arteries. The heart size is normal with a left ventricular forcible apex. The most probable diagnosis is:**

A. Ventricular septal defect

B. Patent ductus arteriosus

C. Atrial septal defect

D. Coarctation of aorta

Patients with COA have cold legs and feet or have pain in their legs with exercise (intermittent claudication). Patients may experience dizziness or shortness of breath, fainting or near-fainting episodes, chest pain, abnormal tiredness or fatigue, headaches, or nose-bleeds. Arterial hypertension in the arms with low blood pressure in the lower extremities is classic. In the lower extremities, weak pulses in the femoral arteries and arteries of the feet are found.

Answer: D i.e., Coarctation of aorta

8. **A seven days old baby presents with complaints of vomiting and diarrhoea. Examination reveals cataract in both the eyes and jaundice. What is the most probable diagnosis?**

A. Rh incompatibility

B. Galactosemia

C. Congenital rubella syndrome

D. Congenital syphilis

Infants affected by galactosemia typically present with symptoms of lethargy, vomiting, diarrhea, failure to thrive, and jaundice. The presence of presenile cataract, noticeable in galactosemic infants as young as a few days old, is highly associated with two distinct types of galactosemia: GALT deficiency and to a greater extent, GALK deficiency.

Answer: B i.e., Galactosemia

9. **A two years old child is admitted with history of fever for two weeks and convulsions for the last one day. CSF examination shows CSF pressure elevated to 30-40 cm H_2O, clear CSF, lymphocytic pleocytosis (250 cells/mm3), elevated protein and low chloride levels. What is the most probable diagnosis?**

A. Pyogenic meningitis

B. Tubercular meningitis

C. Acute encephalitis

D. Subacute sclerosing panencephalitis (SSPE)

Fever and headache are the cardinal features of tubercular meningitis; confusion is a late feature and coma bears a poor prognosis. Meningism is absent in a fifth of patients with TB meningitis. Patients may also have focal neurological deficits. The CSF in TBM usually has a high protein, low glucose and a raised number of lymphocytes. Acid-fast bacilli are sometimes seen on a CSF smear, but more commonly, M. tuberculosis is grown in culture. A spiderweb clot in the collected CSF is characteristic of TB meningitis, but is a rare finding.

Answer: B i.e., Tubercular meningitis

10. A five years old child was diagnosed with nephrotic syndrome, 18 months back. He was treated and successfully went into remission at that time. Following, the initial episode, the child has had 3 relapses, each of which was successfully treated with oral prednisolone (60mg/m^2/24h) until remission, followed by 40mg/m^2 single dose, alternate days for four weeks. What is the diagnosis?

A. Nephrotic syndrome, infrequent relapses

B. Nephrotic syndrome, frequent relapses

C. Nephrotic syndrome, steroid dependent

D. Nephrotic syndrome, steroid resistant

Infrequent relapse nephrotic syndrome are defined as patients having less than two relapses within 6 months or less than four relapses within 12 months of response.

Answer: A i.e., Nephrotic syndrome, infrequent relapses

11. A 7 years old girl presents to you with non-specific abdominal pain, mild abdominal distension, and not growing well. The child weighs 14 kg and height is 95 cm. Systemic examination is normal. The haemoglobin was 7.5 g/dL (microcytic hypochromic RBCs) and has not responded to iron therapy. Which of the following will be the first investigation you will like to do for diagnosing the condition?

A. Bone marrow aspiration

B. Tissue transglutaminase antibodies

C. Lower GI contrast examination

D. Colonoscopy/sigmoidoscopy

Coeliac disease is a long-term autoimmune disorder that primarily affects the small intestine. Classic symptoms include gastrointestinal problems such as chronic diarrhoea, abdominal istension, malabsorption, loss of appetite and among children failure to grow normally. This often begins between six months and two years of age. Non-classic symptoms are more common, especially in people older than two years. For most children and adults, the best way to screen for celiac disease is with the Tissue Transglutaminase IgA antibody, plus an IgA antibody in order to ensure that the patient generates enough of this antibody to render the celiac disease test accurate.

Answer: B i.e., Tissue transglutaminase antibodies

12. A seven years old boy weighing 20 kg presented with bleeding from upper GI tract (haemetemesis) for last 18 hours. On examination, PR-86/m, RR-16/m and BP-100/70 mmHg; and spleen is palpable 5 cm below costal margin. There is no other abnormality. Liver function tests are normal. What is the next best step in management?

A. Fluid resuscitation with crystalloids

B. Intravenous vasopressin

C. Intravenous propranolol

D. Transdermal nitroglycerine

Esophageal varices result can from portal hypertension, regardless of the age group. The increased resistance to blood flow through the portal system is due to prehepatic, intrahepatic, and suprahepatic obstruction, but the most common causes of portal hypertension in children include portal vein thrombosis (prehepatic) and biliary atresia (intrahepatic).

Answer: B i.e., Intravenous vasopressin

13. A seven years old girl presents in emergency room with hypertension, lethargy, headache, seizures, and

visual disturbances. Fundus examination reveals haemorrhages and exudates. Which of the following treatment regimen will be the most appropriate for this child?

A. Sublingual nifedipine

B. Intravenous labetalol infusion

C. Intravenous minoxidil

D. Furosemide

Labetalol is effective in the management of hypertensive emergencies, postoperative hypertension, pheochromocytoma -associated hypertension, and rebound hypertension from beta blocker withdrawal.

Answer: B i.e., Intravenous labetalol infusion

14. **On routine newborn screening at day 3 of life, the baby was found to have TSH level 40mU/L. What should be the next step?**

A. Repeat thyroid profile within one week

B. Start child on thyroxine immediately

C. Repeat thyroid profile after four weeks

D. Repeat thyroid profile/ start thyroxine, if the child has clinical features of congenital hypothyroidism, otherwise wait and watch

TSH concentrations in children are normally higher than in adults. In 2002, the NACB recommended age-related reference limits starting from about 1.3 to 19 μIU/mL for normal-term infants at birth, dropping to 0.6–10 μIU/mL at 10 weeks old, 0.4–7.0 μIU/mL at 14 months and gradually dropping during childhood and puberty to adult levels, 0.3–3.0 μIU/mL

Answer: A i.e., Repeat thyroid profile within one week

15. **A five years old girl is brought to you with history of fever for seven days associated with rash, anorexia, myalgia and petechial haemorrhages. Which of the following investigations will be most appropriate for making a diagnosis of dengue fever?**

A. Detection of NS1 antigen

B. Platelet count

C. IgG capture ELISA

D. Detection of IgM antibodies for dengue

Detection of NS1 (non-structural protein-1) during the febrile phase of a primary infection may be greater than 90% sensitive however is only 60–80% in subsequent infections. Tests for dengue virus-specific antibodies, types IgG and IgM, can be useful in confirming a diagnosis in the later stages of the infection. Both IgG and IgM are produced after 5–7 days. The highest levels (titres) of IgM are detected following a primary infection, but IgM is also produced in reinfection. IgM becomes undetectable 30–90 days after a primary infection, but earlier following re-infections.

Answer: D i.e., Detection of IgM antibodies for dengue

16. **An eight years old boy was diagnosed to have P. vivax malaria and was treated with appropriate dosages of chloroquine. The fever subsided but recurred after 3 weeks. Peripheral smear was again positive for P. vivax. This child should now be treated as a case with:**

A. Relapse

B. Recrudescence

C. Either relapse/recrudescence

D. Fresh infection

The plasmodium parasites, which are responsible for malaria, can persist in the blood without causing apparent symptoms for a few months (recrudescence). Relapse in this context occurs due to activation of hypnozoites in the liver.

Answer: C i.e., Either relapse/recrudescence

17. **A two days old neonate is brought with cyanosis, single second heart sound, and pansystolic murmur on the left sternal border. ECG reveals left axis deviation, right atrial overload and left ventricular hypertrophy. What is the most likely diagnosis?**

A. Tetralogy of Fallot

B. Tricuspid atresia

C. Transposition of great arteries

D. Total anomalous pulmonary venous connection

Tricuspid atresia presents with progressive cyanosis, tachypnea over the first 2 weeks of life, holosystolic murmur due to the VSD, left axis deviation on electrocardiography and left ventricular hypertrophy (since it must pump blood to both the pulmonary and systemic systems) and normal heart size

Answer: B i.e., Tricuspid atresia

18. **A three years old girl is brought with complaint of not being able to ever stand or walk. She achieved head control at one year of age. Examination reveals generalised hypotonia, brisk knee jerk, and ankle clonus. What is the likely diagnosis?**

A. Cerebral palsy

B. Spinal muscular atrophy

C. Congenital hypothyroidism

D. Congenital myotonic dystrophy

Abnormal muscle tone, delayed motor development and persistence of primitive reflexes are the main early symptoms of CP. Symptoms and diagnosis typically occur by the age of 2, although persons with milder forms of cerebral palsy may be over the age of 5, if not in adulthood, when finally diagnosed. It is a developmental disability.

Answer: A i.e., Cerebral palsy

19. **A 5 years old boy is brought to the Emergency Room following a crushing injury. The ECG reveals peaked T waves, prolonged PR interval and widened QRS complexes. Which of the following treatments should be administered immediately?**

A. Sodium bicarbonate infusion

B. Intravenous bolus procainamide

C. Insulin infusion

D. Intravenous magnesium sulphate

With mild to moderate hyperkalemia, there is prolongation of the PR interval and development of peaked T waves. Severe hyperkalemia results in a widening of the QRS complex, and the ECG complex can evolve to a sinusoidal shape. Insulin (e.g. intravenous injection of 10–15 units of regular insulin along with 50 ml of 50% dextrose to prevent the blood sugar from dropping too low) leads to a shift of potassium ions into cells, secondary to increased activity of the sodium-potassium ATPase. Its effects last a few hours, so it sometimes must be repeated while other measures are taken to suppress potassium levels more permanently. The insulin is usually given with an appropriate amount of glucose to prevent hypoglycemia following the insulin administration.

Answer: C i.e., Insulin infusion

20. **A seven years old boy presents with acute onset of mild intermittent pain in the right groin and a limp. Abduction and internal rotation of the hip were restricted on the affected side. There was no fever. Radiographs of the pelvis were normal. The most likely diagnosis is:**

A. Transient monoarticular synovitis

B. Legg Calve Perthes disease

C. Slipped capital femoral epiphyses

D. Osteochondritis dissecans

Transient synovitis causes pain in the hip, thigh, groin or knee on the affected side. There may be a limp (or abnormal crawling in infants) with or without pain. On clinical examination, the child typically holds the hip slightly bent, turned outwards and away from the middle line (flexion, external rotation and abduction). Active and passive movements may be limited because of pain, especially abduction and internal rotation. The hip can be tender to palpation.

Answer: A i.e., Transient monoarticular synovitis

21. **A child is brought with history of ingestion of an unknown substance. On examination child has excess salivation, lacrimation, miosis, gastrointestinal cramps and emesis. What was the most likely substance ingested?**

A. Carbamates

B. Phenothiazine's

C. Opioids

D. Tricyclic antidepressants

Carbamate insecticides target human melatonin receptors, along with inhibiting Acetylcholinesterase.

Answer: A i.e., Carbamates

22. **A term newborn presents with respiratory failure, which is refractory to mechanical ventilation, surfactant replacement therapy, glucocorticoid administration and extra corporeal membrane oxygenation. The most likely diagnosis is:**

A. Surfactant Protein B deficiency

B. Primary ciliary dyskinesia

C. Persistent tachypnea of infancy

D. Lymphocytic interstitial pneumonitis

Surfactant protein B is an essential lipid-associated protein found in pulmonary surfactant. Without it, the lung would not be able to inflate after a deep breath out. It rearranges lipid molecules in the fluid lining the lung so that tiny air sacs in the lung, called alveoli, can more easily inflate.

Answer: A i.e., Surfactant Protein B deficiency

23. **A child after snakebite develops petechiae and ecchymosis on the skin. In addition, child develops bleeding from venipuncture site and oliguria. The most likely snake species is:**

A. Pit viper B. Cobra

C. Mamba D. Python

Hemotoxic snake includes viperids, Vipers and Russell's vipers. Clinical presentation includes local swelling and pain, ecchymosis, hemorrhagic bullae, renal dysfunction etc.

Answer: A i.e., Pit viper

24. **A six years old boy presents with short neck, low hairline and restriction of neck movements. The child also has Sprengel anomaly, scoliosis, and fused cervical vertebrae. The most likely diagnosis is:**

A. Atlantoaxial instability

B. Klippel Feil syndrome

C. Noonan syndrome

D. Sandifer syndrome

The most common sign of Klipper Feil syndrome is restricted mobility of the neck and upper spine. A short neck and low hairline at the back of the head may occur in some patients.

Associated abnormalities may include scoliosis (side-to-side curvature of the spine), which is abnormal curving of the spine. The spine sometimes appears as a "C" or an "S". Approximately 35% of patients with Klippel Feil syndrome will also have a congenital elevation of the scapula known as Sprengel's deformity

Answer: B i.e., Klippel Feil syndrome

25. **A 10 years old boy presents with recurrent bouts of nasal congestion, itching, sneezing, clear rhinorrhoea and conjunctival irritation. On examination he has conjunctival hyperaemia, allergic gape and a transverse nasal crease. Which of the following drugs is preferred for management of this child?**

A. Diphenhydramine B. Fluticasone

C. Cetirizine D. Ipratropium bromide

Allergic rhinitis is characterized by nasal congestion, frequent sneezing, nasal obstruction and clear or mucoid rhinorrhoea. It is managed by topical nasal steroid spray for prevention and oral antihistamines for symptomatic relief.

Answer: B i.e., Fluticasone

26. **A two years old child presents with partial albinism and susceptibility to infection. Peripheral smear examination reveals giant peroxidase positive lysosomal granules in granulocytes. Which of the following is most likely diagnosis?**

A. Angelman Syndrome

B. Hermansky Pudlak Syndrome

C. Waardenburg Syndrome

D. Chédiak-Higashi syndrome

Chédiak-Higashi syndrome is a rare autosomal recessive disorder that arises from a mutation of a lysosomal trafficking regulator protein, which leads to a decrease in phagocytosis. The decrease in phagocytosis results in recurrent pyogenic infections, albinism and peripheral neuropathy.

Answer: D i.e., Chédiak-Higashi syndrome

27. **A one year old child on exclusive milk feeds presents with constipation. On examination there is no fecal impaction. What is the next step in management?**

A. Oral lactulose

B. Increasing intake of vegetables and cereals

C. Colonic enemas using polyethylene glycol

D. Milk of Magnesia

This is a case of functional constipation. Measures that may help include drinking enough fluids, eating more fibers.

Answer: B i.e., Increasing intake of vegetables and cereals

28. A 10 years old girl is brought to the emergency following a road traffic accident. The child is comatose with GCS score of 4. She is hypertensive, has bradycardia and extensor posturing. CT imaging reveals comminuted skull fractures and intraparenchymal hemorrhage. The initial management should include all of the following measures EXCEPT:

A. Head of bed elevation

B. Mechanical ventilation

C. Intravenous dexamethasone

D. Hypertonic saline administration

In a patient with intra-parenchymal hemorrhage, the head should be elevated to 30 degrees, 1.0–1.5 g/kg of 20% mannitol should be given by a rapid infusion, and the patient should be hyperventilated to a pCO_2 of 30–35 mmHg. These measures are designed to lower ICP as quickly as possible prior to a definitive neurosurgical procedure (craniotomy, ventriculostomy, or placement of an ICP monitor) can be done. Corticosteroids are not recommended in the management of IPH because they have been proven to offer no benefit in randomized trials.

Answer: C i.e., Intravenous dexamethasone

29. A 3 years old boy is brought with complaints of staying aloof. He also has delayed speech. Rest of the developmental milestones were attained normally. The most likely diagnosis is:

A. Selective mutism

B. Attention deficit hyperactivity disorder

C. Autism

D. Phonological disorder

Autism is a developmental disorder characterized by troubles with social interaction and communication, and by restricted and repetitive behavior. Parents usually notice signs during the first two or three years of their child's life.

Answer: C i.e., Autism

30. A 6 years old boy comes to the immunization clinic having received all vaccines as per schedule till 18 months of age. Which vaccine should be administered now?

A. DTPw booster

B. TdaP booster

C. DT booster

D. TT booster

The primary series of three doses of DTP (DTwP or DTaP) should be given in infancy, with a booster dose of a tetanus toxoid containing vaccine ideally at age 4–7 years (DTPw) and another booster in adolescence, e.g., at age 12–15 years (TdaP).

Answer: A i.e., DTPw booster